D1560744

AN EAR TO THE CHEST

AN ILLUSTRATED HISTORY
OF THE EVOLUTION OF THE
STETHOSCOPE

AN ILLUSTRATED HISTORY OF THE EVOLUTION OF THE STETHOSCOPE

M. Donald Blaufox, MD, PhD, FACNM, FACP, FRSM

University Chairman, Department of Nuclear Medicine, Professor of Medicine and Radiology, Albert Einstein College of Medicine and The Montefiore Medical Center, New York, USA

The Parthenon Publishing Group
International Publishers in Medicine, Science & Technology

A CRC PRESS COMPANY
BOCA RATON   LONDON   NEW YORK   WASHINGTON, D.C.

Library of Congress Cataloging-in-Publication Data

Blaufox, M. Donald.
    An ear to the chest: evolution of the stethoscope/
M. Donald Blaufox.
      p.;cm.
    Includes bibliographical references and index.
    ISBN 1-85070-278-0 (alk. paper)
      1. Stethoscopes--History. I. Title.
    [DNLM: 1. Stethoscopes. 2. Auscultation--
instrumentation. 3. Blood Pressure
Determination--history. WB 26 B645e 2001]
    RC76.3 .B575 2001
    616.07'544--dc21

                                        2001036721

British Library Cataloguing in Publication Data

Blaufox, M. Donald (Morton Donald)
    An ear to the chest : evolution of the stethoscope
    1. Stethoscopes - History
    I. Title
    616' .0028

    ISBN 1-85070-278-0

Published in the USA by
The Parthenon Publishing Group Inc.
One Blue Hill Plaza
PO Box 1564, Pearl River
New York 10965, USA

Published in the UK and Europe by
The Parthenon Publishing Group
23–25 Blades Court
Deodar Road
London SW15 2NU, UK

Typeset by Siva Math Setters, Chennai, India
Printed and bound by Bookcraft (Bath) Ltd.,
Midsomer Norton, UK

Contents

To Dr Nolie Mumey

"An active mind and a wide variety of interests keep
you from going stale and growing old."

Preface

The initial concept for the preparation of a book on the evolution of the stethoscope occurred in 1991. At that time, Norma L. Mumey was actively engaged in disposing of the collection of her husband, the late Dr Nolie Mumey. Dr Mumey died in 1984, just short of his ninety-third birthday. Dr Mumey had enjoyed a remarkable career as a surgeon and as a pilot. He had served in the United States Army Aircorps and was the company doctor for Continental Airlines for 32 years. He was extremely active in community and medical affairs throughout his career. Among his many pursuits was a profound interest in medical history, which led him to publish in the field and to acquire an extensive collection of medical artifacts. He was a lecturer in medical history at the University of Colorado. Dr Mumey published a prodigious number of books, most of which were limited editions, which were given out to friends and associates. Among the medical subjects which he wrote about was *An Iconographic Sketch of the Life of René Theophile Hyacinthe Läennec*, which was published in Denver in 1932 in an edition limited to 110 numbered and signed copies. Dr Mumey had replicas of the Laennec stethoscope produced, which he gave out as gifts with his book.

My introduction to this remarkable man and his career came about when Elizabeth Bennion referred me to Mrs Mumey as a potential purchaser of her husband's medical collection. Mrs Mumey had indicated that there was a very large component of the collection devoted to the measurement of blood pressure and Mrs Bennion knew of my interest in this area. After several conversations and correspondence with Mrs Mumey, Dr Norman Medow and I flew to Denver to spend the day with her and to examine the collection first hand. A price was agreed upon and Dr Medow and I divided the collection between us. The day in Denver was indeed a very interesting and pleasant one, including a visit to the Mumey house with an in-depth introduction to this man, whom I had never met, and a pleasant lunch of Kentucky fried chicken with Mrs Mumey. At that time, I discussed with Mrs Mumey my plans to publish a book on the history of the measurement of blood pressure, and the fact that several of the items that were in the estate would be helpful in the preparation of that monograph. She told me of Dr Mumey's plans to publish a book on the evolution of the stethoscope, which was never completed. Subsequently, after I returned to New York, I received a package from Mrs Mumey which contained all of Dr Mumey's notes and preliminary materials for his proposed book on the stethoscope (Figure 1). This was sent to me in the hope that some day I would incorporate them into a publication. The material I received was interesting and valuable. It included a collection of photolithographs which were helpful in identifying many stethoscopes. In addition, there was extensive reference bibliographic material, which Dr Mumey had acquired from the American College of Surgeons, and several other sources. I have tried to identify this material when it has been used in this monograph. All references and articles obtained from this source have been checked with the original material for accuracy and completeness.

My interest in the stethoscope is a logical extension of my interest in the measurement of blood pressure. One can hardly imagine modern

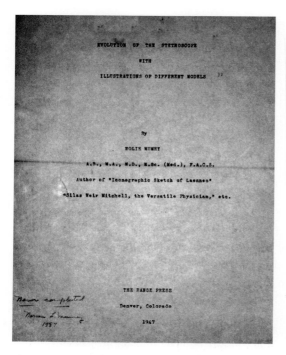

Figure 1 The proposed title page of Dr Nolie Mumey's book dated 1947

This project was never completed as noted by Norma Mumey in 1987 on the bottom left. The printing was planned for a private press. This material along with Dr Mumey's notes were given to the author by Mrs Mumey when part of Dr Mumey's estate was purchased. Some of his previous works are noted on the page.

day measurement of blood pressure without thinking of the stethoscope at the same time. My personal collection of medical artifacts includes a large number of stethoscopes in addition to those acquired from the estate of Dr Mumey. With the successful completion in June 1998 of the monograph that I published with Dr Nasim Naqvi, on the measurement of blood pressure, I turned my attention to a similar volume on the evolution of the stethoscope. The materials I received from Norma L. Mumey have provided a valuable resource for this task, as well as the ready availability of The New York Academy of Medicine and its unparalleled collection of medical literature. The introduction of the stethoscope into clinical medicine is perhaps one of the greatest events in physical diagnosis. This volume is meant to explain how it came about and how it has evolved into the instrument that has become as much a symbol of the physician as the staff of Aesculapius.

M. Donald Blaufox
ALBERT EINSTEIN COLLEGE OF MEDICINE
AND MONTEFIORE MEDICAL CENTER
NEW YORK, USA

Acknowledgements

There are many individuals to thank for helping me successfully complete this monograph. Mrs Norma Mumey generously made her husband's notes and related materials available to me to serve as the stimulus for undertaking this task.

My wife provided additional encouragement as well as proofreading, patience during detours to libraries and antique shops on trips to Europe and all-round support.

Barbara Bartolotta, my secretary, checked the accuracy of all of the references in a dust-laden library, copied patents in the New York Patent Library, and helped to gather the many documentary materials to complete this volume besides completing the extensive typing chores. Elaine Wald also stepped in where a second pair of hands was needed.

Caroline Duroselle-Melish from the New York Academy of Medicine played a vital role in helping me find the many rare but pertinent references used in the volume. Most of the reference material was photocopied there providing first hand documentation of the facts which were often presented in contradictory manner in secondary sources, of which there were few. Her fluency in French was also a great help where my own language skills ran into trouble.

Dinah Alam from Parthenon helped beyond her basic editorial responsibilities by visiting the Wellcome Library for me on several occasions to check out references there.

Dr Erwin Rugendorff helped me with the German literature which has been greatly neglected in previous reviews and also provided the several stamps which have been referred to in the text and made other valuable suggestions.

Bob Lummis reviewed the section on acoustics.

All of the photography for this book was done by the author using a Dimage 2000 digital camera and Photoshop for processing. Some of the illustrations were scanned directly from the pertinent documents. Translations from the French were done by the author except where noted. Some of the materials in Dr Mumey's notes had been translated by personnel from the American College of Surgeons; in most instances these were translated again and modified by the author.

List of Figures

Major events in the evolution of the stethoscope

Date	Inventor*	Event
350 BCE	Hippocrates	Describes the "succussion splash"
1761	**J. Auenbrugger**	**Introduces percussion**
1808	**J. Corvisart**	**Laennec's teacher, translates Auenbrugger, practices immediate auscultation**
1816	**R. Laennec**	**Invents the stethoscope using rolled paper, wood cylinder, experimented with different forms**
1817	F. Double	Discusses immediate auscultation in his text
1819	**R. Laennec**	**Text on auscultation**
1821	**J. A. LeJumeau (Kergaradec)**	**Used stethoscope in obstetrics**
1823	C. J. Hans	Publishes monograph on auscultation in obstetrics
1826	**R. Laennec**	**2nd edition, expanded, modified original model of stethoscope**
1828	**A. Piorry**	**Lighter more convenient instrument with tapered stem, pleximeter**
1829	N. Comins	Suggested a binaural with flexible jointed metal tubes
1830	C. J. B. Williams	Binaural with lead tubes
1832	**W. Stroud**	**Flexible monaural stethoscope**
1840	G. P. Cammann, A. Clark	Introduce auscultatory percussion, solid stethoscope
1841	**H. Landouzy**	**Teaching model with flexible tubes**
1841	G. Bird	Modifies flexible monaural, improved design
1843	C. J. B. Williams	Trumpet-shaped chest-piece
1843–1850	Arnold, Barclay, Billings, Burrow, Cammann, Clark, Dobell, Elliottson, Fergusson, Hawksley, Loomis, Quain, Stokes and many others	Serial minor modifications making the stethoscope slimmer and more portable, use of multiple materials
1851	**A. Leared**	**Binaural stethoscope of gutta-percha**
	N. B. Marsh	**Patented binaural rubber stethoscope**

(Continued over)

Continued

1852	G. P. Cammann	Introduced first practical binaural stethoscope
1859	S. Alison	Differential stethoscope
1866	C. L. Hogeboom	Suggests use of a membrane on chest-piece
1869	F. Knight	Modifies spring on binaural
1876	A. Pinard, Pajot, DePaul	Obstetric modifications, shorter, wider bell
1879	D. Richardson	Uses microphone to amplify stethoscope sounds
1882	Boudet	Invents portable amplified stethoscope
1892	C. Denison	Hard rubber binaural
1894	E. Bazzi, A. Bianchi	Phonendoscope
1894	R. C. M. Bowles	Membrane chest-piece with localizing button
1896	O. H. Sheppard	Modern head-piece design evolved from others
1901	R. C. M. Bowles	Modern diaphragm chest piece
1926	H. B. Sprague	Combined bell and diaphragm
1961	D. Littmann	Criteria for light practical modern stethoscope described
1926–2000	Various inventors	Numerous modifications introduced including a truly practical amplified stethoscope and a portable ultrasound device

*Throughout the text all of the names have been spelled in a consistent manner. It is common to encounter Cammann as Camman, Denison as Dennison, and Alison as Allison, among others. The actual articles cited spell the names in several forms. Occasionally a variant of the spelling has been used in a quotation or a citation. In addition, in the English literature first names are often omitted, the author being given as Dr X, and in the French literature of the 19th century the author is often M. X with the M representing Monsieur or Mr. Anonymous articles also are quite frequent.

1   Introduction

The stethoscope has come to represent the physician perhaps more than any other symbol save the shaft of Aesculapius (Figure 2). It has had a profound influence on the practice of medicine. Some have lamented that the stethoscope distanced the physician from the patient. Others have lauded the dignity it restored to the patient.

Acceptance of the stethoscope after its invention by Laennec was relatively rapid for a profession which is so conservative in nature, although not universal. Public and professional skepticism remained. The London *Times* of 1824 reported:

> A wonderful instrument called the Stethoscope, invented a few months ago, for the purpose of ascertaining the different stages of pulmonary affections, is now in complete vogue at Paris. It is merely a hollow wooden tube, about a foot in length (a common flute, with holes stopped and the top open, would do, perhaps just as well). One end is applied to the breast of the patient. The other to the ear of the physician, and according to the different sounds, harsh, hollow, soft loud etc., he judges of the state of the disease. It is quite a fashion if a person complains of a cough, to have recourse to the miraculous tube, which, however, cannot effect a cure; but should you unfortunately perceive in the countenance of the Doctor, that he fancies certain symptoms exist, it is very likely that a nervous person might become seriously indisposed and convert the supposition into reality.

It is evident from this quotation that the new instrument caused a considerable amount of anxiety among the lay public as well as among practicing physicians. The ongoing debate over the value of the stethoscope and its design is discussed throughout this text.

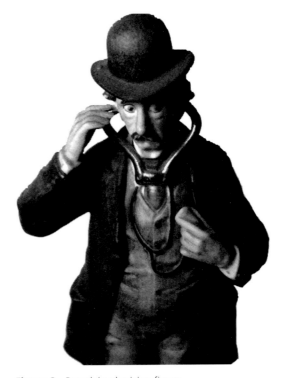

Figure 2   Porcelain physician figure

A rather playful depiction of the physician with his stethoscope. He is holding the chest piece in his left hand and is listening to his heart beat. The statue is marked with a crown and the number 3783 on the base. It is a full standing figure, only the torso is shown. He is wearing a black frock and a gray suit.

An often quoted example serves to illustrate the association of the stethoscope and medicine in a lighter vein. A poem about the stethoscope was composed by Oliver Wendell Holmes about 1848. Although this poem has a satirical note, Holmes was in fact an early supporter of the stethoscope and he won the Boylston Prize for his essay "Direct Exploration" in 1836 which promoted its use. The essay contains a virulent defense of the use of new methods of diagnosis and of the stethoscope. The stethoscope clearly had strong advocates in the United States, England, Germany and France, as well as its detractors. Holmes poked fun at its use in his poem (Holmes 1856):

STETHOSCOPE SONG

BY

OLIVER WENDELL HOLMES

There was a young man in Boston town, He bought him a Stethoscope nice and new, All mounted and finished and polished down, with an ivory cap and a stopper too.

It happened a spider within did crawl, And spun him a web of ample size, Wherein there chanced one day to fall A couple of very imprudent flies.

The first was a bottle-fly, big and blue, The second was smaller, and thin and long; so there was a concert between the two, Like an octave flute and a tavern gong.

Some said that his *liver* was short of *bile*, And some that his *heart* was over size, While some kept arguing all the while, He was crammed with *tubercles* up to his eyes.

This fine young man then up stepped he, And all the doctors made a pause; Said he, "The man must die, you see, By the fifty-seventh of Louis's laws.

"But since the case is a desperate one, To explore his chest it may be well; For if he should die and it were not done, You know the *autopsy* would not tell."

Then out his stethoscope he took, And on it placed his curious ear; "*Mon Dieu!*" said he, with a knowing look, "Why, here is a sound that's mighty queer!"

"The *bourdonnement* is very clear, *Amphoric buzzing*," said all the five.

"There's *empyema* beyond a doubt; We'll plunge a *trocar* in his side." The diagnosis was made out, they tapped the patient; so he died.

Now such as hate new-fashioned toys Began to look extremely glum; they said that *rattles* were made for boys, And vowed that his *buzzing* was all a hum.

There was an old lady had long been sick, And what was the matter none did know; Her pulse was slow, though her tongue was quick; to her this knowing youth must go.

So there the nice old lady sat, With phials and boxes all in a row; She asked the young doctor what he was at, To thump her and tumble her ruffles so.

Now, when the stethoscope came out, the flies began to buzz and whiz; Oh ho! The matter is clear, no doubt; And *aneurism* there plainly is.

The *bruit de rape* and the *bruit de scie*, And the *bruit de diable* are all combined; How happy Bouillaud would be, If he a case like this could find!

How, when the neighbouring doctors found A case so rare had been descried, they every day her ribs did pound In squads of twenty; so she died.

Then six young damsels, slight and frail, Received this kind young doctor's cares; They all were getting slim and pale, And short of breath on mounting stairs.

They all made rhymes with "sighs" and "skies," And loathed their puddings and buttered And dieted, much to their friend's surprise, On pickles and pencils and chalk and coals.

So fast their little hearts did bound, The frightened insects buzzed the more; so over all their chest he found The *rale sifflant* and *the rale sonore.*

He shook his head; – there's grave disease, – I greatly fear you all must die; A slight *post-mortem*, if you please, Surviving friends would gratify.

The six young damsels wept aloud, Which so prevailed on six young men That each his honest love avowed, Whereat they all got well again.

This poor young man was all aghast; The price of stethoscopes came down; And so he was reduced at last To practice in a country town.

The doctor's being very sore, A stethoscope they did devise That had a rammer to clear the bore, With a knob at the end to kill the flies.

Now use your ears, all you that can, But don't forget to mind your eyes, Or you may be cheated, like this young man, By a couple of silly, abnormal flies.

The number and variety of stethoscopes which have been developed defy description. In the United States alone, there have been 318 patents related in some way to the stethoscope during the period 1976–2000.

Although I have attempted to categorize the instruments described in this text as monaural, binaural, etc., to gain some clarity, many do not readily fit this type of rigid classification. For instance Pickering's stethoscope, called "Panarkes," was a combined stethoscope which could be used as a single, binaural and differential stethoscope. It also had a percussion hammer and pleximeter plate (Pickering 1887).

Many unusually shaped stethoscopes were employed in the belief that there was some underlying acoustical principle to justify them. For the most part, until the twentieth century, the modifications were truly dependent on trial and error. G. Tomasinelli, of Italy, modified the stethoscope as late as 1918 so that instead of a round opening the thoracic end was a long bar, resembling a T. He suggested that the sounds heard in a straight line were much more useful than those originating from a circular end (Tomasinelli 1918). There is no justification of this concept (Rappaport & Sprague 1941). Stethoscopes varied greatly in length and in the diameter of the chest piece. Although larger chest pieces produced louder sound, they did not localize the source very well. This was appreciated soon after experimentation began, but the ideal size was quite elusive. The length clearly is an important factor in intensity since the loudness is eight times greater in a 3 inch long tube than in a 26 inch long tube. However, many other considerations played a role in the choice of the length of the stethoscope, including the desire of the physician to distance himself from the patient as a possible source of contagion, the problems of interpreting sounds produced from clothing and friction, and a lack of understanding of the significance of many of the sounds transmitted. The reader will encounter claims about optimum length which ignore to a large extent the physics of sound related to length and are based on more complex considerations. Excessive softness of the wall of the tube affects the transmission through air and, although this was one of the few features most users agreed on, early flexible instruments were limited in quality by the materials that were available for their manufacture. Some more important acoustical principles underlying the use of the stethoscope are discussed later in the section on acoustics to provide the reader with a perspective of the accuracy of the many claims.

I have attempted to include the truly evolutionary examples of the stethoscope in this monograph. Some variations also are described to illustrate the wide variety of approaches which are interesting although they may be of lesser importance. Many examples are contained in the appendix which provides the reader with a comprehensive visual image of the form of the stethoscope as it has evolved during the past 180 years.

There is a lack of standard nomenclature to describe the stethoscope's parts. The terms used in this text are:

ear-piece: the small tips which are placed in the auditory canal

head-piece: the portion that connects the tubing to the earpieces with some form of rigid substance, usually metal

chest-piece, pectoral end, head: various terms used for the end of the stethoscope which is applied to the body

Other parts are described where indicated.

2 Immediate percussion

The story of auscultation is intimately linked to percussion. The two techniques comprise the basic physical examination of the chest. I will not discuss percussion in great detail, but some background is necessary to understand the evolution of the stethoscope.

Percussion was probably practiced to some extent throughout history. Seranus of Ephesus distinguished uterine disease by pressing on the abdomen and listening to the sound, and Aretaeus of Cappadonia described abdominal sounds in dropsy as being drumlike (tympanic) (Davis 1981). Virgil is quoted by Holmes (1836; 1837) as having some knowledge of percussion. After Corvisart published his translation of Auenbrugger's work, percussion became an established method for examination of the patient (Corvisart 1808).

Although percussion is not the subject of this volume, its inclusion is mandated by the role it played preparatory to the description of mediate auscultation. Almost all authors associate the two techniques stating that both are essential to the proper examination of the chest.

Joseph Leopold Auenbrugger (1722–1809) is generally credited with the introduction of this technique into clinical medicine. Auenbrugger was born in Austria and in 1754, when he began to employ percussion, he was a physician at the Spanish Hospital in Vienna. Auenbrugger's discovery is attributed to his boyhood experience of noting how his father employed tapping to determine the fluid level in kegs. His monograph provided a comprehensive description of the method of percussing the chest (Auenbrugger 1761) (Figure 3).

At one point in his book, Auenbrugger mentions that one can feel the difference over the

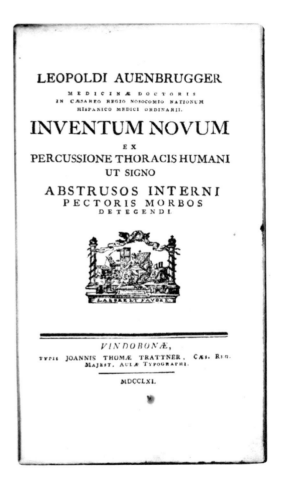

Figure 3 Title page from Auenbrugger's monograph on percussion.

The English title is "New method for recognition of the internal diseases of the lung by percussion of this cavity." It was printed in 1761.

chest at the point where percussion has detected an abnormality. Auenbrugger tapped the patient with his fingertips with the fingers of the hand drawn together if the patient was clothed. He used a glove to percuss the bare skin. He classified the resultant sound as high-pitched, dull or muted. His work was taken up by Maximilian Stoll and by Charles Ludwig, but it did not achieve general use for almost fifty years. The critical role of percussion and its relation to auscultation is a direct result of the interest of Jean-Nicolas Corvisart (1755–1821) who was the teacher of Laennec and physician to Napoleon Bonaparte.

Corvisart translated Auenbrugger's book into French in 1808 (Corvisart 1808). Corvisart states in the text that his translation was based on a Viennese printing from 1763. It is not clear why he gave the date as 1763 rather than 1761. The original Auenbrugger monograph was only 95 pages in Latin; Corvisart's translation contains both the Latin and his own commentaries and was 440 pages in length. A previous French translation by M. Roziere de la Chassagne of the Medical Faculty of Montpellier had appeared in 1770 but it never achieved general acceptance.

Corvisart's great prominence in France was a major factor in moving percussion into the mainstream. Corvisart's method of performing percussion differed from Auenbrugger's: he used the planar surface of his fingers to strike the chest.

Collin, in his monograph *Examination of the Movements of the Chest in Respiration* (1824) devotes the second chapter to percussion and the sounds produced by percussion. He categorizes them into four groups: (1) according to the points of the chest struck upon; (2) according to the leanness, fatness or infiltration of the subject; (3) according to the posture of the patient; and (4) according to the mode of performing percussion. He indicates that the use of slight blows with a stethoscope or other solid body is the best means of producing the sounds. This preference may well relate to his role as an assistant to Laennec who was known to prefer this method, although most physicians did not use it because it was painful to the patient.

After an initial description of normal findings, Collin goes on to describe the changes in disease as dull, obscure, absent or more clear than natural. Clearly by this time percussion had become an accepted and organized diagnostic modality.

3 Immediate auscultation

The earliest recorded reference to breath sounds may be in the Ebers Papyrus (1500 BCE) and is reported to appear also in the Hindu Vedas writings around 1400 BCE. Caelius Aurelianus (500 BCE), da Vinci, Pare, Morgagni, Van Swieten, Hunter and others all have notations in their writings suggesting some awareness of auscultation as a tool for examining the patient (Bishop 1980). Davis (1981) also mentions Caelius Aurelianus (200 BCE) listening to the chest in the diagnosis of bronchitis.

Keele (1963) quotes Hippocrates from *De Morbis* as writing: "You shall know by this that the chest contains water and not pus, if in applying the ear during a certain time on the side you perceive a noise like that of boiling vinegar." The sound in reality is probably respiration or crepitant rales. Hippocrates compared the pleuritic friction rub to the creak of a leather belt. He described the procedure still known today as hippocratic succussion which consisted of shaking the patient and listening at the same time to the thorax to find the seat of an empyema (Meyer-Steineg & Sudhoff 1950).

Hook is quoted by Elliotson (1830) as writing: "And somewhat more of encouragement I have also from experience, that I have been able to hear very plainly the beating of a man's heart, and 'tis common to hear the motion of the wind to and fro in the guts and other small vessels; the stopping in the lungs is easily discovered by the wheezing."

Harvey (1578–1657) refers to sounds from the body in several writings. He remarks: "even for it comes to pass, that while some portion of the blood is drawn out of the veins into the arteries, there is a beating which is heard within the breast." (Harvey 1673)

Prior to Laennec most of the cited references like these are isolated statements in texts or other writings which simply indicate that the author may or may not have applied the ear to the chest (Figure 4). Skoda (1853) writes that "Corvisart was accustomed, in cases where the movements of the heart could not be satisfactorily ascertained by the hand to place his ear over the cardiac region; and thus he practiced immediate auscultation. His pupils followed his example…" Certainly no systematic review of the use of auscultation is referenced.

One of the first suggestions of its regular use is the reference to auscultation in the second volume of the series on *Semiologie* by Double (1776–1881) who, like Laennec, was a student of Corvisart (Double 1817). Another pupil of Corvisart, Gaspard Bayle (1774–1816) used immediate auscultation to study the heart extensively (Risse 1971). Finot (1972) makes a weak case for Double having invented auscultation two and a half years before Laennec. He quotes two paragraphs from Double's text. One indicates that in order to understand a respiratory problem the observer must place one of his ears against the chest and then he can distinguish the sounds. He indicates that he has used this technique every day in his clinical practice. In the other paragraph, Double writes of similar utility for examining the heart, especially to appreciate palpitations. However, on inspection of the original volume from which these quotations are derived, it appears that they are the only significant references to auscultation, along with a few other paragraphs, among many signs that are discussed. Certainly there is no clinicopathologic correlation of this proposed diagnostic test with the disease it reveals.

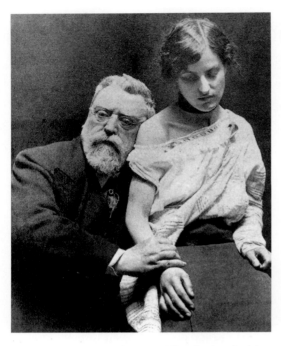

Figure 4 Jaume Ferran (1852–1929), a Catalan physician, demonstrates an idealized reconstruction of immediate auscultation, taken with an esthetic point of view, as part of his major series designed in 1895. This cumbersome method of examination persisted in use through the 19th century in spite of its obvious shortcomings. Courtesy of Fundació Museu d'Història de la Medicina de la Catalunya, Barcelona, Spain

Double was a respected Parisian physician, and this statement and practice surely must have had some influence on the medical community. Perhaps it is the reason that many French physicians adopted the principles of Laennec by using direct auscultation without employing the stethoscope initially. Regardless, although Double may have been the first to formally suggest the value of auscultation, he clearly did not systematize it into an indispensable part of clinical practice. Laennec introduced many new observations with his use of the stethosope including many terms such as rales, fremitus, cracked pot sound, egophony, bronchophony, cavernous breathing and bruit among others.

Immediate auscultation certainly was practiced more frequently, if not routinely, after the publication of Laennec's book, which clarified the significance of the various sounds that were associated with specific pathological conditions in the chest.

An excellent review of the debate over the advantages and disadvantages of mediate compared with immediate auscultation has been published by Reiser (1974). Among the arguments quoted by Reiser for the use of immediate auscultation was the fact that application of the ear to the patient causes no pain nor anxiety and it can be applied more quickly when listening to a larger area. Arguments against immediate auscultation included the problem that physicians frequently had to deal with dirty, unbathed patients, certain areas of the body were not applicable to immediate auscultation such as the axilla, and young women in particular felt uncomfortable by this approach involving intimate physical contact. Groups on both sides argued the relative accuracy of the technique.

The position taken by Louis as stated below was not a rare one:

In opposition to Laennec, it is now allowed that the naked ear perceives sounds as well as when aided by the stethoscope; and, indeed, it often happens that it distinguishes shades of sound which had escaped it when assisted by this instrument. The cases in which we ought to prefer mediate auscultation are very rare, and it is often necessary to have recourse to immediate auscultation to determine with clearness what would otherwise be obscure. (Louis 1837)

However Louis' interest in the stethoscope was probably greater than implied by this statement. According to Barth and Roger (1850), a stethoscope designed by Louis was one of the more practical ones in use at that time.

4   Mediate auscultation

Laennec

Countless volumes have been written about the life of Laennec (1781–1826) and of his momentous invention. In reality the invention of the stethoscope might not have created such reaction if it had not been described in a remarkably detailed text of the pathophysiology of the lung and its diseases. Laennec's first edition in 1819, published when he was physician at the Necker Hospital, a member of the Society of the Faculty of Medicine of Paris and "of many other societies national and foreign," and perhaps more importantly the second in 1826, codified examination of the lung by auscultation. His descriptions of physical findings and the clincopathologic correlation solidified the importance of his discovery. I will not attempt to focus deeply on Laennec's contributions to pulmonology but will concentrate on the stethoscope itself and its remarkable evolution. Laennec also launched modern examination of the heart, but his strength was in diagnosis of diseases of the lung. He correctly correlated the first sound of the heart with ventricular systole, but erroneously believed that the second sound was caused by auricular systole.

According to his good friend Kergaradec (Jean Alexandre LeJumeau), Laennec described his invention as resulting from his recollection of children listening at one end of a beam of wood to hear the sound as another rubbed the other end. An account of the first use of the stethoscope in Laennec's words, which is in countless volumes, appears below. A very different account was presented by Granville (1854). He states that on September 13, 1816, Laennec was dissatisfied with the results of percussion and immediate auscultation in a patient whom he had examined in the routine way. He turned to the students around him and said, "Why should we not avail ourselves of the help which acoustics yield to us of making distant sound more audible. The speaking-trumpet enables the dull of ear to hear the faintest whisper ... the ticking of a watch placed at the end of a long beam, is heard loudly by the ear applied to the other extremity: a tube therefore applied over the lungs or to the chest over the heart ought to instruct us more plainly through our ear." He then took the *cahier des visites* from a pupil, rolled it up lengthwise in the shape of a cylinder and applied it to the various aspects of the chest. "On the following day Laennec had procured proper cylinders made of a thick paste-board ... eight inches long and one and a half in diameter." Granville goes on to state in a footnote: "Why Laennec in his first edition ... should have changed the scene of its first application from the ward of a hospital to the chamber of a fair patient, is not very intelligible to me, except on the score of French *galanterie*. My own notes taken down at the time and on the spot are liable to no misconception." This version has itself been questioned, especially since it was published so many years after the event (Duffin 1998), although it is difficult to understand why Granville would choose to do this. Laennec did make some changes in his own account between the 1819 and the 1826 edition of his work. Granville brought a paste-board stethoscope to England with him when he returned from Paris in November 1817, which may have been its earliest introduction to England.

Another controversial point is whether Laennec knew about the work of the famous physician, physicist and chemist William Hyde Wollaston (1766–1828) at the time of his invention. Wollaston used a long notched stick resting on his foot, with a cushion at one end for the ear to listen to, and counted the sounds of muscle contractions in his foot (Wollaston 1810). Laennec does not mention this in the first edition, and although he devotes several pages to the event in the 1826 edition of his work, he regards its success in counting the contractions of the muscles as being doubtful.

At any rate Laennec's account is quite different:

In 1816, I was consulted by a young woman labouring under general symptoms of diseased heart, and in whose case percussion and the application of the hand were of little avail on account of the great degree of fatness. The other method just mentioned being rendered inadmissible by the age and sex of the patient, I happened to recollect a simple and well-known fact in acoustics, and fancied, at the same time, that it might be turned to some use on the present occasion. The fact I allude to is the augmented impression of sound when conveyed through certain solid bodies – as when we hear the scratch of a pin at one end of a piece of wood, on applying our ear to the other. Immediately, on this suggestion, I rolled a quire of paper into a sort of cylinder and applied one end of it to the region of the heart and the other to my ear, and was not a little surprised and pleased, to find that I could thereby perceive the action of the heart in a manner much more clear and distinct than I had ever been able to do by the immediate application of the ear. From this moment I imagined that the circumstance might furnish means for enabling us to ascertain the character, not only of the action of the heart, but of every species of sound produced by the motion of all the thoracic viscera. With this conviction, I forthwith commenced at the Hospital Necker a series of observations, which has been continued to the present time. The result has been, that I have been enabled to discover a set of new signs of diseases of the chest, for the most part certain, simple and prominent, and calculated, perhaps, to render the diagnosis of the diseases of the lungs, heart and pleura, as decided and circumstantial, as the indications furnished to the surgeon by the introduction of the finger or sound, in the complaints wherein these are used.

In prosecuting my enquiries I made trial of instruments of various composition and construction. The general result has been that bodies of a moderate density, such as paper, wood, or indian cane, are best suited for the conveyance of the sound, and consequently for my purpose. This result is perhaps contrary to a law of physics; it has, nevertheless, appeared to me one which is invariable.

I shall now describe the instrument which I use at present, and which has appeared to me preferable to all others. It consists simply of a cylinder of wood, perforated in its centre longitudinally, by a bore three lines in diameter, and formed so as to come apart in the middle, for the benefit of being more easily carried. One extremity of the cylinder is hollowed out into the form of a funnel to the depth of an inch and half, which cavity can be obliterated at pleasure by a piece of wood so constructed as to fit it exactly, with the exception of the central bore which is continued through it, so as to render the instrument in all cases, a pervious tube. The complete instrument – this is, with the funnel-shaped plug infixed – is used in exploring the signs obtained through the medium of the voice and the action of the heart; the other modification, or with the stopper removed, is for examining the sounds communicated by respiration (Figures 5; A2). This instrument I commonly designate simply the Cylinder, sometimes the Stethoscope.

In speaking of the different modes of exploration I shall notice the particular positions of the patient, and also of the physician, most favourable to correct observation. At present I shall only observe that, on all occasions, the cylinder should be held in the manner of a pen, and that the hand of the observer should be placed very close to the body of the patient to insure the correct application of the instrument (Figure 6).

The end of the instrument which is applied to the patient – that, namely, which contains the

Figure 5 Laennec's first stethoscope

The illustration of Laennec's stethoscope from the first edition (1819) with the legends:

Figure 1   The cylinder reduced in all of its dimensions

  a. The plug or stopper in its place

  b. The inferior body of the stethoscope

  c. The upper half

  d. The auricular extremity which will be applied to the ear

Figure 2   A cut of the stethoscope in its length

  a. A cross-section of the obturator in place

  b. Point of union of the upper and lower half

  c. The upper portion of the stethoscope

Figure 3

  a. The superior or auricular portion

  b. The inferior or pectoral portion

Figure 4

  a. The body of the obturator made of the same wood as the rest of the stethoscope

  b. Brass tube for fixing it into the base of the stethoscope

Figure 5   The superior body of the stethoscope

  a. Its body

  b. Screw thread with which it is connected to the lower, pectoral, half

Figure 6   Actual diameter of the stethoscope

  a. Diameter of the above

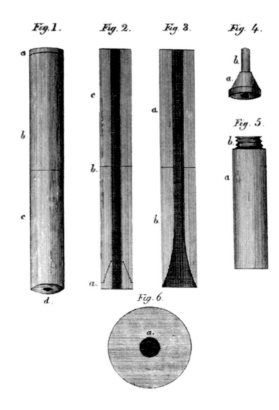

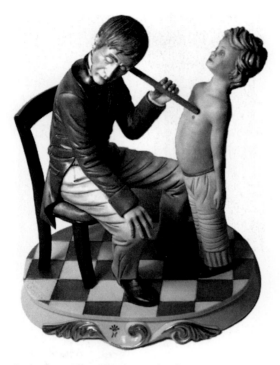

Figure 6 Laennec listening to the chest

A porcelain figure from the Capo-Di-Monte history of medicine collection showing Laennec listening to the chest of a young boy with a monaural stethoscope, signed R. Guidolin. This is a colorful representation with Laennec wearing a deep red coat and sitting on a chair on a red and white tile floor. The stethoscope is modeled to represent a brown wooden tube. The awkwardness of using the instrument comfortably can be appreciated from this illustration.

stopper or plug – ought to be slightly concave to insure its greater stability in application; and when there is much emaciation, it is sometimes necessary to insert between the ribs a piece of lint or cotton, or a leaf of paper, on which the instrument is to be placed, as, otherwise, the results might be affected by the imperfect application of the cylinder. The same precaution is necessary in the examination of the circulation in cases where the sternum, at its lower extremity, is drawn backwards, as frequently happens with shoemakers, and some other artisans.

Some of the indications afforded by the stethoscope, or mediate auscultation, are very easily acquired, so that it is sufficient to have heard them once to recognize them ever after: such are those which denote ulcers in the lungs, hypertrophia of the heart when existing in a great degree, fistulous communication between the bronchia and cavity of the pleura, etc. There are others, however, which require much study and practice for their effectual acquisition.

The employment of this new method must not make us forget that of Auenbrugger; on the contrary, the latter acquires quite a fresh degree of value through the simultaneous employment of the former, and becomes applicable in many cases, wherein its solitary employment is either useless or hurtful. It is by this combination of the two methods that we obtain certain indications of emphysema of the lungs, pneumo-thorax, and of the existence of liquid extravasations in the cavity of the pleura. The same remark may be extended to some other means, of more partial application, such, for example, as the Hippocratic succussion, the mensuration of the thorax, and immediate auscultation; all of which methods, often useless in themselves, become of great value when combined with the results procured through the medium of the stethoscope. (Laennec 1819)

Initially Laennec called his invention *le cylinder* (the tube). Later he chose the name stethoscope from the Greek stethos – chest – and scope – to observe, look at. The word auscultation is much older, from the Latin – to hear. It dates from 1634 in English but its first medical use may have been by Forbes in 1821. The names of the stethoscope and the auscultatory signs were questioned in a thesis for the Faculty of Medicine of Paris by Louis-Marius Rouit of Mane. He suggested the name somascope or echophore since the stethoscope was used for examining more that just the chest (Rouit 1828).

Acceptance of mediate auscultation

The principles of auscultation so well defined by Laennec were accepted rapidly in France but less so in England. Forbes in the first of his several translations of Laennec (1821) states:

> I have no doubt whatever, from my own experience of its value, that it will be acknowledged to be one of the greatest discoveries in medicine by all those who are of a temper, and in circumstances, that will enable them to give it a fair trial. That it will ever come into general use, notwithstanding its value, I am extremely doubtful: because its beneficial application requires much time, and gives a good deal of trouble both to the patient and the practitioner: and because its whole hue and character is foreign, and opposed to all our habits and associations. It must be confessed that there is something even ludicrous in the picture of a grave physician formally listening through a long tube applied to the patient's thorax as if the disease within were a living being that could communicate its condition to the sense without. … I may also observe that my first trials of the instrument were very unsatisfactory, from the doubtfulness and uncertainty of the results obtained. This however, arose entirely from inexperience and from not attending properly to the directions given for using the instrument.

Regardless of Forbes' early concerns Laennec's place was firmly established as one of the greatest physicians of all time (Figure 7).

Forbes' translation played a critical role in the acceptance of the stethoscope in England, A second edition was begun within twelve months of the first and in the preface to the fourth edition written in 1834 the material is presented with

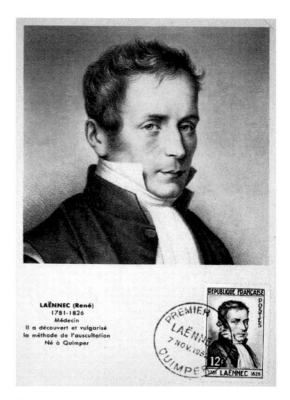

Figure 7 Stamp celebrating Laennec

The legend reads Laennec (René) 1781–1826 Physician. He discovered and popularized the method of auscultation. Born in Quimper. The first issue stamp is from Quimper dated November 7 1952. Courtesy of Dr Erwin Rugendorff.

none of the anxieties evidenced in the first edition. Another contemporary translation was that of F. H. Ramadge, edited by Theophilius Herbert (Ramadge 1846). This was taken from the greatly expanded work contributed by Gabriel Andral and Meridith Laennec (Laennec and Andral 1837) and faithfully follows that version as does the last edition of Forbes. Forbes in his first translation rearranged Laennec's treatise into a section of pathology and a section of diagnosis, both of which had been integrated by Laennec in his first edition.

James Hope (1801–1841), who worked as Physician to St George's Hospital, is credited with having influenced the acceptance of the stethoscope by the London medical community (Bluth 1970). Hope had spent two years studying on the continent after graduating from Edinburgh in 1825 and spent time in Laennec's clinic. He suffered from tuberculosis during this time and died of the disease in 1841, but he managed to publish a major contribution to the study of the heart *Treatise on the Diseases of the Heart and the Great Vessels* (1842) in which he reported his systematic studies of the heart valves and myocardial contraction.

Hope's efforts in support of the stethoscope are the subject of several letters to the editor in the English medical literature. T. W. Pocock of Knightbridge wrote an account in the *London Medical Gazette* (1838). He reports an occasion when Dr Hope used a blackboard during a ten-minute period to explain the method of discriminating valvular disease with the aid of the stethoscope. Six patients from St George's Hospital, who were selected for the demonstration, were then presented to four students, one of whom was Mr Pocock. Out of sixteen diagnoses arrived at by the students, only one was incorrect. The letter is followed with each of the students' diagnoses. Dr Hope wrote a letter to the editor following this in which he states: "an intelligent student, familiar with the anatomy of the heart and with its situation in reference to the surface,

will learn the diagnosis of the several valvular diseases in two hours, if they be demonstrated to him on six or eight well marked cases, presenting all the varieties of valvular disease." Hope also established an annual prize for proficiency in auscultation which he presented at the end of his sessions.

The whole proceeding noted above was in itself marked by controversy. In 1839, Drs R. J. Graves and W. Stokes, among the most eminent physicians of their time, wrote about a similar episode in a note on "Dr Clutterbuck versus the Stethoscope." Dr Clutterbuck in a lecture had severely criticized the use of auscultation equating it to mesmerism and homeopathy (Clutterbuck 1839). Graves and Stokes responded forcefully and noted Hope's practice of conducting brief teaching sessions on the use of the stethoscope in the diagnosis of heart disease. They wrote their commentary for: "the junior student, who might be deterred from studying an important and now indispensable part of his profession, by the statements above quoted." However they also remarked on the accuracy of the student's diagnoses in these sessions: "but that these conclusions were correct, we have only Dr Hope's word for" and expressed concern that Hope might have caused some harm by exaggerating the power of the technique (Graves & Stokes 1839).

William Stokes (1804–1878) was born in Dublin and he entered Edinburgh Medical School in 1823. There he came under the influence of S. Scott Alison, whose work is described below. Before he left Edinburgh to return to Dublin in 1825, he had written and published a book entitled *The Use of the Stethoscope* (1825).

A review of his book in the *Lancet* (1825) provides some skepticism of Stokes' endorsement of the instrument. The reviewer writes: "But does it (the stethoscope) really deserve the extravagant praise of its admirers or the fastidious contempt of its enemies? We are pretty certain, it neither merits the one nor the other." The review essentially endorses the utility of the stethoscope while being rather critical of Stokes, partly because of his youth and lack of experience at the time he wrote the volume. He was 21 years old.

Stokes became a leading authority in diseases of the lungs and in 1837, he published *Diseases of the Chest*, in which he endorsed the use of auscultation in bronchitis and other diseases of the chest. In 1842, he became Regius Professor of Physic at Dublin University.

Another early text on the stethoscope originated in Germany from Karl Gastav Schmalz (1775–1849) who was one of the first Germans to use the instrument. The introduction to his text contains an extensive discussion of auscultation and percussion (Schmalz 1825). He used a Laennec-type stethoscope for both pulmonary and cardiac auscultation. He used it also for abdominal and joint auscultation.

An anonymous author reports that in 1826 the stethoscope was employed almost universally in France and extensively in Germany, but not as frequently in England as it deserved (Anon 1826). Schoenlein (1793–1864), a prominent physician who was personal physician to the Kaiser in Berlin, lectured on the stethoscope and auscultation in 1841. At that time, according to Losse, many physicians in Germany were still not using the method because they feared the introduction of technology into medical practice (Losse 1991). However, there is an extensive German literature on auscultation which is rarely quoted in English or French texts. These monographs, referred to throughout this volume, suggest that there were greater German contributions to the field than is generally acknowledged.

One of the first reports of the use of the stethoscope in the United States was by John Bell, a New York City physician (Bell 1824). At this time, Bell noted, only a few American physicians were using percussion and auscultation. Reports of the invention of the stethoscope appeared in several sources in the United States as early as 1821 (Smith 1978). The 1821 Forbes translation of Laennec was published in Philadelphia in 1823.

We can gain some insight into the acceptance of auscultation in the United States from the translation of Collin's monograph (1829). Victor Collin was an assistant of Laennec and first published his monograph in 1824. Ryland, a fellow of the Massachusetts Medical Society from Salem, Massachusetts, substituted the author's introduction with one of his own in his translation of this brief volume. He writes:

> Although the Stethoscope is well thought of by most practitioners, yet it is introduced into practice by a very few only, and ignorance, and prejudices, and perhaps in some instances honest doubts have conspired to decry its use… The use of the Stethoscope has become familiar to many of the most enlightened and distinguished practitioners of Europe. In England it is ordered to be used generally be the army surgeons, who are required to report their observations; in this country it still remains a novelty.

By 1830, acceptance had grown significantly although there were still many detractors. A monograph by John Elliotson (1830) of the Royal Hospital of St Thomas strongly supports the use of the stethoscope in cardiac disease. In his introductory remarks he states, "It has more than once happened to me, to be unable to form any opinion as to the nature of a disease without auricular examination." Although he generally uses the term auscultation and the ear, it appears that he is referring to that with the aid of the stethoscope: "… and applying the stethoscope, the sound proved as dead in some part as if the thigh had been struck, and no respiration could be heard, or the voice has rushed through the instrument, or an unnatural sound was heard in the heart and the whole mystery at once cleared up."

As late as 1844 Henry Bennet wrote,

> In France, at the present time, although auscultation is universally practiced as an essential, indeed, indispensable means of diagnosis, the stethoscope is either entirely discarded in auscultation of the

lungs, by the most eminent men of the day and consequently by the great mass of practitioners, or otherwise is only employed in a very limited manner. In England, on the contrary, wherever auscultation is resorted to, either in private or hospital practice, you nearly always find that the stethoscope is used. (Bennet 1844)

Although this article strongly supports the use of auscultation and percussion, it is a much more restrained endorsement of the use of the stethoscope.

In the United States, Bowditch (1808–1892), who had studied under Andral, Chomel and Louis in France, returned to write an important text on physical diagnosis. At that time, although quite familiar and adept with the stethoscope he wrote, "in the vast majority of instances of disease, the ear is sufficient. I find a stethoscope needed most in diseases of the heart." (Bowditch 1846) He also wrote, "All I seek in a stethoscope are lightness, smallness and a good sized earpiece." Rather remarkable statements from an individual who chose to title his book *The Young Stethoscopist*.

A manual of physical diagnosis by Souligoux (1868) contains continued discussions of the merits of both immediate and mediate percussion and both forms of auscultation. He takes the diplomatic view with auscultation, indicating that he thinks each approach has its merits and disadvantages and one should use them to suit the problem. However he firmly endorses the use of the pleximeter for mediate percussion, which is discussed later in this monograph.

Stethoscopes were sold in London by Weiss as early as November 1819 and the next year they were imported from Paris by Treutell and Wurtz who were booksellers who sold them with Laennec's book for two francs. Grumbridge was one of the earliest British makers, and a woodturner named Allnutt sold them in Piccadilly for four shillings (Bishop 1980).

Weiss' catalogue of 1863 lists eight stethoscopes all of which were monaural except for Alison's Differential. It also illustrates a pleximeter and a percussion hammer. The number of choices of stethoscope continued to increase at a geometric rate, but the number of truly significant modifications, as noted in the chronological table, were remarkably few until the binaural stethoscope was invented (Table 1).

5 Mediate percussion

Piorry

The work of Pierre-Adolphe Piorry (1794–1879) brings together percussion and auscultation in an integrated manner. Piorry, who was Professor of Physiology and Pathology of the Faculty of Medicine of Paris and a member of the Royal Academy of Medicine, is credited with the invention of the pleximeter for percussion. This instrument was struck with the finger or a hammer providing a more reproducible surface for percussion. He first reported his invention in 1826 at the Académie Royale de Médecine in Paris (Piorry 1826). Piorry also modified the stethoscope significantly, providing the first model with a narrow tube instead of the thick cylinder used by Laennec (Figures A1; A4).

These two diagnostic methods later diverged although they re-emerged in the concept of auscultative percussion, introduced by Cammann and others, which is discussed in a separate section of this volume. In the second chapter of his volume of 1828, Piorry discusses percussion and the contributions made to this diagnostic method by Auenbrugger, Stoll and Corvisart. He notes: "most authors recommend joining the fingers with their extremities on a well circumscribed area for tapping. Others, tapped on the thorax with the flat of their fingers joined together." (Piorry 1828) Auenbrugger, he notes, used a glove and he indicates that Laennec used his stethoscope for percussion. He goes on to discuss the various techniques of percussion and finally the inconveniences of direct thoracic percussion, which include some discomfort to the patient, disturbance of the underlying condition, the danger of having the patient unclothed, and fatigue in assuming the position necessary to undergo percussion. He also mentions several other conditions which make direct percussion inconvenient, including the patient's illness in certain circumstances and a variety of other potentially misleading signs for the abdomen as well as the lungs.

In the third chapter he introduces the concept of mediate percussion, which he describes as using a small plate or pleximeter, which is struck to obtain the sound. He notes that lead, leather, wood, horn and ivory can all be used successfully as pleximeters, but he preferred ivory because of its better characteristics. He modified the form of the stethoscope as well and adapted it to be combined with the pleximeter (Figures 8; A1; A4). His was the first significant modification of Laennec's form of the stethoscope and it was quickly followed by numerous others.

The obvious use of the finger as a pleximeter took some time to come into vogue because many clinicians felt it would not be as reproducible as the pleximeter and it could be painful to the examiner. However in the *British and Foreign Medical Review* edited by John Forbes and John Conolly (1837) it is noted that by then the fingers were the commonly employed mode of percussion and that this approach was introduced by a Dr Skerrett who is said to have been using it at the time Piorry was working on his pleximeter. Blakiston in his textbook on diseases of the chest (1848) noted that it was usual to place the forefinger of the left hand on the chest and strike it with the first and second fingers of the right hand. The percussion hammer was introduced by M. Anton Wintrich (1812–1882) in 1841. He wrote an extensive text on the diseases of respiration in which he devoted a major portion to

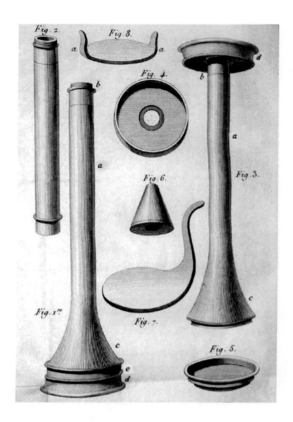

Figure 8 Piorry, stethoscope and pleximeter

The figure is taken from Piorry's original plate in his textbook (1828). The figure has been modified in size for presentation in this text.

Figure 1   The stethoscope in its entirety

    A. The body of the instrument of cedar reduced 1/4

    B. The auricular extremity made of ivory and presented with a threaded end

    C. The thorax extremity

    D. The cover of ivory screwed on to the pleximeter

    E. The pleximeter of ivory itself screwed on the stethoscope

Figure 2   The cylinder of the same dimension as the body of the stethoscope and which can be joined to the instrument if it is judged useful. [This apparently was to distance the physician from the patient, although the indication is not stated.]

Figure 3   The stethoscope put together in a manner for service

    A. The body of the instrument

    B. The auricular extremity

    C. The thorax extremity

    D. The cover screwed on the stethoscope

Figure 4   The cover by itself

Figure 5   The pleximeter in ivory detached from the rest of the instrument

Figure 6   A conical fitting which can be placed in the thoracic extremity of the stethoscope

Figure 7   Pleximeter, a form with a curved handle

Figure 8   Pleximeter with handles of ivory and wood. One can make this portable by means of hinges placed at points AA

auscultation and percussion (Wintrich 1854). The percussion hammer which he illustrates is of a type that was used well into modern times, with an India rubber tip. He also mentions the use of the stethoscope for percussion in this text, citing Laennec. The stethoscope he illustrates is a simple transitional one of the time but is somewhat unusual because either end can be used for application to the chest and the ear piece is separate and can be inserted into the end which is not applied to the chest.

Skoda

Josef Skoda (1805–1881), who was born in Pilsen, Bohemia, and became a leading professor of medicine in Vienna, is noted for his treatise on percussion and auscultation first published in 1839. The volume went through several editions including an English translation (Skoda 1853). He believed that the stethoscope was indispensable and should be used by all physicians, but he also urged the use of immediate auscultation, and for physicians to practice both. According to Skoda the choice of the composition of the wood of the stethoscope received much attention but it did not really matter for "the greater part of the sound traverses the air in the stethoscope and not the wood." He used a stethoscope which was one foot long and thought Piorry's to be too short, although he probably did not use the extension which would have relieved that objection (Figure A1).

Flint

An American who played an important role in the refinement of auscultation and percussion in the examination of the chest was Austin Flint (1812–1886). Flint studied with Dr James Jackson who was a firm supporter of the use of the stethoscope. Flint practiced in Buffalo, Chicago, Louisville, New Orleans and New York. A stethoscope which belonged to him is contained in the collection of artifacts of the New York Academy of Medicine. He published numerous volumes on physical diagnosis and was a highly influential practitioner. *A Manual of Percussion and Auscultation* went through eight editions (Flint 1876). The stethoscope in the New York Academy of Medicine collection is a Cammann's design. He mentions using the finger as a plexor in his manual, but notes that in a busy ward practice this could be painful because of repeated examinations and a pleximeter may be preferred. W. H. Welch, at a memorial for Austin Flint at the New York County Medical Association, remarked that Austin Flint "did more by his writings and his teachings than anyone else in [America] to render popular the methods of exploration by physical signs." He was sometimes called "the American Laennec."

6 The evolution of the monaural stethoscope

Acoustics

The evolution of the stethoscope can be understood better with some basic knowledge of acoustics. The two major forms of sound transmission which need to be considered with respect to the stethoscope are air and bone conduction.

The first stethoscope was made by rolling a pad of paper into a tube. It is fortunate that Laennec used a roll of paper to create his first stethoscope. It is very difficult if not impossible to roll a paper so tightly that it does not have a small central bore. Had he used a solid he might have given the stethoscope up as a bad idea. The central bore greatly facilitated his ability to hear breath sounds. Sound is conducted through various media according to their density and compressibility. Sound travels faster through wood than through water and air. It has frequency and intensity, energy and velocity. The ability of the observer to hear sound is dependent on both the frequency and the intensity. Humans can discern sound which has energy of about 10^{-16} watt per square centimeter (10^{-11} erg/cm^2 sec) and between 20 and 20 000 Hz. Most physiologic sounds are in the range of 20–1000 Hz. Although sound in wood travels faster than in air, the wood absorbs more energy. In addition, sound may be reflected and refracted as it moves from one density to another. The greater the difference between the two materials through which sound is being transmitted, the greater the reflection. Sound from the chest will be reflected most by a solid, less so by air, and least by water. Because of this it is necessary when using a monaural stethoscope to press it very tightly against the ear and the body part being examined. This presents a number of difficulties which are discussed later in the text.

The act of pressing the ear against a wall to hear what is on the other side reduces the loss of sound which would occur if it had to pass through the wall and then through air to reach the ear. This concept was appreciated by some of the inventors of stethoscopes but certainly not all. Laennec's decision to place a bore through his stethoscope made it a practical instrument. He originally worked with a solid block, because he is said to have recollected children scratching at one end of a wooden plank and listening at the other end, but found it unsuitable. A major mechanism of conduction of sound with a solid stethoscope is through the vibration caused in the skull at that frequency.

The density of the material times the velocity of sound through it provides a measure of specific acoustic resistance of the medium. For water it is about 3800 times that of air: it takes a pressure 60 times that of air to produce the same intensity of sound in water. The velocity of sound in air is 1128 feet per second, in water it is about 4600 feet per second and for hard solids it ranges from about 3300 to 20000 feet per second. Compressibility and elasticity also play an important role in the conduction of sound and its intensity. It was the closed column of air created in the cylinder that made the stethoscope a success and which serves as the basis for modern stethoscopes. A very tight interface was necessary between the ear and the instrument and between it and the body to ensure transmission through the air column. However, the acoustical considerations of a column of air in a tube are quite complex. Numerous other considerations including the composition of the instrument enter into the theoretical design of the stethoscope, very few of which were understood or appreciated as the instrument evolved. Most of the design changes were based on convenience, rather than acoustical principle.

Some understanding of the concepts of acoustics during the time that the stethoscope was evolving rapidly may be gathered from a publication by Andry (1844), who was a student of Laennec. Andry has a section in his manual *Some Laws of Acoustics Applicable to Auscultation*:

When sound waves spread in a mass of air limited by a cylindrical tube, following the direction of its axis, the amplitude of the vibrations remains constant, and consequently the intensity of the sound suffers no diminution in spite of the extent of the space covered. Everyone knows that by applying the ear to the end of a beam, he perceives distinctly the drop of a pin at the other end. This property of solid bodies, to transmit any noise faithfully and without any noticeable modification of timbre, explains the intention of the "end-pieces" which fill up so freely the lower cavity of the stethoscope. They conserve the cavity, however, and the central opening which pierces the stethoscope. Laennec observed that, if an altogether-solid body is the best instrument for exploration of the heart, and may serve in necessity for respiration and rales, the central tube is indispensable for exploration of the voice, and gives, just as the widening of the lower part of the tube, more intensity to the respiratory sounds themselves. Laennec recommends, therefore, the use of the end-piece when one wishes to auscultate the voice of the patient and the heart-beat, and its suppression on studying the respiration and rales.

If it is true that the sounds transmitted to the ear by a solid body, whatever its length, arrive almost identical, it is on the condition that these sounds are accompanied by a blow applied more or less directly to the extremity of the conducting body; if, on the other hand, this extremity is not directly struck, the propagation under discussion occurs in inverse ratio to the length of the course. Auscultate successively with several stethoscopes of unequal dimensions; take, for example, the stethoscope of Laennec, one of the halves alone, and then whole; then take cylinders of wood of different lengths and you will recognize that the sounds of the heart, no doubt due to the blows which accompany them, are transmitted a distance that will astonish you. If they are perhaps weakened by this distance, this weakening itself should cause us to think, as shall be established later, that the entire cause of these sounds does not reside in a blow.

The second law of acoustics, especially applicable to these latter sounds, which Laennec had in mind when he counseled the suppression of the end-piece to hear them, follows: When the sounds, instead of traversing a cylindrical tube, are projected against the parabola of funnel-shaped tube, widened at one end and narrowed at the other, the intensity of the sounds increases, increasing the amplitude of the excursion of the waves, the oscillations acting more energetically on the surrounding particles of air in the direction in which the extraordinary increase of velocity has been communicated.

The sound is thus amplified by the widening of the lower end of the stethoscope ... it may be amplified, and at the same time the timbre may be modified, by the nature of the material from which the stethoscope is made, the sound received by the ear being a complex sound of sorts, the result of the mixture of the primary sounds with secondary sounds produced by the vibrations of the conducting body itself.

This principle is of special interest, not so much for its application in the fabrication of the stethoscope, in the choice of such or such material, or whether wood is to be preferred to metal, and whether among the woods, spruce or cedar, etc., but for that other indication pointed out by Laennec himself, and mentioned here in advance by the author, namely, that in projecting in some fashion, by thought, the body conducting the sound into the midst of the organs, we should have the best calculation of the density, not only of the tissue producing the sound, but also those neighboring it, certain stethoscopic signs being able thus to obtain a high practical value from this consideration.

Although there are certain laws of acoustics which it is necessary to observe in the matter of auscultation, one should guard against believing that the stethoscope must represent one of the most perfect acoustic instruments. The sounds, which the stethoscope is called upon to transmit to us, are not so imperceptible that minute precautions must be taken to hear them. What does it matter whether a metal ring or an ivory disc attenuates by ever so little the conductive property of the cylinder! And by the sole fact of such a fitting, is the stethoscope of Piorry, as Landouzy claims, inferior to that of Laennec? Not at all. Light, convenient, widened out below in the form of a truncated cone in such a manner that the sound may not be reflected before it reaches the ear, it may, even without its end-piece, which the author considers a useless addition, answer all the essential indications. Become habituated to its use, exercise your ear by frequent use of this instrument. In two words, there is the main fact. Of all acoustic conditions, there, without contradiction, is the indispensable one.

(Translated by American College of Surgeons, Department of Literary Research, 1937).

Later investigators had the advantage of accurate measuring devices to more accurately define the factors affecting stethoscope performance. In 1941 Rappaport and Sprague published an extensive review of the factors affecting auscultation and they later constructed an elegant device for evaluating the effect of the tubing on the efficiency of the stethoscope (Rappaport & Sprague 1951). They concluded that although at that time a $^3/_{16}$ inch bore was common, a $^1/_8$ inch caliber was much more efficient in the physiologically important range of sound (100–1000 cycles per second). The efficiency increased as the tubing length decreased until the point where it became too short to handle properly, about 10 inches being optimal. The smaller the air volume of the instrument the greater the sound intensity and the wall of the tubing should be rigid enough to reduce wall motion. Other analytic reports

appeared in the literature around this time (Johnston & Kline 1940).

Also important in considering the underlying principles for stethoscopes is the difference between bone conduction of sound and air conduction. Modern stethoscopes and all of the flexible ones depend primarily on air conduction for their function. The principles noted above apply to these types of instrument. The monaural stethoscopes whether perforated or solid have a component of transmission of sound by bone conduction. The sound is conveyed by the solid part of the instrument to the skull where the vibrations are perceived as sound. This greatly complicates the specifications of the design and helps to explain the many varied approaches and theories presented in this text.

Landes used more precise methods to evaluate the acoustic properties of monaural stethoscopes (1931). He used an elaborate device with a sound transmitter, a monaural stethoscope and a microphone at the aural end. He noted that monaural stethoscopes did not transmit all frequencies uniformly resulting in distortion of the sound. However, his experimental design permitted mainly the detection of air transmission and did not account for bone transmission. Martini (1920) described the sound transmission through the solid part of the monaural stethoscope mathematically. He noted that the sound was heard better as the connection to the ear-piece was increased in diameter. Although he discusses the properties of the monaural stethoscope in detail, he does not account for the portion of sound heard through bone conduction. He does indicate the need for a very tight connection with the ear. Tobler (1930) investigated numerous monaural stethoscopes as well as binaural ones of differing design. His experimental design, like that of Landes, used a microphone for the detection of the sound and also did not account for bone conduction. However, he did remark that low pitched (205–870 Hz) sounds can be heard well even with the lumen of the stethoscope obstructed. Higher pitched (1161 and

1470 Hz) sounds were not conducted as well in this manner. Since most physiologic sounds are in the range of 20–1000 Hz, the lack of sensitivity of wooden monaural stethoscopes for higher pitched sounds would have less biologic significance.

The properties of an ideal stethoscope from the modern point of view were nicely summarized by Littmann (1961):

1. An open chest-piece with a maximum diameter convenient for manipulation and with the least practical volume and a depth to prevent occlusion by underlying tissue for low pitched sounds.
2. A closed chest-piece of the largest convenient size, least internal volume and a plastic diaphragm to filter out low pitched sound without overall attenuation for all but the lowest pitched sounds.
3. Tubing of firm inert material with a small smooth lumen and thick enough to exclude external noise. Starting as a single bore and then dividing at the head-piece.
4. As short as practicable with an inner diameter of or close to ⅛ inch and a comfortable spring for the head-piece to occlude the auditory canal.
5. It should be light, convenient to carry and of inert long lasting materials.

The story below will explain how we reached these ideals over a period of about 150 years.

Early modifications

Some insight into the stimuli for the evolution of the stethoscope can be gained from an article by C. Theodore Williams (Williams 1907):

Sir Charles Scudamore visited Laennec to try the wooden stethoscope with an aperture. However, he could hear nothing on account of the large size of the tragus of his ear. Laennec consequently hollowed out the ear-piece and then Sir Charles was able to hear.

Laennec continued to experiment with the form of the stethoscope, introducing several modifications: none was a major improvement on the original design. Laennec made many of his stethoscopes himself and the lathe which he used was purchased by Recamier at auction some years later.

Using the monaural stethoscope was not easy. The manner in which auscultation was performed utilizing a monaural stethoscope can be appreciated by the article of B. Louis, which was reprinted from the *Presse Medicale* in the *London Medical Gazette* (Louis 1837).

The person to be examined should lie on his back, or sit, according as we wish to auscult the anterior or the posterior part of the chest; he must lean neither to the right nor the left; his shoulders must be in the same plane, and his symmetrical muscles in the same state of relaxation or tension as the position of the patient.

This concept served as the stimulus for the development of the differential stethoscope and its early popularity.

The contraction, tension, and relaxation of the muscles, have a marked influence on the results of auscultation, and when the corresponding points of the thorax are examined in comparison with each other, as we must always do if we want to draw rigorous inferences, we might imagine differences that did not exist, merely from the bad attitude of the patient.

The auscultator, too, must select a convenient position, as Laennec recommends, and take care that the respiratory sounds are not intercepted by thick clothes, and particularly that the patient does not retain any which might produce a fallacious sound, as, for instance, silk coverings. He must also find out which is his best ear, as experience shows that almost every observer has one ear finer than the other.

This belief contributed to the delay in adopting binaural stethoscopes.

All these precautions, which at first sight may seem over-punctilious, are absolutely necessary to prevent our falling into gross errors.

In opposition to Laennec, it is now allowed that the naked ear perceives sounds as well as when aided by the stethoscope; and, indeed, it often happens that it distinguishes shades of sound which had escaped it when assisted by this instrument. The cases in which we ought to prefer mediate auscultation are very rare, and it is often necessary to have recourse to immediate auscultation to determine with clearness what would otherwise be obscure.

The patient and the observer being properly placed, auscultation, to be successfully practised, requires another condition, namely, the ear, if unaided, is to be exactly applied to the chest; if the stethoscope is used, the whole of its circumference is to be applied to the parietes of the thorax, so that if the patient is so wasted that the intercostal spaces leave a cavity under the stethoscope, it must be filled up by compresses placed upon the thorax.

It is clear that the proper use of Laennec's stethoscope required meticulous technique. This certainly contributed to the early controversy over its use. Laennec's ability to use it so well could not have been as casual as his description of its first application. He must have experimented a great deal to become adept with it. This is supported by his description of the many modifications he employed before arriving at the final design. He states in the 1819 edition of his text that the first instrument he used was a cylinder of paper of three quires, compactly rolled together and kept in shape by paste. Because there was always a longitudinal aperture he states that this led to an important discovery, namely its value in exploring the voice. He felt that without the aperture the stethoscope was best for examining the heart and could be used for respiration and rhonchus, but was better for the latter when perforated and excavated into a funnel shape at one end to a depth of 1½ inches. Glass and metals provided inferior results, as did goldbeaters skin.

Paper, lighter wood or Indian cane were the best materials to use. This lead to the one he finally used of wood, 1½ inches in diameter, and 12 inches long, perforated longitudinally by a bore three lines wide (one line = 1/12 inch) and hollowed out into a funnel shape to 1½ inches. It was divided in two for the purpose of carrying it and sometimes using the shorter piece. An obturator was inserted in the aperture to use for the heart or voice. He further states that the dimensions are critical and the only time the shorter piece is useful is if the patient is not easily reached with the longer instrument.

Laennec type

Laennec's stethoscope went through a number of modifications which did not greatly change its general form. Laennec himself continually experimented with the instrument to improve it. In the first edition of his text of 1819 he used the design shown in Figure 5.

The second edition of 1826 illustrates an instrument whose major modification was a rounded plug instead of the screw to join the two halves and a rounded stopper at the end which allowed the user to reduce the opening of the end which was applied to the chest when listening to the heart (Figure 9a). In his translation of the text with Andral's notes from the fourth edition, Forbes (Forbes 1838) illustrates a version which he notes was then in common use. In this version the obturator and the cavity which contained it at the thoracic end of the stethoscope were returned to the original conical rather than rounded shape and the brass retaining tube is omitted. The joint between the two halves is made similarly and there are horn or ivory rims at each connection. In addition the ear-piece is flared slightly (Figure 9b).

The sequential modifications of Laennec's stethoscope revolved mainly around the joints, although he did experiment with the size which ultimately was 12 inches long and 1½ inches in diameter. When he decided to divide the tube in half the first model was joined by a screw joint, which Keele attributes to Haden (Keele 1963) although no primary source is given. The second, which is shown in the 1826 edition of his text, was simply a rounded plug in arrangement (Figure 9a). Other versions included one which returned to a connection by a brass tube to the obturator and was attributed to Charles Thomas Haden (1786–1824), who is said to have worked at the lathe with Laennec (Sheldon & Doe 1935). This modification used a flare at the end with an ear-piece and was about 6 inches in length. It essentially omitted the auricular half, converting the pectoral half into a single complete unit. It was intended for use with ambulatory patients and children (Huard & Niaussat 1982). Figure A3 is a modified Laennec which very closely resembles a form attributed to Haden in a photoengraving from the Mumey collection. The source of this attribution is not given. A biographical note of Haden by Thomas Alcock indicates that Haden was one of the first people in England to use the stethoscope, but it does not mention any of his work on modifying the device (Alcock 1827). Laennec had commented earlier on simply using one half of the stethoscope in certain cases. There were many other versions which Laennec experimented with, but these were the most successful.

Piorry type

A good understanding of the thought behind Piorry's modification of Laennec's stethoscope can be derived by a translation of his explanation for the first plate of his text, which shows the instrument (Piorry 1828).

> I thought to adopt the pleximeter to the stethoscope and the union of these two instruments would prove not only the substitution of my

method to that of Laennec but would clarify with each other the results furnished by the two means of investigation.

> Persuaded that the extreme inconvenience of the long cylinder of wood, which was used by Laennec and the many obstacles to auscultation, which have to be surmounted, I searched to determine whether it would be possible to modify the length and the weight of the object to render it more portable.

> I recognized that a reduction in the diameter in the cylinder did not alter the property of conduction of the sounds, which were preserved by the conical cavity, which terminated the instrument. On the other side, the modification made is often easier to use. It seemed to me as a consequence the stethoscope, which I have modified, replaces very well the cylinder of Laennec but I do not have the pretension that it has any advantage over the other, other than its convenience.

He mentions in a footnote that, although it might seem that dividing his stethoscope into two pieces would be still more convenient, he has found that it does not conduct the sound as well (Figure 10).

Piorry's first book describing the pleximeter (Piorry 1828) was dedicated to the memory of Auenbrugger, Corvisart and Laennec. Piorry summed up his work in a later volume, *Treatise of Pleximetry*, which was published in 1866. This work includes material from the *Treatise of Mediate Percussion* (1828), *Procédé operatoire de la percussion* (1833), *Traite de diagnostic* (1835–1836), *Traite de medicine practique* (1842–1852) and *Atlas de plessimetisme* (1851). It contains a much more detailed discussion of pleximetry, including a discussion of the difference between those sensations which can be felt during pleximetry and those which can be heard. Figure 10 shows a drawing of his stethoscope with pleximeter, which is now quite different from the stethoscope of his first publication.

He refers to a stethoscope which he dates at 1826, which is quite different from the plate in his original publication of 1828. It resembles more

Figure 9a Later modifications of Laennec's stethoscope.

The Stethoscope, as altered by Laennec, and delineated in the second edition, published in 1826 (from Forbes 1838). It is altered in size for this text.

- D. Longitudinal section of all the parts united, one third of the actual dimensions
    - a. Stopper in its place
    - b. Point of junction of the two parts
    - c. Upper or auricular half
- E. The stopper removed
    - d. Its body, made of the same wood
    - e. Brass tube for fixing it into the base of the stethoscope
- F. Pectoral or lower half of the stethoscope
    - f. Its body
    - g. Its upper extremity reduced so as to fit the cavity in the other half; directed to be covered with thread or leather, in order to make it fit accurately

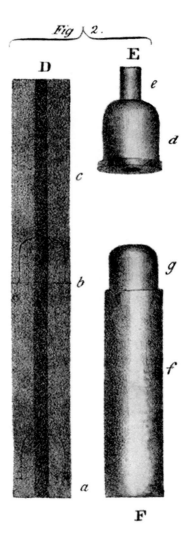

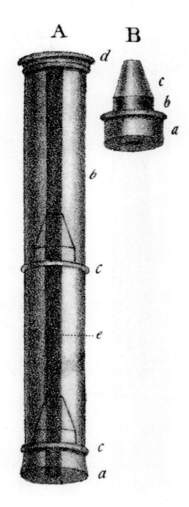

Figure 9b Later modifications of Laennec's stethoscope.

The stethoscope as now in most common use, being a modification of the two forms proposed by Laennec (from Forbes 1838). A very similar instrument is attributed to Grumbridge and dated at 1823 by Bishop (1980). In this modification, the extremity only of the plug (b,c), and consequently its containing cavity, are made conical, according to the first form of Laennec, while a portion is left of equal diameter (B, b) to enable it to retain its hold, without the brass tube.

A. The whole instrument with the two portions adjusted and the plug infixed, drawn so as to exhibit both its exterior and interior configuration. (The figure in the plate is not drawn to the exact proportions of the instrument, being only about one-fourth of its length, while it is one-third of its diameter.)

    a.   The plug in its place

    b.   The upper half of the instrument

    c.   Rims of ivory or horn surrounding the pectoral extremities of either half

    d.   A cap of the same material surrounding and covering the whole auricular extremity of the instrument

    e.   The central bore

B. The stopper (constructed to fit either the upper or lower half of the instrument) removed

    a.   Portion exterior to the funnelled cavity when the plug is in its place, of the same diameter as the stethoscope

    b.   Outer portion of the plug, of equal diameter throughout

    c.   Conical portion of the plug

closely the monaural stethoscopes in common usage at the time of this current volume (Piorry 1866). He also notes that this form had been falsely attributed to Louis, but was really his own invention. In the same figure, he shows an illustration of the stethoscope, which he published in the *Atlas of Plessimetisme*, in which he has used the pleximeter to serve as part of the chest-piece and which has a much narrower tube than his original model (Figure 10). He mentions the advantage of this instrument which makes possible simultaneous auscultation and percussion.

In the same section of his book, Piorry comments on having heard of the operation of auscultative percussion in America in which one listens while another percusses, apparently referring to the work of Cammanns. He criticizes this technique because it requires two people, emphasizing that his method can be performed with one examiner and that the French utilized this technique as early as his original experiments in 1826. He also shows illustrations of several other pleximeters, which are now graduated with linear scales for measurement as well.

Other monaural stethoscopes

After Piorry demonstrated that a reliable stethoscope could be made of a narrower tube, the remaining modifications in monaural stethoscopes were simply further refinements of the shape and composition and not innovations. A note by Andral in the Forbes translation of the fourth French edition (1838) reads:

> The stethoscope has undergone various modifications of form since the time of Laennec, but I am of the opinion the one last used and recommended by him is still the best, with this only alteration, of having the stopper made conical in place of being rounded ... [Regarding] the modification of the stethoscope, now very commonly used and originally introduced by M. Piorry, too

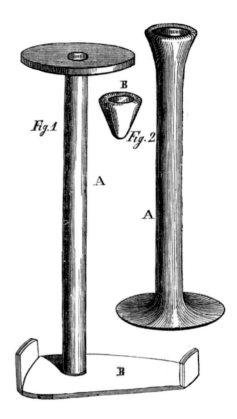

Figure 10 Piorry's "stetoscope and plesthetheoscope"

Taken from a later edition in which the form of the stethoscope has changed (Piorry 1866). This later stethoscope was composed of either copper or nickel silver and the pleximeter as well was made of metal (Figure 1). It is dated by Piorry as being from 1851. The form shown in Figure 2 is noted in the text as originating in 1826 and presumably is the same as the one noted in Figure 8 although the shape is presented quite differently except for the obturator.

much has been sacrificed to portability and elegance…. [It is] faulty in having the conducting power of the wood impeded by screws and a thick cap of ivory.

The stethoscope for which Andral is stating a preference in shown in Figure 9B.

Effect of material technology

During the last decade of the nineteenth century technological developments arising from the industrial revolution provided greater opportunities for the refinement of medical instrumentation. The process to make vulcanized rubber was invented by Charles Goodyear (1800–1860) in 1839. Before that, suitable material for a practical binaural or flexible stethoscope simply did not exist. Many refinements to improve the quality of this product were the result of industrial development after John B. Dunlop (1840–1921), a veterinary surgeon from Belfast, made a pneumatic tire for his son's tricycle in 1887 which he patented in 1888. Before this, the manufacture of a reliable flexible tube was a complex and uncertain process. This new material offered the possibility of making tubes which were far better and would not deteriorate easily. This allowed the development of simple but essential components for medical instrumentation. As the industrial requirements for a better quality, longer-lasting and multipurpose rubber, and other materials, were fulfilled, the stethoscope was able to evolve into its modern form. During the twentieth century, the introduction of synthetic plastics further opened the possibilities for modification of stethoscope design. The simple wooden tube and later the metal tube were the most practical materials in the early part of the nineteenth century. The earliest flexible tubes used for stethoscopes were soft metals such as copper, tin or lead. True flexible tubing initially was made of woven silk and unrefined

cautchouc (rubber). Later, reliable flexible tubes were available (Table 2).

Table 2 Some events in the development of material technology relevant to the stethoscope

18th C	Gutta percha
1820	Charles Macintosh introduces rubberized fabric; Thomas Hancock introduces an elastic product
1839	Charles Goodyear develops vulcanization to resist temperature changes
1869	John Hyatt invents celluloid
1888	John B. Dunlop patents pneumatic tire
1910	Leo Hendrik Baekeland introduces Bakelite
1928	Dupont introduces nylon, plastics industry grows rapidly

Further modifications of the monaural stethoscope

It would not be possible to review all of the suggested modifications to the monaural stethoscope. The instruments included here provide a perspective of the approaches taken by several contributors. The illustrated appendix contains many of the important monaural stethoscopes devised and serves the purpose of introducing the reader to the evolution of the instrument from that point of view (Figures A5–A24).

Most of the monaural stethoscopes, unlike the binaurals, were designed with only one ear-piece or chest-piece. Modifications were meant to make it easier to carry by dividing in two or similar conveniences.

One of the earliest modifications in the chest-piece of the stethoscope was introduced by C. J. B. Williams (1805–1889). He modified the bell-shaped chest-piece to a trumpet or bugle shape because the bell edges were uncomfortable to the patient and this shape provided better contact with the chest wall. He also suggested making the aural end trumpet-shaped and movable. Williams experimented with a variety of materials and preferred mahogany and walnut to larch and cedar, but finally settled on ebonite because of its strength (Williams 1873).

Hawksley introduced a stethoscope made of gunmetal. Hawksley's monaural stethoscope consisted of a hard rubber ear-plate, screwed into a rigid metal tube which flared at its other extremity into a bell-shaped chest-piece, or which was fitted with a detachable bell made of vulcanite or of ebony.

H. Veale reported a monaural stethoscope which he named the "Medical Officers' Stethoscope". It was 6½ inches long with a wooden cylinder and either ivory, ebony or boxwood ends. The unique aspect of it was that it had two chest-pieces: one was 1½ inches in diameter and the other only 1 inch. Both the chest-piece and the ear-piece were concave on one end and convex on the other and could be screwed onto the stem either way. There was considerable disagreement about whether the ear-piece should be flat, concave or convex. Veale enumerated his concept of the requirements for a perfect stethoscope at the time: "it should be portable ... a good conductor of sound ... its ear piece should be of a shape to fit any ear ... its chest end should be capable of being adapted to any surface, and ... any case." (Veale 1880)

Walter Garstang modified the stethoscope in 1856 in an effort to have the sounds transmitted more accurately to the listener. His instrument, in contrast to Veale's, was 9 inches long. It was made of polished cedar. The tube was perfectly smooth internally.

There also was a wide variation in the preferred length of the stethoscope. Very long ones are occasionally encountered, thought to be used by physicians dealing with very poor, unclean patients. However, many practitioners thought a longer stethoscope provided better sound, sometimes because fewer adventitial sounds were heard. Piorry provided an extension to his stethoscope for this purpose to accord the user his preference.

In 1881, Whittaker designed a disarticulating stethoscope, contrived chiefly for convenience in carrying (Whittaker 1881). One half of the stem was contained within the other half, the screw thread keeping it in place. The smaller tube was unscrewed for use and applied the reverse way to the larger tube, and fixed by the screw. This formed a stem similar to the ordinary stem of a stethoscope. The ear and chest-pieces were designed to fit one within the other for easier transportation. When required for use, they were separated and fixed firmly to their respective ends of the stem. Many similar designs were used (Figure A15).

Hudson's manual of physical diagnosis offers some insight into preferences in monaural stethoscopes (Hudson 1887). He illustrates six monaural stethoscopes but states that Barclay's is the one in most common use (Figure A17) and also the simplest in form. It is interesting that he expresses some doubt of the value of the central perforation and indicates that Cammann's auscultator is just as valuable.

The number of varieties is boundless. Modifications continued to be introduced throughout the nineteenth century and even into the twentieth. The stethoscopes were made folding in two parts, in three parts, of wood, metal, ivory, tortoiseshell, gutta-percha, calibrated, modified to serve as a reflex hammer (Figure A82), long, short and medium length (Table 1).

Gerhardt (1833–1902) who was a prominent German clinician, wrote a major text on auscultation and percussion which went through several editions. He felt that the flexible stethoscope (discussed below) did not provide results as good as the standard monaural of the time. His opinion was that stethoscopes made of rubber, horn or similar substances gave the same results, but none were better than wood. He also felt that it did not matter how the ear-piece was shaped or if the tube was short or long, thick or thin; the results depended on the skill of the physician (Gerhardt 1866;1890).

Flexible monaural stethoscopes

After Piorry, the first truly different version of the monaural stethoscope was the flexible one. Initially many physicians simply used the flexible hearing aids which were in common use at that time as stethoscopes. Many instrument collectors today will argue whether a flexible tube was a hearing aid or stethoscope, but in practice physicians used whatever was convenient and it often was a hearing aid.

A number of individuals claimed to have introduced the flexible stethoscope. Drs. Burne and Golding Bird engaged in a public debate in the *London Medical Gazette* over who was first. However, a letter in this publication from Francis Sibson, Resident Surgeon, General Hospital near Nottingham, dated August 13 1841, claimed that the invention of the true flexible stethoscope should be attributed to William Stroud. The type of stethoscope used by Sibson was 2 feet long with a funnel-shaped wooden chest-piece and no ear-piece (Sibson 1841). He reported that this was superior to using a solid stethoscope and conducted sounds better than the traditional ear trumpet, which, as noted, also was used to double as a stethoscope. It is truly remarkable that it took at least 14 years or more to move from a monaural flexible stethoscope to a binaural stethoscope. Part of the delay was the lack of a suitable material, but flexible hearing trumpets were available before the flexible monaural stethoscope was introduced. Johann August Drucker patented the first flexible hearing tube in 1819.

C. J. B. Williams (1805–1889), a noted English authority on chest disease, also reported that Stroud was the first to use a flexible stethoscope, some time around 1834. Williams was concerned that the flexible stethoscope conducted sounds in an inferior way to the rigid stethoscope. He admitted that the flexibility permitted the stethoscope to be applied to the patient in various positions which prevented the use of a rigid stethoscope. Although Williams often used a flexible stethoscope, he felt that a good auscultator should also use a rigid stethoscope in order to be more accurate. He presents an interesting discussion of the construction and use of instruments in percussion and auscultation in his article in the *London Medical Gazette* (Williams 1842). He argues here that the central bore of the stethoscope is essential for its function, a fact which was disputed at the time. He also takes the position that the wooden walls of the stethoscope help to convey the sound to the central bore providing an additional advantage over a flexible stethoscope which is dependent solely on the air column.

Another flexible stethoscope was introduced before 1839 either in France or Belgium. Raciborski notes in his monograph on auscultation and percussion:

> M. Montdezert modified the ordinary stethoscope in a manner appropriate for the exploration of the posterior surface of the trunk of a patient lying on the back by giving it a flexible tube made of gold-beater's skin containing a wire of iron rolled in a spiral. (Raciborski 1839)

William Stroud (1789–1858), who practiced at 29 Great Coram Street, published a report of his stethoscope in September 1841 in the *London Medical Gazette*. In that report he cites Comin's introduction of a "flexible stethoscope" which was in fact a jointed stethoscope (Stroud 1841–1842). His refinement was stimulated by attendance at lectures by Laennec in Paris. He states in his article that he used one of the flexible tubes used by deaf persons and, on applying it to the chest of the master of the shop in which he saw it, determined that at a distance of several feet he could hear respiratory and cardiac sounds. He then proceeded to develop a truly flexible stethoscope which he reported in his article in 1841. Stroud's invention actually consisted of three instruments: one was a cardioscope with a leather pleximeter, which was to explore the heart and arteries. It was a cylindrical stick made of cedar with two circular disks of ebony. It was essentially a small solid Laennec with a disk at each end, intended for examination of the heart. The flexible stethoscope itself consisted of an aural end, a pectoral end, and a tube which was made of caoutchouc-cloth lined with a spiral and elastic iron wire, the coils of which were in close contact with each other. This was used for pulmonary auscultation (Figures 11; A25).

Stroud cites Bird's use of a flexible monaural stethoscope which he gave to him. Golding Bird, in a letter to the *London Medical Gazette* (Bird 1841) earlier that year dated Dec 5 1840 wrote:

If a wooden stethoscope be preferred, undoubtedly the simpler the construction the better; it should be constructed of one piece of light wood, in the manner recommended by Dr Billing (*Principles of Medicine*, third edition, p. xvii), excepting that the ear-piece should be rendered very slightly convex, and somewhat larger than he has suggested. One of the length of four inches, having a cup shaped cavity, with a carefully rounded margin an inch in diameter at one end, the other extremity being slightly convex, and about two inches in diameter, possesses, in addition to its extreme portability, every advantage which a solid stethoscope can offer. Nothing exceeds, or even equals, the simple application of the naked ear to the chest for all purposes in which the examination of sounds over an extended surface is alone required; the stethoscope being only necessary for the purpose of localizing sounds, and, for appreciating those depending upon impulse, a simple cylinder of wood will answer just as well as a perforated instrument.

For the isolation of all the sounds generated during respiration, on the action of the heart, whether in health or disease, no form of stethoscope can equal, for convenience of application, as well as for permitting the due appreciation of sounds, one furnished with a flexible tube, providing it be so arranged as to permit the acoustic vibrations to be propagated to the ear through the column of air it includes. For this purpose Dr Clendinning, and I have been informed also, Dr Stroud, have for some time past employed the

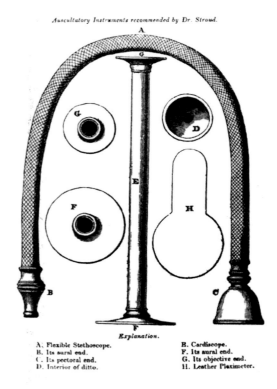

Figure 11 Stroud's flexible stethoscope

Stroud's stethoscope as illustrated in his article from 1842. The stethoscope consists of A. Flexible stethoscope; B. Aural end; C. Pectoral end; D. Interior of pectoral end; E. Cardioscope; F. Aural end; G. Objective end; and H. Leather pleximeter. It was a multipurpose device which could be modified in form as needed.

common snake hearing trumpet. This instrument is much longer than is necessary, and hence is inconvenient in application, as well as from its diminishing the intensity of sound by causing it to traverse an unnecessarily long column of air: the little tube introduced into the meatus is also very disagreeable in practice, and not infrequently productive of pain and uneasiness to those using it.

Bird discusses his modification of the stethoscope (Figure A25) in the same article:

The end which is applied to the chest consists of a thin cup of ebony, an inch in diameter, and carefully rounded at its edges: a flexible tube, from sixteen to twenty inches in length, formed of a spiral iron wire, covered with caoutchouc, and bound tightly round with silk or velvet, having an internal diameter of about one-fourth of an inch, is fixed into the apex of this cup: the other end of the tube is cemented into a perforated ebony ball, on the top of which is screwed a slightly concave plate of ivory two inches in diameter, also perforated in its centre.

When this instrument is used, the ebony cup should be held, between the fingers and thumb of one hand, against the walls of the chest, and thus, with the utmost facility, and without producing unnecessary pressure, a tolerably airtight approximation is effected. The ebony ball at the other end should be held in the other hand, and the ivory plate closely applied to the ear. In this manner, we have a column of air, bounded at one extremity by the vibrating surface of the chest, and at the other by the membrana tympani, which thus becomes placed in the position most favourable for assuming vibrations throughout its whole extent. The cup of ebony has its vibrations damped by the pressure of the fingers grasping it, whilst the covering of silk or velvet performs a similar office, with sufficient accuracy, for the spiral wire forming the tube of the instrument, whilst from the convenient position in which the physician can place himself with regard to the patient, the necessarily close approximation of the end of the stethoscope to the surface of the chest may be effected. In addition to this, the intensity of sound

does not appear to be sensibly diminished by the flexure of the tube, and thus we can auscultate the sides and back of the chest by a very slight movement of the body of a patient whilst in the recumbent position…

Bird's primary objection to Stroud's instrument is the ear-piece for which he preferred using a flat disk rather than a plug to insert into the ear.

Shortly after Stroud's report, C. W. Pennock reported using a "new flexible stethoscope" (Pennock 1844) in the United States. He stated that "this device entirely supersedes the objectionable European instrument." The device was reported in the July issue of the *American Journal of the Medical Sciences* by Ludlow (1844) following Pennock's commentary in March. The major improvements were a tube of brass, a perfectly conical bell of a defined thickness, and the use of a flattened brass wire for the construction of the tube itself. The tube was covered by elastic cloth and webbing (Figure A26).

A flexible stethoscope was also described in Germany in 1875 by Voltolini from Falkenberg who reported that he had been using it for twenty years. It consisted of an acorn-shaped ear-piece made of horn joined to a wooden (fir) bell-shaped chest-piece by India rubber tubing (Voltolini 1875).

A model of flexible stethoscope which achieved considerable popularity was introduced by Paul (1881a). It could be used as a monaural, binaural or teaching device. His description of his invention also serves to illustrate the rationale for the continued use of monaural stethoscopes after the binaural was well developed.

I have the honor to present in my name a new model of flexible stethoscope furnished with a reinforced trunk. For the 19 years that I have substituted the flexible stethoscope for the rigid stethoscope, I have been able to demonstrate that one cannot pretend to recognize pathologic bruit of the heart and the vessels unless one has determined very exactly the topography, the timing and the tone. The flexible stethoscope is simple and yet better than the binaural stethoscope, permitting one to make understood a pathologic bruit to a large number of observers. One should therefore share the same observation, which is a necessary condition to arrive at the same interpretation. This instrument is, therefore, very good. I come to submit to you an improvement in the ring shaped nozzle, which Dr Russel of Geneva has invented for his transfuser. My stethoscope when so modified, has remarkable acoustic qualities. Because the adaptation permits a reproducible pressure on the skin and the presence of the cavity of the bell forms a reinforced compartment, the sound which one hears takes an intensity and a clearness which is remarkable. If one adapts to this new chest-piece a metallic tube with two branches to make the stethoscope binaural, one arrives at an intensity unknown up to now in the auscultation of cardiac and vascular bruits. The suction nozzle permits the further automatic fixation of the stethoscope at the point chosen to auscultate and the pupils are able to come successively to take the acoustic tube without displacing the apparatus. It permits one to listen not only to the bruits in children and in adults but also the bruit of the fetus. Therefore, the superior acoustic quality and facility for demonstration. These are the qualities of this new stethoscope constructed on my indications by M. Galante.

(Translation from M. Constantin Paul, D'Instrument, Academy de Medicine Bulletin, Paris 1881a).

Paul went on to write a book *Diagnosis and Treatment of Diseases of the Heart* which was translated into English in 1884. The use of his stethoscope figured prominently in this text (Figures 12; A67).

Other individuals continued to make modifications to the flexible stethoscope. Frederick P. Henry, Physician to the Episcopal Hospital of Philadelphia, presented a modified monaural stethoscope in 1876. It consisted of the ear-piece of an otoscope at one extremity, and the ordinary trumpet shaped chest-piece of the stethoscope at

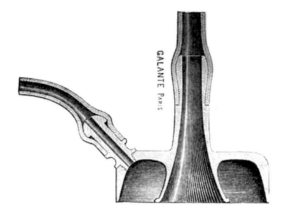
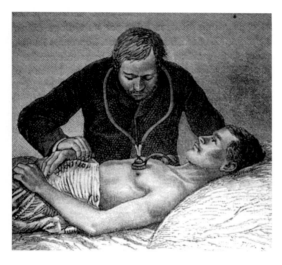

Figure 12 Paul's stethoscope

A. cross-section of the chest-piece shows the double chamber with a connection for a bulb to evacuate the air and create a suction chamber to hold it in place by air pressure. B. A lithograph showing the physician examining the patient without the need to hold the stethoscope in place (Paul 1884). It is shown with two flexible ear tubes in place, but numerous modifications were used (see Figure 26).

the other. The two end pieces were connected with three feet of fine black India rubber tubing of French manufacture. The internal diameter of the tube was about one-quarter of an inch (Henry 1876).

A truly unusual addition to the flexible monaural stethoscope was introduced in 1901 by W. E. Scott. This instrument had a flexible tube which was placed in one ear and an earplug for the other ear to keep out extraneous sound. The earplugs were made of metal and both were connected by an elastic band which held them in place. The stethoscope head was held with a belt on the person so that both hands could be free for percussion or other manipulations (Figure A27).

7 The evolution of the binaural stethoscope

An obvious question is why physicians did not move more quickly toward the development of the binaural stethoscope. Part of the explanation lies in the need for the introduction of suitable flexible materials. But another was the great concern of an imbalance between the ears. S. Scott Alison (1859) expressed this concern when he wrote about his differential stethoscope: "It is to be observed, that for the differential stethophone to have its properties made available, it is necessary that both ears of the observer should be alike in acuteness."

Long after the invention of a practical binaural stethoscope there remained a preference for the monaural variety. Finlayson (1891), in the section on auscultation of his clinical manual, describes primarily the use of the monaural stethoscope in the examination of the chest but he also indicates: "A binaural stethoscope with a single bell is also frequently used, and is said to intensify the sounds." An article by Syers (1902) strongly condemns the use of the binaural stethoscope: "I am convinced that much of the faulty diagnosis of chest disease which is so frequently seen at the present day is the result of the habitual use of the binaural stethoscope."

The Kny–Scheerer Co. catalog of about 1912 has 14 pages devoted to different types of stethoscope. There are 78 varieties of monaural stethoscope offered including ones made of ebony, metal, ivory, celluloid, hard rubber and aluminum. The variety is remarkable and some even used membranes on the thoracic end. There are 53 binaural instruments listed with an equal variety of sizes, shapes and materials (Figures 13a and 13b). The French Boulitte catalog of 1923 lists a simple binaural stethoscope with the comment:

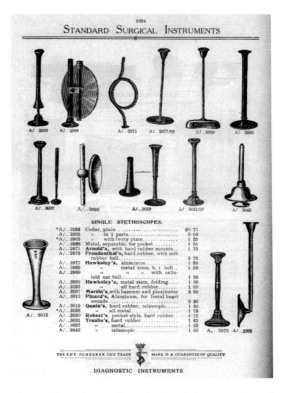

Figure 13a   A page from the Kny–Scheerer catalog of 1912 illustrating the monaural stethoscopes in vogue at that time. The names vary greatly from catalog to catalog. Sometimes the name of the manufacturer is used, in other cases it is the name of the inventor and often the instrument is simply named after some prominent physician.

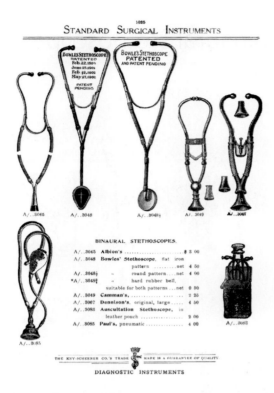

1085
STANDARD SURGICAL INSTRUMENTS

BINAURAL STETHOSCOPES.

A/..3045 Albion's .... $ 3 00
A/..3048 Bowles' Stethoscope, flat iron
                pattern ....net 4 50
A/..3048½   "   round pattern ...net 4 00
*A/..3048¾ "   hard rubber bell,
        suitable for both patterns ...net 0 50
A/..3049 Camman's, ... 2 25
A/..3067 Dennison's, original, large 4 50
A/..3083 Auscultation Stethoscope, in
        leather pouch 2 00
A/..3085 Paul's, pneumatic 4 00

THE KNY-SCHEERER CO.'S TRADE ✠ MARK IS A GUARANTEE OF QUALITY
DIAGNOSTIC INSTRUMENTS

Figure 13b   A page from the Kny–Scheerer catalog of 1912 illustrating the binaural stethoscopes in vogue at that time. The more popular binaural devices showing the reluctance to abandon the older Cammann's and Denison's. Oertel's, Sansom's, Snoften's and Bianchi's versions are shown on other pages.

"This instrument, very practical, is being employed more and more."

Perhaps the ultimate demonstration of the continued late adherence to the monaural form is from the article by Louis Lowenthal (1918). In this note he describes a monaural stethoscope which has been modified with a piece of India rubber tubing that fits in the other ear so that it can be used either way (Figure 14). A similar concept was described earlier in the German literature by Hecker of Weissenburg (1903). An example of this can be seen in Figure A83. The example shown has a horn pectoral end and a boxwood chest-piece as modified by Hecker. He states that he had been using this for twenty years and that he made the modification to make it less fragile. Hecker mentions another monaural with the secondary tube that was described by Dr Heermann of Posen.

More than fifty stethoscope patents were granted in the United States between 1872 and 1920, and among them were three which were for monaural instruments, the latest being June 26 1906. Physcians were still using monaural stethoscopes as late as 1915. An example is Arnold's phonophore which was made in both binaural and monaural models. It was claimed to be especially helpful when listening to faint high-pitched sounds. It had soft rubber ear-pieces, a heavy metal and rubber tubing, and a resonating steel chest-piece. The sharp edges of the chest-piece were covered with a rubber cushion for the comfort of the patient (DaCosta 1915).

The use of the monaural stethoscope persisted even beyond these dates. George P. Pilling and Son of Philadelphia, who were deeply committed to stethoscope manufacture, patented a monaural stethoscope in 1933 (US Patent 1,932,227). It was made to swivel at both the auricular and chest end and was invented by Charles J. Pilling and Bruno Wiegand of Philadelphia. It was made of hard rubber and metal and meant to be both more portable and adjustable in position when examining the patient.

The first binaural stethoscope

Arthur Leared (1822–1879) claimed to have invented the double stethoscope some time before 1851. However, C. Theodore Williams reported that his father, C. J. B. Williams, constructed a binaural stethoscope in 1829 (Williams CT 1907). This was described as a clumsy affair, made of lead because of the lack of suitable flexible materials. A report to the Royal Medical and Chirurgical Society by C. J. B. Williams in 1873 was at variance with his son's account. He showed a binaural stethoscope with metal tubes and wooden ear- and chest-pieces which he reported he designed thirty years before (Williams CJB 1873). The argument over precedence is discussed somewhat vitriolically by Leared in a letter to the *Lancet* dated August 2 1856 (Leared 1856). In this letter he claims precedence by having registered his invention with the executive committee of the Great Exhibition of London in 1851. The description of his invention was sent to the committee on January 28 1851. He also states that in fact he had already used the instrument for one or more years. He goes so far as to suggest that his idea might have been pirated by Marsh, who patented a binaural stethoscope in 1851, and he discounts Williams' instrument as never having been published (Leared 1856). A picture of Willams' version was included in the article written by his son (Williams CT 1907) (Figure 15). Leared gained wide recognition for his invention, although the only original publication by him about it appears to be the listing in the catalog of the great exhibition (Leared 1851). Leared completed a thesis for the degree of MD at the University of Dublin in 1860 entitled *On the Sounds Caused by the Circulation of the Blood*. In this thesis he illustrates the device he constructed to carry out his studies. The stethoscope he used in these experiments is the standard monaural of the time (Leared 1861). This certainly would cause one to wonder about the utility of his invention.

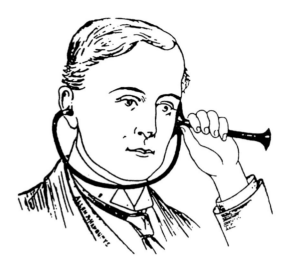

Figure 14 Lowenthal's modified monaural

The brief description of this in the literature perhaps epitomizes the reluctance to abandon the monaural stethoscope while beset by the increasing evidence of the advantages of the binaural (Lowenthal 1918a and b). The concept shown is almost identical to that presented by Hecker (1903) fifteen years earlier.

41

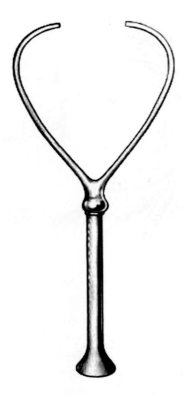

Figure 15 C. J. B. Williams' binaural stethoscope

C. T. Willams indicates that his father C. J. B. Willams (Willams CT 1907) constructed this stethoscope in 1829 using a chest-piece of mahogany and two bent lead pipes for ear-pieces since rubber was not yet available. C. J. B. Williams himself leads us to believe it was actually from about 1840 and the tubes were made of an unspecified metal.

An article published by Comins in 1829 reviews the general reception of the stethoscope in England and seems to clearly establish that he was the first to suggest a binaural instrument (Comins 1829). Comins modified the monaural stethoscope for use at the Royal Infirmary. He cites the invention of the stethoscope as the most important invention in medicine since the introduction of vaccination by Jenner. According to Comins, a problem with the monaural stethoscopes then in vogue was that the patient frequently had to change position in order for the physician to complete the examination. The chest-piece of his device consisted of a concave piece of ivory, which was screwed to the cylinder of the tube and an ear-piece which was made to cover the ear. The innovation of Comins' stethoscope was that it was jointed allowing the observer to listen from a variety of positions without having to require the patient to move. It also could be extended by adding an additional tube to increase the distance between the observer and the patient. It is evident from Comins' comments that the patients were forced to assume a wide variety of positions when the standard monaural stethoscope was used and that the stethoscope was pressed very tightly against the chest to the point of causing discomfort. Comins also states: "Laennec's, like almost every other invention, has been opposed; but the quick sale of his works proves that his discovery, like that of Jenner, necessarily and rapidly overpowers opposition." The role of the stethoscope at that time is made clear by his article:

It is often indispensable in pneumonia, pleuritis, bronchitis, measles, scarlatina, croup, fever, confluent smallpox, latent catarrh, phthisis, diseases of the heart, hydrothorax, doubtful cases of pregnancy, etc.... It has been shown also, that it affords to the surgeon most important information, previously to deciding on the operations for empyema, or for the extraction of foreign bodies from the trachea; in detecting haemorrhage into the pleura; in ascertaining the state of the lungs previously to the operations for cancer of the breast, carries of the ribs, white swelling, etc.

Comins frequently refers to his instrument as a flexible stethoscope, although in reality it was an articulated monaural which could be modified for binaural use.

Its importance lies in the fact that many authors attribute the invention of the binaural stethoscope to Comins since he states in his article,

It has occurred to me that both ears might be simultaneously and advantageously employed in stethoscopic examinations. The instrument adapted to this purpose consists of a tube, connected at its middle at right angles to the cylinder, to be applied to the patient, and connected at its moveable extremities to two tubes, moveable also on the principle that has been described. It admits of easy adaptation at once of the patient, and to both ears. (Figure 16)

The introduction by Golding Bird and by Stroud of stethoscopes in which the rigid stem of the ordinary form was replaced by a flexible tube paved the way for the development of a practical binaural stethoscope. Although these were still monaural stethoscopes, they introduced the concept of using a flexible tube and demonstrated that such an arrangement could transmit the sound reliably (Bird 1840–41).

Arthur Leared of London, England, designed the binaural stethoscope noted above some time before 1851, about the same time as Marsh, although, as noted above, he strongly claimed precedence. Leared's "double stethoscope made of gutta-percha" was exhibited in the Great Exhibition of 1851 in London. An instrument which is said to be Leared's is illustrated in Aitken's textbook (Aitken 1866; 1868; 1872) (Figure 17).

Aitkens' text (1866) illustrates much of the confusion of the time over the development of the binaural stethoscope. He responds to Leared's letter to the editor noted above and states:

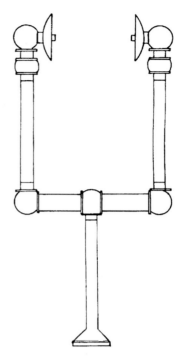

Figure 16 Comins' stethoscope

The figure shows Comins' stethoscope assembled for binaural use. In his original article although he suggested this form as an option, Comins shows the individual parts consisting of the ear-piece, connecting tube and pectoral end joined with flexible connections, but only one aural tube is shown (Comins 1829 from Sheldon, Doe 1935).

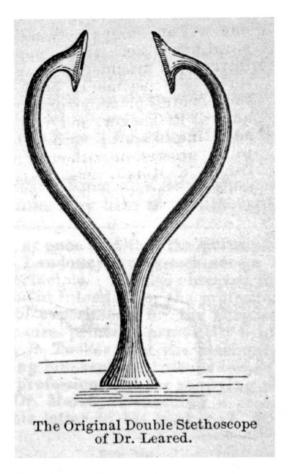

The Original Double Stethoscope
of Dr. Leared.

Figure 17 Leared's stethoscope

Leared's stethoscope is shown as it is illustrated in Aitken's text of 1872. It was composed of gutta-percha and the ear-pieces held in place by the tension of the semi-elastic material.

"An American, however, took the idea home and having made some minor alterations, a stethoscope with two tubes was patented in America as "Dr Cammann's self-adjusting double stethoscope," obviously confusing Marsh and Cammann. (Aitken 1866). Many English catalogs illustrate Cammann's stethoscope with the name 'Leared's. Aitken must be given credit for discovering the error of his statements in the 1866 edition of his text and retracting them with a more accurate discussion of Cammann's invention in the next edition (Aitken 1868). Alison (1861) provides a more detailed description of Leared's stethoscope:

> It is composed entirely of gutta percha. It has two tubes and a body end or hollow cylinder, which received the distal ends of the tubes. The ear extremities of the tubes have the ear-pieces of the common stethoscope (monaural). To use this instrument ordinarily in practice, one would require three hands, for it possesses no self-adjustment, such as renders Cammann's so valuable.... Thus, while it must be admitted that Dr Leared greatly preceded Dr Cammann in making known the principle of bin-aural auscultation, it is to this latter gentleman we are indebted for an easy, efficient and very agreeable method...

Aitken provides a similar description, adding that the elasticity of the gutta-percha tubes helped to keep the instrument in place in the ears (Aitken 1866).

Nathan B. Marsh of Cincinnati, Ohio, patented his binaural stethoscope (U.S. Patent #8,591) on December 16 1851 (Figure 18). His patent specifications described the instrument as a "stethoscope and ear trumpet." As can be seen in the figure this was at best a very crude invention. It consisted of an India rubber tube with a bell formed by flaring out the rubber or by attaching a bell made of different material such as bone, horn or wood. The ear-pieces consisted simply of a U-shaped tube of rubber joined to the chest tube with a solution of gutta-percha in chloroform or any other material to make it airtight.

The justification for the patent was: "The double branch connected with the maintrunk so as to enable persons to use both ears simultaneously." Although no ear-pieces were described he suggested tapering the ends of the tube which went into the ear to facilitate its insertion.

Cammanns' stethoscope

All of the contributions described above set the stage for the adoption of the binaural stethoscope, but it was Cammann's stethoscope which was the first truly practical binaural device. George P. Cammann (1804–1863) graduated from Rutgers Medical School and practiced in New York City. The chest-piece of his invention was made of ebony and it was attached to two tubes composed of gum elastic and metallic wire which in turn were connected to two metallic tubes of German silver with ivory knobs at the aural extremity. A movable elastic band was arranged to adjust the ear-pieces and to keep them in position. The bell-like expansion of the chest-piece was 2½ inches in diameter, gently curving outward, to present a rounded edge to the chest. Several examples are shown in Figures A28–A31. The tubing was covered with woven silk.

Although it appears clear that Comins first suggested the binaural stethoscope in 1829, the first truly practical device was Cammann's. A public debate over infringement of patent followed the introduction of the Cammann's device. Marsh had patented his invention. But Cammann was opposed to physicians' patenting their inventions, believing that they should be freely available to the public, a concept which unfortunately is no longer shared by the medical community. Aitken in the 1868 edition of his text quotes James Leaming who was the literary executor of Dr Cammann's estate and his clinical assistant when the work on the stethoscope was done. According to this account, in the spring of 1852 H. W. Browne brought one of Marsh's

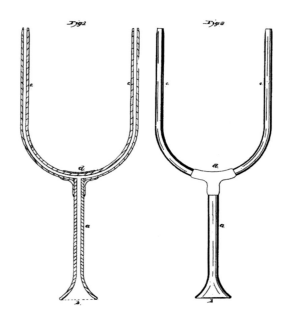

Figure 18 Patent of Marsh's stethoscope

The figure here is taken from Marsh's original patent application. The structure is as described in the text. He described it as either a stethoscope or an ear trumpet. It was made of India rubber although the bell could either be flared from the rubber or made of horn or wood and inserted in the tubing. Marsh is said to have suggested a membrane over the bell, but it is not mentioned in the brief version of the patent nor is it shown in the accompanying diagram.

stethoscopes to Dr Cammann's class at the Northern Dispensary. Cammann noted that the principle was not a new one and he recalled Landouzy's polyscope of which he had an example. Landouzy's original description mentioned using tubes of soft metal such as copper or tin, but it appears by this time he had begun using gum elastic for the tubing. He began a series of experiments with the assistance of H. W. Browne and C. P. Tucker which culminated in the "self adjusting binaural stethoscope." Aitkens accompanies his editorial note with an illustration of Cammann's stethoscope which is a later model using the elastic band without the earlier spring to maintain the ear tension.

The debate is understood best by reviewing this letter of Dr Cammann's to the correspondence section of the *New York Journal of Medicine* (Cammann 1857).

Being informed that Dr Marsh, of Cincinnati, complains of my having infringed the patent of his double stethoscope, I would state that,

1. Dr Marsh's instrument and mine differ essentially one from the other both in principle and construction.
2. I wholly disclaim any intention of interfering with the rights and interests of Dr Marsh. I have never received any advantage from the sale of my stethoscope, but presented it free to the profession. Dr Marsh has remained perfectly quiet for two years from the first appearance of the double self-adjusting stethoscope, and now, when the period has elapsed within which I might have secured myself by patent, if so inclined, his aim and endeavor seem to be not to dispose of his *original patented instrument*, but to avail himself of mine with all its *improvements and adaptation to practical purposes*. Is the Profession, then, prepared, on the *ipse dixit* of Dr Marsh, to sustain him in the sale of my stethoscope under restrictions, when he has not taken the usual course to establish his legal right so to do. He certainly cannot acquire the moral right to receive the benefit of other men's labors.

3. Dr Marsh's stethoscope appears to be but a modification of other instruments long known in Europe and now in my possession.

The above statement, including the opinion that my stethoscope is not an infringement of Dr Marsh's patent, is made under advice of eminent counsel.

New York, Dec 2 1856 G. P. Cammann

Before this, an editorial had appeared in the *New York Medical Times* (Editorial, 1855) which formally introduced Cammann's stethoscope to the medical consumer. It read:

The stethoscope of Dr Cammann presents, as will be seen by the engraving, an objective end, made of ebony, the extremity of which is about two inches in diameter, two tubes composed of gum elastic and metallic wire, two metallic tubes of German silver, two ivory knobs at the aural extremity, and a movable elastic spring, so arranged as to adjust it, and keep it in its proper position.

H. Landouzy, of Paris, previous to 1850, formed a stethoscope having a number of gum elastic tubes,

[He was mistaken here, Landouzy described using tin or copper, perhaps later it was changed to rubber]

by means of which several persons could listen at the same time. Dr N. B. Marsh, of Cincinnati, 1851 patented a stethoscope with two gum elastic tubes, and a membrane over its objective end. Dr Cammann does not, therefore, claim any originality on account of the two branches of his instrument, but on account of other advantages which it possesses. The instrument of H. Landouzy was not found of any practical use.

The objections to that of Dr Marsh are:

1. That the aural extremity is composed of roughly cut India-rubber, without anything to adapt it to the ear, which both causes irritation and does not exclude sounds from without.

2. That it required both hands to keep it in position.
3. That it gives a loud, muffled, and confused sound, caused by reverberation within the instrument, in consequence of the drum at the objective and the inequality of the diameter of the bore. These circumstances render it of but little practical value.

The only resemblance between the instrument of Dr Cammann and that of both Drs Landouzy and Marsh is, that each is composed of more than one tube.

On reference to the engraving of the stethoscope of Dr Cammann, which represents the instrument of one-third its size, it will be observed that the bell-like expansion of the objective extremity will be two and a half inches in diameter, with a convolvulus excavation, gently curving outwards, to present a rounded edge to the chest, in order to prevent causing pain to the patient. The bore of the instrument is two and a half lines in diameter, care being taken to have it made smooth and even.

The tubes are made of German silver, with a double curve towards the aural extremities, which curves require to be constructed with great care, so that the ivory knobs may rest closely upon the external openings of the ears. When applied, it is necessary that the orifices of the knobs should point upwards, Some of the instruments are constructed with a spiral, and others with an elastic spring, as shown by the plate. Some of them are so arranged that they can be disjointed, to render them more portable.

One point, heretofore *sub judice,* is settled by this instrument, viz, that the sound is conducted entirely through the air, and not at all through the media, as these were, for experiment's sake, changed nine or more times, without affecting in the least the intensity of the conducted sound. On making the objective end solid, all sound was lost.

The advantages claimed for the instrument by Dr Cammann are listed:

1. That being applied, it adjusts itself closely to both ears, excluding all external sound.

2. It leaves both hands of the examiner free.
3. It gives sounds pure, and greatly increased in intensity, though differing in quality from those hitherto afforded by auscultation, the pitch being lower. This intensity is produced by both ears being acted upon at once, by the ear-pieces of the instrument fitting closely into the meatus of both ears, and by the smoothness and careful construction of the bore of the stethoscope as to curves, etc., according to the law of reflected sound.
4. Sounds not heard throught the instrument in common use can be detected by this.
5. Sounds which are doubtful by ordinary instruments are made perfectly certain. Even when disease is seated in the central part of the lungs, they can be detected, when the ordinary stethoscope will fail to render them recognizable. The same advantages are obtained in examining the morbid sounds of the heart.

The great increase of intensity of sound by this instrument renders it valuable to those with impaired hearing.

In the use of this stethoscope it is necessary that the chest should be uncovered, to prevent all friction between it and the clothes; otherwise the sound thus generated is conducted with such intensity as to embarass the examiner. A short practice may be required to become familiar with it, in consequence of the increased intensity of the sounds produced by it, and the difference between them and those afforded by ordinary auscultation. Many of the recognized physical signs of thoracic disease will be so modified as to be new to the examiner, but a short experience will enable him to appreciate them, and give them their true value.

These stethoscopes are manufactured and sold by Messrs. George Tieman & Co., No. 63, Chatam Street, who pay particular attention to their construction – a point very essential to an instrument of this kind.

The figure shows a stethoscope which is at variance somewhat with what most collectors today consider to be the earliest Cammann (Figure 19; Figures A28–A31). An identical article

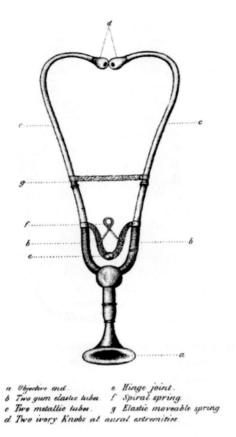

a *Objective end.*
b *Two gum elastic tubes.*
c *Two metallic tubes.*
d *Two ivory Knobs at aural extremities.*
e *Hinge joint.*
f *Spiral spring.*
g *Elastic moveable spring.*

Figure 19 G. P. Cammann's self-adjusting double stethoscope, 1855

This is probably the earliest marketed version of the instrument. The major difference between this and later models is the spiral spring in addition to the gum rubber to help adjust the tension between the ears (NY Medical Times, 1855; Pollock 1856). The gum rubber had to be slid up or down the ear-pieces or reduced in size to adjust the tension. The head-piece and the rest of the instrument was a dramatic advance over what had been suggested previously.

without the figure appeared in the Practical Medicine section of the *New York Journal of Medicine* the following May (NY Medical Times, 1855); the previous one had appeared in January.

Cammann's stethoscope was rapidly recognized in Europe and was often referred to as "the American model." James Pollock (1856) reported on its use very early in the *Lancet*. He reasserts the claim that Williams used a double stethoscope with a metal tube and also Landouzy's invention in 1841 (H. Pollock (1933) gives the date as 1850) of a multiple-tubed stethoscope. He was also aware of Marsh's patent and of Leared's double instrument made with gutta-percha. Cammann gave one of his early instruments to a Dr Coulson of Castle Donington, England, who loaned it to Pollack. Although Pollack pointed out many strengths of the Camman, he also expressed the usual reluctance to abandon his current practice of using monaural stethoscopes. His great foresight is attested by the statement in his concluding paragraph: "...it is little likely that advances in our knowledge of chest affections are to come through improvements in mechanical devices." However, in spite of his reservations about Cammann's model, he notes that he asked the instrument maker Coxeter to make some.

Modifications of Cammann's stethoscope

Many modifications followed Cammann's invention. Another binaural stethoscope was invented by Dr S. A. Skinner and improved by Dr C. C. Tafton. An ad for this stethoscope is included in a catalog of surgical apparatus manufactured by Watkins, CA and Co. 1858 at the National Library of Medicine in the United States. The device is particularly interesting because it has a spring within the tubing to hold the ivory ear-pieces in the ears and a rod extending from the junction of the ear-pieces which was held in the mouth to help keep it in place. It was quite long and had a bell-shaped chest-piece.

The details of the material used are not given (Figure 20).

Scott Alison (1859–1861) devised a differential stethoscope which was closely related to the binaural. It consisted of two flexible monaural stethoscopes, connected by a joint for adaptation to the two ears at the same time. Although it was binaural, it really was conceptually two monaural stethoscopes being used at the same time. The differential stethoscope is discussed later on page 66. Some manufacturers sold a later version in which by changing the chest-piece one could easily switch between a Cammann's type stethoscope and an Alison. Considerable confusion was caused by the multiple claims for precedence in the invention of the binaural stethoscope. The 1887 catalog of Lynch and Co. lists Leared's stethoscope for 19 shillings and sixpence, but the illustration shows a Cammann's with an option for an Alison differential (Lynch & Co. 1887).

Frederick Irving Knight (1841–1909) is an excellent example of the ultimate acceptance of auscultation. After earning his MD degree from Harvard in 1866 he studied at several European hospitals. Knight settled in Boston where he devoted his attention to diseases of the throat and chest and became Instructor in Auscultation, Percussion and Laryngoscopy at Harvard University (Atkinson 1878). It is remarkable that his professorship was based on these highly regarded diagnostic techniques rather than any disease or organ system. This professorship suggests a broader acceptance of auscultation in the United States at this time. However, Knight himself in an article dated 1869 qualifies this acceptance writing "…the double stethoscope is very little used, even in this country, where it was invented, except by graduates of Harvard and Bellevue, and almost never, I believe abroad" (Knight 1869). The same article quotes Austin Flint's acceptance of the binaural. A major problem with Cammann's stethoscope was the awkwardness of using the elastic band to adjust the tension on the ears. Knight introduced the adjustable spring arrangement

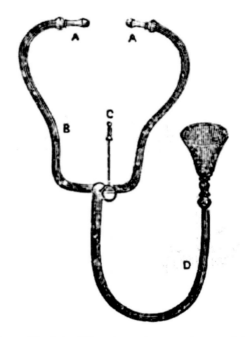

Figure 20 S. A. Skinner's stethoscope improved by C. C. Tafton

This appeared in an 1858 catalog of G. A. Watkins and Company of Springfield, Vermont. Although this stethoscope is dated after Cammann's, note the greater similarity to Marsh's invention (Figure 18).

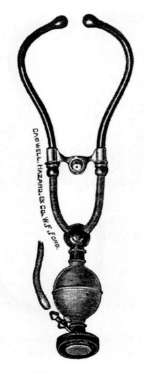

Figure 21 D. M. Cammann's stethoscope

This illustration, taken from the *New York Medical Journal* (Cammann 1886) shows a chest-piece with Cammann's modification of Paul. The rim is left open to allow for the suction to the chest. The central bell is covered with a diaphragm and the ear-pieces are closed so that the entire instrument can be filled with water. Although he acknowledged the water-filled stethoscope was not very good for ordinary auscultation, Cammann reported that it was much better for ausculatory percussion.

which is seen in Figure A35 on a Denison model and was incorporated into several other designs of the period. Although the design was named after Knight, he attributes its invention to Moses G. Farmer.

D. M. Cammann (1852–1928), the son of George P. Cammann (not to be confused with George), was an instructor in diseases of the chest and physical diagnosis at the New York Polyclinic. He devised a modified binaural stethoscope which increased the intensity of the sounds conveyed to the ears (Cammann DM 1885b).

The chest-piece of D. M. Cammann's stethoscope was a circular chamber, open on the side which was applied to the chest. The inner and outer walls of this chamber were circular and about half an inch apart. The inner wall was the extremity of the tube leading from the chest to the ear. The outer wall was also the outer wall of the chest-piece, which arched above and joined the inner wall, thus forming the roof of the chamber. The chamber is connected by a small tubular opening to a rubber bulb. By pressure and relaxation of pressure by the hand upon the bulb, the air in the chamber was exhausted, and the stethoscope was held against the chest by pressure of the external air. It was essentially a modification of the cup of Paul in which the cup surrounded the tube instead of being separate from it. Paul's stethoscope is shown in Figure 12. The advantages presented by this modification were that it left the hands of the user free and it provided better contact with the chest. A model modified to be filled with water was used for auscultatory percussion (Figure 21; A67).

By the year 1887 Hudson could write: "owing to the greater convenience, attractiveness, and applicability of the binaural of Cammann, which, in this country at least [United States], is almost synonymous with stethoscope, so little is any other used or known." (Hudson 1887) He goes on to say its use is discouraged by many English and Continental physicians, their criticism being that it intensifies sounds and alters the pitch and quality. Even as late as this he was compelled to include a section on the reasons for using the stethoscope rather than the ear.

Snelling spent five years between 1866 and 1870 modifying Cammann's stethoscope (Snelling T G, 1870–1871). A useful modification was an India rubber rim which was attached to the rim or lip of the chest-piece of the stethoscope. This made it possible, with gentle pressure, to make the contact airtight by the elastic expansion of the India rubber ring, thus making it easier to listen to the true sounds of the region being auscultated. A rubber bell (Snelling's Bell) was sold as an insert for the Cammann's chest-piece in later years. Sharp and Smith, the instrument company, marketed a "perfected Cammann" stethoscope (Figure A57).

Denison's good stethoscope

Another popular binaural stethoscope was invented by Charles Denison (1845–1909), who was born in Royalton, Vermont. He graduated from the University of Vermont in 1859 and, while in Hartford in 1873, he suffered pulmonary hemorrhages. He then moved to Denver where he became Professor of Diseases of the Chest and Climatology at the University.

Denison experimented with several modifications of the stethoscope (Denison 1885). He observed that a stethoscope made entirely of metal, or with metal tubes only, had a metallic quality to the sounds it transmitted. Stethoscopes made of gutta-percha, wood or celluloid had a more natural sound.

Based on these observations he used hard rubber instead of metal for the arms of the ear-piece with double flexible tubes made so as to give a smooth inner surface to the coiled wire between them which was added to hold the shape. The size of the lumen was largest at the attachment of the bell and gradually decreased in diameter to the ear ends.

All of the joints, bells, tubes and arms were constructed on the principle of a slightly conical tube, and each portion fitted evenly and tightly into the other. The fastenings of the flexible portion to the hard rubber were made so that there would be no interruption in the transmission of sounds from the chest to the ear.

There was a choice of four fittings. The smallest bell ending was for use in detecting valvular lesions and for auscultation with infants. This was actually the ending into which the other bells fit. The medium-sized bell was the one to be most generally used. A soft rubber bell was made to fit inside the medium bell so that its flexible edges projected about a quarter of an inch. This provided a good seal on the skin. It is usually mistaken now for hard rubber when found because of the changes in rubber with time. The largest bell had a rim three inches in diameter. It was especially constructed for stethoscopic percussion. This instrument was manufactured by Charles Truax & Co., 81 Randolph St., Chicago, Illinois (Figure A35).

Denison's stethoscope (1896), like Cammann's was modified by several people, some of whom attempted to reduce the cost of the instrument by using cheaper materials and manufacture, which resulted in poor stethoscopes. Consequently, after making several improvements in his instrument, Denison published a list of the essential requirements of a good stethoscope with a strong condemnation of the copies.

His concern about changes and the principles of his design are in his own words from the *Medical Record*, Oct 22, 1892:

> I have been promising myself for some time to write in protest against the frauds of instrument-makers in the manufacture of the stethoscope which bears my name. My instrument was not patented, as it should have been, for the purpose of needed regulation as to the quality of work and reasonableness of price. Therefore it is essential for an instrument-dealer to order a lot made by an

irresponsible Manufacturer, and sell them to unsuspecting medical men, as the real article, at an unreasonable proceed. This has been done in two instances in New York, and one in Chicago, to my knowledge. In consequence, my attention has been called to the most awkward and imperfect imitations, under the name "The Denison Stethoscope," and I have been chagrined to see joints uneven and loose, tubes impervious or partly occluded and especially the flexible portion made with inflexible rubber tubing, with no regard whatever to my directions.

In London, Down Brothers have made a pretty [good] instrument, excepting their poor adjustment of the spring, but in this country [the USA] George Tiemann & Co. are the only ones whose make I can recommend. They have come nearer than any other Manufacturer that I know of in following the requirements of a perfect binaural stethoscope which desiderata I will state as follows:

1st. THE SMOOTH INNER CALIBRE, large size, and gradually decreasing from the bell to the ear-ending, in imitation of the speaking tubes used for deaf persons. The law of sound is like that of light transmission, i.e., the angles of incidence and reflection are equal; and that transmission is aided by the trumpet-shaped bell and gradually decreasing size of the smooth inner surface of the tubes.

2nd. THE CONTINUOUS TRANSMISSION OF SOUND – This must be natural, so hard rubber or celluloid are preferable to metal for the tubes, as the latter gives a high pitch and metallic sound to the sounds heard. The joint between he bells and the main tube, and between the arms and the flexible tubes, are made by the even and perfect fitting of slightly conical tubes into each other making the whole instrument as if of one piece, as far as the transmission of sound is concerned. Probably the larger part of the sound is transmitted through the stethoscopic substance than through the hollow cavity.

3rd. THE CONSTRUCTION OF THE FLEXIBLE TUBES – The coiled wire for these tubes, which lines the usual rubber tubes and is itself lined with smooth soft rubber, is made

to impinge at each end of each tube against the gutta-percha, so that a nearly perfect transmission of sound is obtained. This is the part that Tiemann & Co. alone have succeeded in rightly making, and is an important feature of my stethoscope.

4th. THE EAR ENDINGS as lately made are acorn shaped, with openings so turned as to be directed directly toward the drums of the ears. This is a compromise from what I wanted, which was to have the lower and forward side of these tips bulge as to fill the space behind the tragus, and leave the hole above and back immediately in front of the auditory canal. The difficulty of fitting variously shaped ears with perfectly adapted ear-tips is considerable with any other than the even conical pattern, I think ought to be overcome.

5th. THE SPRING ATTACHMENT to pull together the arms is adjustable so that all the pressure of the ear-tip can be obtained that the listener can stand with comfort. This much pressure is desirable for perfect transmission of sound.

6th. THE ORDINARY BELL ENDINGS are as follows: The stationary bell, with slightly flaring rim one and one-eighth inch in diameter, which is large enough to use in examination of infants and in the detection of valvular lesions. The medium-sized bell, which has a rim one and one-half inch in diameter and sufficiently flaring to give a good impinging surface against the chest, is the size ordinarily used. The soft rubber bell, rather thin and flexible, is intended to crowd into the medium sized bell, giving a one-fourth projecting rim or soft rubber for use on uneven surfaces, as in much emaciated consumptives.

7th. THE LARGE BELL FOR STETHOSCOPIC PERCUSSION – This is not, as has been assumed, for use held against the chest-wall, but for gathering the waves of sound emitted from the open mouth during expiration while forcible percussion is being made over portions of the lung where softening, bronchiectasis, or excavation is suspected. The concussion of the air contained in the thorax carried with it the succession, the cavernous, or the cracked-metal sounds which accompany the three above-named conditions, and by holding this large bell two inches from the patient's mouth, and percussing during expiration, they are distinguished better than can be done in any other way. Indeed, in thin chested persons with superficial excavations connected with a main bronchus, the fingernail percussion will nicely and accurately outline the limits of the excavation. The cracked-pot or hollow sounds are altered in various ways, a slushy or succession quality being some-times imparted to either, according to the amount of moisture or breaking down which complicates the condition. I believe that the importance of the question of the first breaking down of lung tissue elevates this stethoscopic percussion to a first place in the area of physical diagnosis. It is certainly coequal with ordinary percussion, and second, if at all, only to auscultation.

The test I suggest of a good stethoscope is not, as assumed by Dr Valentine in his article in the MEDICAL RECORD of July 16th, to hold the medium sized bell against to face of a watch, but put the watch on a show-case or table, cover it with the palm of the hand, then press the bell against the back of the hand. The clearness with which the working of the machinery is heard is the criterion of perfection in the instrument. By this test seven-eighths of the other stethoscopes sold fall short of their proper utility. I am willing to have my instrument, if properly made, tried by this test and if anyone will improve on mine as much as I have improved on the ordinary kind, I will have his make if it costs $50. I do not believe, however, that there is room enough in the perfect reproduction of auscultation sounds for so much improvement, unless it would be a telephonic stethoscope, which would necessitate an electric battery accompaniment.

Portability and cheapness of construction are not cardinal points in a good stethoscope. Utility should be considered first, last, and chiefly. Yet the former points should not be lost sight of in making my instrument. It should be as short and compact as flexibility and convenience of use will allow, and should be proportioned in its different parts as shown in the accompanying cut.

Denison continued to experiment with improving the stethoscope (Denison 1896). He introduced interchangeable ear-pieces to suit the observer and other minor changes.

Other binaural models

A variety of other stethoscopes were introduced during this period including Bartlett's stethoscope with metal ear tubes instead of India rubber, Davis', Ford's and Knight's. Most of these modifi-cations were relatively minor. Examples are shown in the appendix (Figures A32–A34).

The continued reluctance to fully abandon the monaural stethoscope is illustrated by that of Cousins, who modified it (1882) so that it could be used as a simple, a binaural or a differential stethoscope (Figure 22). A similar modification was introduced by Aydo Smith (1884). Cousins also advocated using his stethoscope with the long shaft between the teeth or pressed against the forehead and with the tubing in place.

An interesting concept was presented by Mark Knapp, of New York, who complained of the buzzing sound heard through most stethoscopes (Knapp 1895). He thought that the buzzing came from the sound waves in the atmosphere, striking the metallic ear-pieces. He wanted to retain metal for the stethoscope, which he thought was a good conductor, but eliminate the buzzing, so he cov-ered his metal instrument with rubber. It was manufactured by Tiemann & Co., which was the premier instrument maker at that time as noted by Denison.

Numerous other models were introduced during the last quarter of the nineteenth century and the first quarter of the twentieth. The most important innovation was the introduction of Bowles' chest-piece and the simplification of the head-piece. It became possible with improving technology to replace the woven silk and rubber tubing with a flexible rubber and then plastic. The bell portion evolved into its modern form from the earlier versions. The major change here related more to the manner in which the bell was

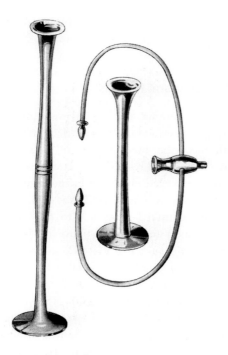

Figure 22 Cousins' Stethoscope

The parts shown are: 1. The long single stethoscope adapted for subclavicular auscultation (9″) and for keeping the patient's head away from the examiner; 2. The ordinary short stethoscope adapted by dividing the long in half; 3. The double stethoscope which is made complete by joining it to the shaft of the short single tube (composed of elastic tubes with wooden ear plugs). This was one of many designs to satisfy the belief that no single type of stethoscope was ideal for all the possible clinical situations which might be encountered (Cousins 1882).

constructed rather than the actual shape. The major evolutionary changes are outlined in Table 3.

The Bowles' stethoscope

One of the most enduring modifications of the stethoscope came from Robert C. M. Bowles of Brookline, Massachusetts, who patented five modifications between 1901 and 1904 (US Patents #677,172, #693,487, #700,728, #734,159 and #773,274). They were based largely on his patent of Oct 2 1894 (US Patent #526,802). The 1894 patent used an ear-piece like the later Cammann's and a chest-piece with a buttonlike projection. In this version a diaphragm was placed within the bell or funnel so that it did not make contact with the body. A projecting rod or stud actually made contact and it was similar to the Bazzi–Bianchi design. The projecting rod was popular at the time and another interesting stethoscope that used it was the amplifone (Figure A58). The concept of the modern Bowles stethoscope head really took shape when the projecting button was dropped in the 1901 patent. However, in his patent of 1894 he notes that the main features were "a stethoscopic instrument provided with a diaghragm firmly secured at its rim." He noted that the diaphragm had to be thin and could be made of metal, hard rubber, celluloid, silk, mica or other suitable substance. The major step forward was the recognition that the diaphragm should be on the surface of the chest-piece so that it could make direct contact with the body. The early patent obviated this by still using a localizing button. Several other inventors had used membranes of various types including Pratt in 1887, Papendell in 1898 and Wigmore in 1897 (US Patents #370.711, #599,064 and #581,929) among others. Bowles' chest-piece prevailed not only because of its practicality but also because of its marketing by Pilling. By 1901 the button was removed and the diaphragm formed the air chamber with the back of the chest-piece (Figures 23; A37–A41). In the 1902 patent Bowles recognized the need to use both a bell and a diaphragm and introduced the awkward version shown in the appendix (Figures A42; A43). The remaining patents were minor modifications including one in which he used a sliding spring on the head-piece so that the pressure on the ears could be adjusted.

This design dominated the stethoscope market during the twentieth century. The diaphragm served not only to prevent the tissues of the chest from projecting into the shallow cup of the chest-piece while it was pressed against the chest, but it also enhanced the detection of high pitched sounds.

A major advantage of the Bowles design was that the chest-piece was very flat, and thus the auscultator could listen to the posterior portions of the lungs without turning over an extremely ill patient, or requiring him to sit up. This was an advantage, but it was not as good for low pitched sounds. This problem was later resolved as noted by the introduction of the Sprague combined chest-piece. The Bowles' stethoscope also was modified in one version so that six to twelve observers could auscultate at the same time.

Before 1904 the Bowles' stethoscope was manufactured in two sizes; one of 2-inch diameter and one of 1³/₈-inch; the smaller size for smaller areas, such as above the clavicle, the apices, etc. Having to use two sizes proved inconvenient, so Bowles modified the stethoscope by constructing a diaphragm of pear or flat iron shape (similar to Figure A73). With this instrument, he was able to obtain the maximum sound transmission of the larger style stethoscope, yet he also had the adaptability of the smaller instrument (Bowles 1904) (US Patent #773,274).

A further modification is discussed by Faught in his book:

A special stethoscope has recently been devised [1913] which is a great aid in performing the

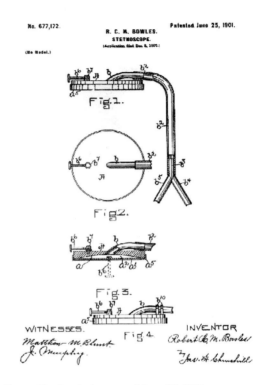

Figure 23 Bowles' patent of June 25 1901

The major innovation was the diaphragm with a small air chamber. The idea of a localizing rod had not been fully abandoned at this time and can be seen as b6 and b7 which could be screwed into the diaphragm where shown in Figure 3. This was totally abandoned later to achieve the modern form.

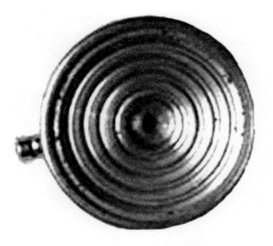

Figure 24 Pilling's grooved sound chamber

The grooved sound chamber as described in Pilling's patent of 1909 is shown. The diaphragm at this time had achieved the modern form and the grooved sound chamber is described as being a means to accumulate and deflect the sound waves and direct them through the tube to the ears. This is shown with the diaphragm removed to expose the sound chamber.

auscultatory method (of blood pressure measurement). This … is a Bowles stethoscope with a button-like projection from the face of the diaphragm, which greatly facilitates application to the artery below the sphygmomanometer cuff. This is secured in position by a narrow cuff fastened with a friction buckle. This little apparatus is self-retaining and allows the operator the freedom of both hands with which to manage the sphygmomanometer"

(Faught 1913). This was reminiscent of the earlier 1894 model (Figures A85–87).

Pilling who had worked closely with Bowles introduced a modification in 1909 in which the internal chamber was grooved in a concentric circular fashion to transmit the sound better (US Patent #910,854) (Figure 24). Some other concepts are shown in Figures A69–A73.

Another popular version of the diaphragm stethoscope head was Fleischer's, which was marketed by the Becton-Dickinson Company of Rutherford from the 1920s until the middle of the twentieth century (Figures A85; A86). The major difference in this design was the chamber which was dome-shaped and directed toward a small hollowed-out section next to the hole which led to the connection to the rubber tubing on the side. The connector was frequently fitted with a Luer-Lok for easy interchange of headpieces. Andrew W. Fleischer merged his firm, which was interested in sphygmomanometers and stethoscopes, with Becton-Dickinson in 1921 and continued to work on the development of the stethoscope. In 1925 Fairleigh S. Dickinson received the patent for the Luer-Lok to secure hypodermic needles to syringes. These two products merged in the instrument described above and shown in the appendix.

All the competing designs had modifications in the design of the sound chamber under the diaphragm as a major justification for the patent. However, they all relied on some type of thin membrane to modify the sound, or a simple bell configuration. The concept of putting the two approaches together to optimize the detection of high- and low-pitched sounds began to take shape as the realization grew that no single design was optimal for all frequencies.

Sprague's modification

"Because of the variable qualities of different cardiac murmurs," Dr Howard B. Sprague of Boston designed a combined stethoscope chest-piece (Sprague 1926). The bell type chest-piece was most useful for low-pitched murmurs, while the Bowles' type chest-piece registered high-pitched murmurs more accurately. Sprague, who was working with Paul Dudley White at the Cardiac Clinic of the Massachusetts General Hospital, put these two chest-pieces together by connecting them with a three-way valve. By simply turning the valve, one or the other chest-piece was connected to the ear-piece, and the other was shut off. Thus it was possible to listen to both the high and low pitched cardiac murmurs without changing instruments. This very versatile chest-piece has been used in many versions and modifications combining the advantage of the Bowles diaphragm for high-pitched sound with that of the well-established bell for low-pitched murmurs. It was designed in collaboration with, and patented by, the George P. Pilling Company of Philadelphia and continues to be sold today (Figure 25).

Sprague's article appeared in June 1926. A patent was applied for by Otto Rieger of St Petersburgh, Florida (US Patent #1,671,936), in January 1927 for a very similar device using a yoke lever to switch between the bell and the diaphragm, both of which were somewhat different from the one used by Sprague. The major claim of the patent was the location of the bell and diaphragm at right angles to each other and a common control to switch from one to the other. The patent was granted in May 1928 and was assigned to George P. Pilling and Son of Philadelphia. The device used by Sprague was

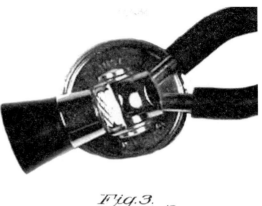

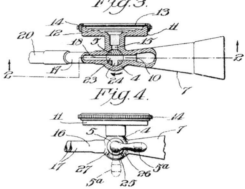

Figure 25 The Sprague stethoscope

A. Sprague type stethoscope which was used by the author during his internship is shown. It consists of a standard bell and a Bowles type diaghragm (It is often call the Sprague-Bowles chest-piece) and a U-shaped switch to open or close each chamber. The patent filed by Pilling and the article by Sprague describe a simple lever arrangement to switch chambers (Sprague), The yoke arrangement was suggested by Rieger in his patent. Otherwise, except for some minor differences in the design of the diaphragm chamber and the bell, the two are virtually the same. B. A cut taken from the Pilling patent of Sprague's invention shows the lever and the mechanism to switch from one chamber to the other. In this patent the lumen is a T shape; Rieger suggested that the two channels form a V shape to create less deflection of the sound.

patented on April 1929 one year later, having been filed by Pilling in May 1927, a few months after Rieger. This design used a lever instead of a yoke to switch from one chamber to the other, and the bell resembled Ford's and the diaphragm Bowles'. The claims for the stethoscope were almost the same as Rieger's. Pilling, in their catalog of 1932, list both instruments as well as a revolving dual head (the Swivel-Bowles) but they emphasize the Sprague-Bowles with a brief overview of its use. The Rieger-Bowles and the Sprague-Bowles were patented, but not the Swivel.

A similar concept to the Sprague device was proposed earlier by P. A. Aurness, in 1907, who called his instrument the duplex stethoscope (Aurness 1907). His modification consisted of a metal shell, which formed two focalizing chest-pieces with a common central body and connection to the ear tubes. An adjustable hollow plug, attached to flexible transmission tubes, made possible the use of the large or small chest-piece simply by half turning the plug. The chest-pieces were covered by a membrane, and were made of copper, zinc, or lead.

As early as July 1910 a patent was granted for a double diaphragm head in which there was a valve to switch from a larger to a smaller diaphragm, using the same principles as the Sprague and the Rieger (N. Fuchs, US Patent #965,174). A similar design is found in the Astatique (Figure A68).

A stethoscope was also described with a double head which could be revolved in a manner similar to the Aurness device to present either a diaphragm or a bell as early as 1915. This became a very simple and popular approach (Med and Surgical Appliances 1915).

All types of claim were made that the perfect stethoscope had been devised. For instance, T. C. Blackwell modified the binaural stethoscope so that it was "mathematically correct throughout." The combined sectional areas of the two smaller tubes equaled the sectional area of the larger tube. The lumen of the tube remained the same from chest-piece to ear. Therefore there was nothing to interfere with the sound waves. He claimed that with this modification all exaggeration of sound was avoided, and the exact sound produced was conveyed to the ear (Blackwell 1911).

A later and somewhat unusual stethoscope is the Capac Binaural. Although it has been suggested that this is not a medical stethoscope, there is a detailed discussion of it in an article by Stephen Morris (1967). According to Morris, this was first made available in 1935 with a lightweight and a heavier model each having concave and conical screw-in ends. The head incorporates an annular interior diaphragm. It came with a combination of head frames and chest-pieces (Figure A51).

Stethoscopes without rigid head-pieces

Many stethoscopes which were composed of the chest-piece and two flexible rubber tubes to conduct the sound to the ear were introduced with the increasing availability of good quality rubber. When practical binaural head-pieces became available, virtually all of the various chest-pieces were offered with the option of either flexible tubes or metallic head-pieces. In that regard the division here is somewhat artificial, but it is meant to provide some idea of how the inventors or the instrument manufacturers introduced their products.

An early model was developed in 1877 by John Brown which consisted of a cup shaped ebony chest-piece with two small holes to secure perforated pegs. These pegs were connected to the ear-pieces with about twelve inches of India-rubber tubing. He also suggested a double stethoscope with one chest-piece and four ear-pieces for two observers (Brown 1877).

Arthur Ernest Sansom (1839–1907) was a prominent stethoscopist who was born at Corsham, entered King's College at the age of sixteen and received an M.D. in London in 1866. He spent some time in Paris studying with Piorry. His book *Manual of the Physical Diagnosis of Diseases of the Heart* went through several editions. In the edition of 1881 he comments:

> The binaural stethoscope is extremely valuable. For the cardiac auscultation of infants and children it is indispensable... The practical conclusion is, use both forms of stethoscope, the ordinary and the binaural. I have my own stethoscope so constructed that the same cup and stalk can be screwed into the ordinary wooden ear-piece...

At this time he was using a stethoscope which he indicates may have been introduced by Professor Stern of Vienna. This had India-rubber conducting tubes which fitted into a vulcanite or wooden extremity, which was a monaural stethoscope thus adapted to binaural use. He also recommended graduated marks on the tubing to serve as a chest measure.

Sansom later improved his binaural stethoscope making the upper portion of the tube of metal instead of India rubber, so that only the lower part was flexible. The ear-pieces were of rubber. The chest-piece was reversible so that the examiner could use a large or small oval for application to the chest wall. It had an India rubber cushion (Sansom 1892).

John R. Philpots (1892) described a stethoscope composed of two pieces of India rubber tubing, each 2 feet 2 inches long, which had vulcanized ear-pieces at the upper ends and the lower ends made of vulcanite for insertion into the chest-piece. The chest-piece was 7/8 inch long and 5/8 inch wide and was cup-shaped.

Many other modifications were introduced to the binaural stethoscope during this time period. In some the tubing entered the chest-piece separately; in others it was fused into a single tube at or near the point where the chest-piece was connected. The Bazzi-Bianchi phonendoscope was a very important contribution from Italy which may well have been the first practical membrane or diaphragm chest-piece. It achieved widespread use at the end of the nineteenth and the beginning of the twentieth centrury.

The Bazzi-Bianchi stethoscope

The most popular of the binaural stethoscopes with flexible ear connections was the phonendoscope which was invented by Dr Aurelio Bianchi, of Florence, Italy (Figures A59; A60). Bianchi studied at the University of Siena, and later at the Instituto Superiore of Florence. He was Professor of Pathology at the University of Parma. His instrument consisted of two principal parts: the resonator and the conducting tubes of soft rubber. The resonator was composed of three parts: the resonator proper, a removable membrane and a staff of metal tipped with a hard rubber button. It shared the membrane concept with Bowles' chest-piece but it was much larger and heavier with an emphasis on auscultatory percussion (Figures 26; A59; A60).

An early unnamed version of the phonendoscope (the *estetosopia*) was introduced in August 1885, at the XI Congreso de la Asociacion Medica Italiana (Eleventh Congress of the Italian Medical Association) (Bianchi 1925). Ten years later, it was presented under the name of "phonendoscope" (a device to bring sounds from within the body to the outside) to the Congreso Internationale de Roma, which met in October 1895.

Bianchi's initial work was stimulated by dissatisfaction with the reliability of percussion and an article describing Cammann and Clark's use of auscultatory percussion. Their method had fallen into disuse because it required one examiner to percuss and one to auscultate. He worked in association with Eugenio Bazzi, a distinguished Italian physicist (Manges 1904). The first phonendoscope was manufactured by Martin Wallach's Nachfolger at Cassel, Germany. It weighed 8½ ounces. In the United States it was promoted by the George Pilling Company which published an English

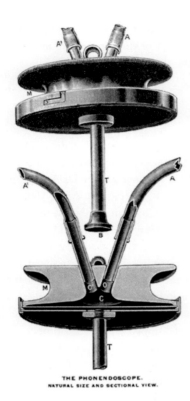

THE PHONENDOSCOPE.
NATURAL SIZE AND SECTIONAL VIEW.

Figure 26 The Bazzi-Bianchi phonendoscope

The phonendoscope has the form and size of a large pocket-watch, Its anterior part, which in the watch corresponds to the face, is formed by two superimposed laminae: the internal one more delicate and sensitive, the external one more resistant and easily removable to expose the other. The external lamina has a hole in its center, into which may be screwed a small rod with a button on the end B, of variable length T, which serves to localize the examination to a point, and which may have different forms and sizes for the diverse examinations of the internal organs.

translation of Dr Bianchi's lectures in 1900 (Bianchi 1900). This monograph provides a detailed description of the invention and the use of the phonendoscope.

The following remarks are taken from Bianchi's description of his instrument (Bianchi A, 1894):

> To have a good means of examining the murmurs and sounds of the organism is a desirable and necessary thing. The author has always thought therefore that the search for an improvement of the means of investigation has been useful and has devoted himself to it until the present. In 1880 and in 1882, he offered the microphone and the biauricular stethoscope and showed the advantages over the ordinary stethoscopes, although there were defects.
>
> Therefore, with a distinguished physicist, Dr Eugenio Bazzi, professor of physics in the Technical Institute of Florence, he studied the subject and the fruit of the long experience of the eminent professor and the multiple observations of the author is the instrument presented today, which is called the phonendoscope, or rather the investigator of internal sounds.
>
> The phonendoscope, applied to the medical sciences, serves indiscriminately for the auscultation of all the spontaneous and provoked sounds which the human organism develops, with superior intensity and with more exact localization than the ordinary stethoscopes used until now, and without alteration of the timbre of the sound. It serves thus:
>
> 1) for the auscultation of respiratory murmurs, circulatory murmurs and the murmurs of the organs of digestion, in health and in disease;
> 2) for the auscultation of muscular, articular and osseous sounds;
> 3) for auscultation of the murmurs of the uterus in gestation and of the product of conception;
> 4) for the auscultation of the sounds of the circulation in the capillaries (dermatophonia) and of the auricular and ocular sounds;
> 5) for the auscultation of sounds provoked artificially by the approximative or exact delimitation of the dimensions, position and displacement of the organs and of the liquid contents of the principal cavities;

6) for the internal auscultation of the ear, the uterus, the bladder, the stomach and the intestines.

The posterior part of the phonendoscope has two central holes for fixation of the auricular tubes, and two rings in which, when it is not in use, the rod may be placed. Furthermore, toward one side of its margin, it has a hinged hasp. The periphery of the phonendoscope is hollowed out like a pulley and may contain the auricular tubes, wrapped around the throat of this instrument when not in use. The auricular tubes are finished on one end with small metal tubes for fixing in the holes of the phonendoscope, and on the other with ear-pieces with curved shank for fixing in the auditory canal.

In order to use the phonendoscope, it is necessary simply to place the instrument with the portion of the laminae over the body to be examined, in the suitable spot, and to introduce either one or both of the tubes in the ear. In such a manner the two hands remain perfectly free and may be used at the indicated points in the examination.

To have a little practice with the phonendoscope, it is necessary to begin by auscultation with only one ear and then to make the comparison between the direct auscultation and the biauricular type. After a few comparisons, one will readily appreciate the superiority of phonendoscopic auscultation over the ordinary stethoscopic and direct auscultations.

The phonendoscope serves for the examination of extensive areas and those well localized, offering different grades of sensitivity. For the examination of extensive areas, it is enough to place the lamina over the part to be explored. For the examination of localized areas, as for example the sounds of the heart, the arteries, etc., it is necessary to screw into the center of the external lamina the little stick with the button, and apply it to the part, using mild and gradual pressure.

Then for sensitivity, different gradations may be obtained in the following manner:

Minimal sensitivity is had on applying the phonendoscope with both laminae and only one tube in the ear.

Medium sensitivity is obtained by applying the two laminae with the two tubes in the ears.

Maximum sensitivity may be had by removing the external lamina and applying the instrument with only the internal lamina, but with the two tubes in the ears.

The sensitivity of the instrument is such that the slightest alterations of sound are appreciated, and thus the delimitation of the visceral areas is of extreme facility, although this previously was not striking, by simply pressing and sliding with the apex of the index finger from the outside toward the same viscus over which the phonendoscope is placed.

A few admonitions are necessary:

First of all, avoid friction of the laminae, the walls and the tubes against the clothing or other objects during the observations.

Then make a gradual and gentle pressure on the explored part to assure the most direct contact possible.

Protect the internal lamina from shocks and from too strong pressure.

Always affix the two tubes to the phonendoscope, and then one may be used.

The phonendoscope, in differentiation from other stethoscopes, permits of:

1) executing rapidly and surely the functional examination of one or more organs;
2) being able to make a brief but exact examination even over the clothing, because the instrument holds fast and compressed;
3) being able to stand away from the patient, with marked hygienic value to the doctor and with greater comfort and dignity for the patient himself;
4) not being disturbed by noises which may occur in the examination room;
5) being able, by using only one hand and with no disturbance of the patient, to produce the sounds which will accomplish an exact delimitation of the viscera;
6) not altering in any way the elevation of the sounds and their reciprocal relations;
7) giving to the learned person who uses it the same superiority regarding the study of the murmurs and sounds of the organism, that

there is for the eye which is equipped with a magnifying glass in comparison with the eye which has none".

(translation by the American College of Surgeons, 1934)

Some other modifications

Herman B. Baruch of Mt. Sinai Hospital in New York modified the phonendoscope by attaching the distal end of the rubber tubes to the ear-piece of an ordinary stethoscope (Baruch 1896). However, the instrument is commonly encountered in the medical antique marketplace and I have only seen it with the flexible rubber tubing.

A modification of Bianchi's stethoscope is described in the Boulitte catalog of 1923, in which an obturator is added to the back of the instrument which can be opened to hear low-pitched sounds better. This also appears in several other later catalogs. The phonendoscopic end also was made to revolve so that an ordinary chest-piece could be used for the intercostal space or other purpose (Medical and Surgical Appliances 1915).

In 1906, Edmund F. Woods recommended a new stethoscope for its simplicity, lightness and durability. The bell was made from very hard metal, nickel plated, and so thick that it shut out all outside sounds. The tubes led directly from the bell to the ears without a Y connection. He reported that it conveyed the heart and lung sounds without the humming sound so noticeable in other stethoscopes of that day (Woods 1906).

About 1928, J. Kilpatrick Reid and W. Owen Morris suggested a model in which the ear-pieces were separate, and were made to twist well into the ears where they would remain firmly in place. The chest-piece was of light composition, and caused no pull on the ears. The lumen of the transmitting tubes was constant throughout. The chest-piece was protected by a rubber cap, which ensured comfort for the patient and also added clearness for the transmission (Reid & Morris 1928).

Several other examples of binaural stethoscopes using flexible tubes and no head-piece are shown in the appendix (Figures A57–A73). As noted above, during the early part of the twentieth century and at the end of the nineteenth, virtually all of the stethoscopic chest-pieces could be purchased with or without a head-piece.

Modifications in the bell

One modification of the bell (Gordon 1929) consisted of a circular metal base 1.4 inches in diameter to which was attached a projecting soft rubber ring. The central portion of the reverse side of the base extended upward to serve as a finger rest and also as a point of attachment for the steel and rubber transmission tubes which protruded at right angles from the chest-piece. The advantages of this instrument were the rubber ring which was not cold to touch and yielded to the irregularities of the chest wall, and the finger rest which facilitated holding the bell in place.

Numerous other modifications of the bell were introduced. They differed in size and shape but were all essentially the same concept (Figures A36; A44–A49; A50; A53).

The movement back to a design in which a single connection from the chest-piece bifurcated to join two tubes or in which a Y adapter was used at some point to allow for one tube to enter the chest-piece, ultimately dominated the design of the connecting tubing because of its practicality.

8   Stethoscopes of special purpose

Numerous modifications were introduced to expand the range of use of the stethoscope. Perhaps the ultimate example was the "Panarkes" of Pickering (Pickering 1887). This instrument could be used as a monaural, binaural or differential stethoscope. In addition it also had a percussor, hammer and pleximeter. Physicians commonly put things like thermometers in the central bore of their monaural stethoscopes. On the same page of Pickering's report is a description of another binaural which can be converted to a monaural stethoscope by removing the chest-piece and screwing on an ear-piece (Batten 1887).

Stethoscopes also were used to examine virtually every organ in the body either through auscultative percussion or auscultation of associated sounds. There are articles and chapters in textbooks dealing with auscultation of the eye, brain, ear, abdomen, bone and joint, and countless other efforts to expand the range of the stethoscope. In many of these situations some modification of the stethoscope was suggested to enhance its value. While most of these applications have fallen into disuse, the more important types of use are discussed below. Other applications can be found in References and Suggested Reading at the end of this text.

Teaching stethoscopes

The stimulus for development of a teaching stethoscope is well-described by Landouzy (1841).

> The difficulty of popularizing the admirable discovery of Laennec has caused me to ponder on a means to make perceptible at the same time to several students, the stethoscopic signs, and I believe that I have found it in the manner of propagation of sound. If, one places his bare ear at any point on the external wall of a solid or hollow cylinder (or a stethoscope), he will perceive the communicated sounds almost as clearly as if the ear were placed at the extremity of the cylinder ... Therefore I constructed a stethoscope of tin-plate, 120 cm long, with several mobile articulations, so that it could be bent in different directions, according to the position of the patient or the physicians, and with 10 flexible appendages, so that when the conical base of the cylinder is applied against the organ, each one may readily perceive the sounds by means of these conducting appendages.
>
> The results were entirely in conformity with my theory, and ten persons, auscultating at the same time without disturbing each other, heard simultaneously, in a very distinct manner, the sound of the systolic murmur.
>
> One immediately sees the advantages which may be obtained from this new mode of auscultation for practical teaching in the schools of medicine, and especially in the large faculties.
>
> Certainly I would not be accused of exaggeration when I say that of the sixty (and sometimes more) students in the clinic who surround a patient, there are not more than six who are able to verify themselves the phenomena perceived and pointed out by the professor. Whether because the patients, worn out by the explorations of the doctor or interns, refuse to allow themselves to be auscultated again, or the students because they do not wish to lose any of the facts of the doctor's examinations, leave the bed at the same time as the professor; there is always only a very small number who can apply themselves to a complete examination, and there are many students who, not being able to follow the special courses of the chiefs of

63

clinic or interns, terminate their medical studies without knowing auscultation, and are forever deprived of one of the surest sources of diagnosis.

The new method which I have indicated seems proper to obviate this serious difficulty, since by means of a long tube on which each student may place his ear or stethoscope, or by means of a hollow cylinder, equipped with several conducting appendages which may be applied to the ear, it requires no more time for sixty observers to auscultate a patient than it would for six to do so separately.

... it is understood also that when the sounds are very faint the polyscope will not give advantageous results, but the best proof that organic sounds, without being intense, may be heard by several auditors, is the fact that I caused the uterine murmur and fetal heart-beat to be heard simultaneously by the students at the Hotel-Dieu.

I recognize that in simultaneous auscultation, the sounds lose much of their intensity, due directly to the number of appendages to the stethoscope. This stethoscope should therefore be used only for the intense organic sounds.

I have named this the "stethopolyscope" or the "polyscope".

In his conclusions Landouzy states that the best stethoscope is one with a thin wall made of light wood such as fir. He indicates that a long one is preferable to a short one to avoid adventitial sounds and he suggests a thin membrane on the end if one wishes to use a glass or tin stethoscope in certain cases. His suggestion of a long stethoscope certainly raises question of the validity of calling longer stethoscopes "poor house stethoscopes," although this term was probably appropriate in some cases as most physicians did not want to get too close to their patients.

Another concept of a teaching stethoscope was illustrated by Paul in his textbook. This figure shows most of the possible combinations which can be used in moving from monaural to binaural and from single to multiple observers with various length connections and the option of differential stethoscopy (Figure 27) (Paul 1887).

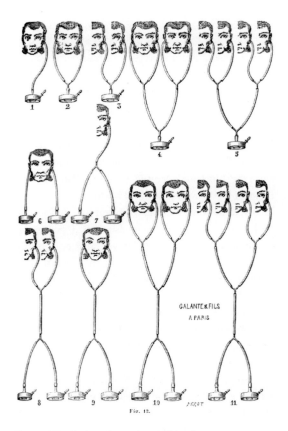

Figure 27 Paul stethoscope combinations

The top row shows a Paul stethoscope for monaural or binaural use with one, two or more observers. The bottom row shows similar combinations for the differential stethoscope. These combinations reflect the many approaches in vogue at that time when no single approach had been accepted as the ideal.

A double stethoscope to teach auscultation at the London Hospital was described by Herbert Davies in 1861. He called it the "class of consultation stethoscope". The teacher and one pupil could auscultate at the same time (Davies 1862). There were numerous other teaching stethoscopes. As technology improved it became an increasingly simple matter to add bifurcations to the tube to increase the number of observers. Several of the stethoscopes described in the text were also modified to serve as teaching stethoscopes.

Obstetrical stethoscopes

Francois-Isaac Mayor described fetal heart sounds in 1818, but it was Kergaradec who first introduced the use of the stethoscope for this purpose.

The concept of modifying the stethoscope specifically for use in obstetrics did not arise directly from Laennec. In the second edition of his text he states: "I had personally not thought of applying auscultation to the study of the phenomena of pregnancy. This fortunate idea is entirely due to my compatriot and friend doctor de Kergaradec." (Laennec 1826). Kergaradec read a memoir on mediate auscultation applied to the study of pregnancy to the Academie Royale de medicine on Dec 26 1821. He originally used the stethoscope which had been designed by Laennec. At that time he noted the double pulsation caused by the fetal and maternal heartbeats (Stofft 1981).

There was a great deal of early interest in the use of the stethoscope in obstetrics in Germany. C. J. Haus published a monograph on auscultation in obstetrics in 1823, shortly after Kergaradec's report (Haus 1823). By 1838 a treatise *Die geburtshülfliche Auscultation* by H. F. Naegele (1810–1851) had appeared (Naegele 1838). He used a slightly modified form of the Piorry stethoscope, which was about seven and a half to eight inches long, six to seven lines thick with a bore of four lines. The pectoral end was a conical cavity one inch,

four lines, deep and one inch, four lines, in diameter at its base. He states clearly in his text however that he did not believe that the specific instrument used was critical: "the auscultation of the abdomen may be practiced almost equally well with any stethoscope." Naegele's book, which was based on 600 cases, was translated into English in 1839 (Naegele 1839) and received a favorable review in the *London Medical Gazette* of 1840.

Another, earlier, advocate of the stethoscope in obstetrics was an Englishman with a similar name, David C. Nagle of Trinity College in Dublin. He reported on numerous uses of the "cylinder" in obstetrics, including the identification of twins, and he debated the value of the placental soufflé, but he made no suggestions about the design of the instrument (Nagle 1831; 1832).

By about 1876 a modification of the stethoscope for obstetrical use was introduced and named after Adolphe Pinard (1844–1934). It is not clear what role he played in its design. Although he mentions the use of the stethoscope in his book on clinical obstetrics (Pinard 1899) he does not describe it. The earliest modifications for obstetrical use were in shortening the tube and expanding the bell end.

An 1889 French text *Histoire des accouchements chez tous les peuples* by G. J. Witkowski illustrates three fetal stethoscopes in use at that time. All are very similar. Pinard's is the longest, Pajot's the shortest and Depaul's version is between the two (Figures A74–A78; A81). In his text Witkowski quotes Pajot as stating: "Stethoscope for obstetrical teaching, [the] more it is short, [the] less it rocks. For the trained physician the choice of instrument is insignificant." Depaul (1811–1883) who was Professor of Obstetrics at the Faculty of Medicine of Paris, devotes a chapter of his textbook to auscultation. In this section he discusses the merits of mediate versus immediate auscultation and comes out firmly in favor of the use of the stethoscope. He also states: "I will not describe to you the stethoscope; you all know this instrument, I am showing you the one that I currently use. I recommend one that is long enough, 15–16 centimeters, and take care that the ear-piece is not too concave; 5–6 millimeters is sufficient to accommodate the ear." He cautions against choosing one which is too short. It is interesting that the stethoscope he appears to be describing is that which has been named after Pinard which is about 6 inches long or 15 centimeters. He also mentions the use of a vaginal stethoscope of Nauche (metrescope), after the idea of Maygrier (Depaul JAH, 1872–1876).

The Hillis-DeLee obstetric stethoscope was introduced in 1916 (DeLee 1917) and became a very popular modification. It was intended to allow the observer to hear the fetal heart during the last part of the second stage of labor. An attachment for the stethoscope was devised which consisted of a metal and leather band like that used on an ENT head mirror, passing from front to back over the top of the head. The Y of the binaural stethoscope was fastened to the front plate of the band by means of a short spiral spring and a universal joint. This could be set with a thumbscrew permitting proper adjustment of the ear-pieces and also holding the stethoscope in position at right angles to the forehead (Hillis 1917). The head–piece could be folded and carried in the bag or pocket (Figure A79).

Falls and Hunter devised a stethoscope with a stopwatch wired to a small flashlight cell and bulb. The bulb flashed every 15 seconds, to help count the fetal heart rate. Later, Falls invented another type of head stethoscope with an ordinary pocket watch, with a second hand, attached to the headband just above the bridge of the nose. A magnifying mirror was mounted on a ball and socket joint clamped to the horizontal bar that supported the bell of the stethoscope. The image of the watch could be seen in the mirror to time the heart rate (Falls & Hunter 1924).

Morris Leff, of New York, introduced a bell, consisting of a metal weight three inches in diameter weighing two pounds. Its undersurface was concave with an opening which was continuous with the stem of the instrument. The hollow stem was connected with an adapter to the binaural head-piece. Two advantages of this instrument were: (1) the weight was sufficient to keep it in place on the abdomen without extra pressure; and (2) the fetal heart sounds could be heard while there were noises in the room (Leff 1930) (Figure A80).

The variety of approaches to auscultation in obstetrics was truly remarkable. A vaginal stethoscope was devised to diagnose pregnancy at an earlier stage. It had an elongated tube, the bell of which could be introduced into the vagina. It was claimed that pregnancy could be diagnosed by about the fourteenth week. The vaginal stethoscope is of no value for hearing the heart tones after the twentieth week because by that time the uterus has risen so high into the abdomen and the fetus is so large that the distance of the heart from the lower uterine segment is too great (Falls 1926).

Another vaginal stethoscope of the diaphragm type (Turman 1934) was used to locate the placenta. It consisted of a metal diaphragm, attached by a short piece of rubber tubing to a metal tube. Ear-pieces were attached at the opposite end of the metal tube. There were steel bands on the anterior and posterior surfaces of the tube which made it possible to extend or flex the head of the diaphragm in order to auscultate the anterior or posterior wall of the lower uterus.

Differential stethoscopes

The differential (double) stethoscope was introduced in 1858 by Dr S. Scott Alison, Physician to the Brompton Hospital for Diseases of the Chest. It could be thought of either as a binaural stethoscope with two chest-pieces or two flexible monaural stethoscopes joined together and using both ears. The purpose was to allow sounds produced at two different points of the chest to be heard at the same time. It made it possible to compare sounds from two different sources which was considered at that time to be critical to the examination.

What Alison actually did was to take two Cammann's stethoscopes and place an individual chest-piece at the end of each instead of terminating the two tubes in the same chest-piece. This provided a right stethoscope for the right ear and a left stethoscope for the left ear. The stethoscope was often sold with the option to buy extra tubes to convert from a standard binaural to an Alison's and back.

If a respiratory sound was heard with the right stethoscope, the right cup was then lifted and the left cup applied at a different point. This permitted the observer to determine any difference between the sounds in loudness, volume or duration. When used in this manner, Alison's stethoscope is simply a convenient way of making comparisons, provided the observer's auditory acuity is equal in the two ears. However, when the two stethoscope heads are used simultaneously, being applied at different points on the chest wall, the more important feature according to Alison is apparent. When there is a significant difference in the intensity of two sounds on different points over the chest, the presence of the abnormal sound can be more easily appreciated. Alison explains that the result is not that a louder sound is heard with one ear and a less intense sound with the other ear, but rather that the louder sound is heard with the ear connected to the bell on that side, while the other ear hears nothing. A relatively quiet respiratory murmur in the right chest and a relatively loud murmur in the left chest, observed simultaneously, results in the loud sound being heard with the one (left) ear and the absence of sound to the other (right) ear. It is this "eclipsing" or "suppression" of the weaker of the two sounds which Alison claimed as the unique feature of his instrument. "Consecutive observations with the single stethoscope may leave a doubt as to the relative loudness of the two sounds, but the double stethoscope at once resolves this doubt, for if a difference exists it is announced absolutely by the apparent non existence of any sound on the feebler side." (Alison 1861) (Figure 28a/b)

Several standard textbooks (Gairdner 1862; Fuller 1867; Bennett 1868; Aitken 1872) endorsed its use and Geo. L. Carrick (1872) wrote: "I feel I can never conscientiously pronounce an opinion on the condition of a patient's lungs without having carefully examined them by the differential stethoscope."

Other differential stethoscopes were introduced by Lyons (1862), Spencer (1874), Boston (1927) and Masserman (1931).

Spencer put forth a long discussion about the requirements for a proper differential stethoscope arguing that it was necessary that both ears hear the sounds. His device resembled Alison's; however he introduced a joint so that both chest-pieces communicated with both ears. One or other chest-piece could be shut off by occluding a thin rubber tube near the pectoral end allowing sounds to be compared by both ears, which probably was an advantage (Spencer 1874).

Boston's version consisted of two Bowles chest-pieces connected by rubber tubing with a central Y bivalve switch attachment. Through this switch, sound from either chest-piece could be excluded or allowed to pass to the ears. Thus, sounds from two locations could be compared without moving the instrument; first by listening to one disk, then turning the switch and listening to the other disk (Boston 1927).

As experience with auscultation accumulated the need for simultaneous comparison fell into disuse. Subsequently the term "differential" was applied to a stethoscope having only a single chest-piece used in precordial examinations. Successive, not simultaneous, observations and more quantitative comparisons of relative sounds were made.

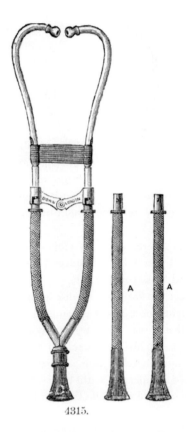

4315.

Figure 28a Alison's differential stethoscope

It can be seen from the illustration that this is essentially a Cammann's stethoscope with two separate chest-pieces. As noted in the text it was not uncommon for the physician to carry an extra single chest-piece to convert this to an ordinary binaural. A cut from Down Bros catalog of surgical instruments, 1900, illustrates the Cammann's stethoscope with an option to buy the two extra tubes and chest-pieces (A) which converted the head-piece to an Alison Differential. The text cites the binaural as "Original model" (known as Alison's or Leared's) at a price of 16 shillings; the differential ends were offered for an additional 5 shillings.

Single differential stethoscopes

The Oertel stethoscope consisted of a chest-piece to which a metal tube was attached. There was a slit in the tube which could be opened. The length of the opening could be read on a scale. A second tube slid over the one with a slit; thus the slit could be made any length up to 1.6 inches. A Y tube was attached to the end of this tube which in turn was attached to the head-piece of a binaural stethoscope. The chest-piece was placed over the apex of the heart and the slit opened until the first sound could not be heard. The slit was then shortened until the sound could be heard. The length of the slit provided a quantitation of the volume of the sound which could be compared to another parameter such as the aortic valve. This instrument had to be used in a quiet room or in a room with a constant level of sound. Oertel also designed a more conventional chest-piece (Figures A61; A62).

The Bock differential stethoscope consisted of a conical chest-piece attached to a circular box which was divided into two compartments by a thick metal diaphragm which was pierced by a small hole. A cone of metal was inserted into the hole and could be rotated until the opening was completely closed. The pointer on the circular box was set at 100 when the opening was completely closed. Like the Oertel device, the first heart sound was measured by finding the point at which it was no longer heard and then comparing it with the intensity of the aortic valve. The Bock stethoscope could be used in comparatively noisy surroundings (Leyton 1916; 1918). This instrument was popularized by Leyton and is referred to as Leyton's Differential in many instrument catalogs (Figure 29).

Amplified stethoscopes

Numerous electric stethoscopes were introduced as amplification of sound and the microphone became perfected and generally available. An early stimulus occurred in 1878 when an electric stethoscope was used to send a signal 100 miles. But it took more than 100 years to achieve a truly practical model.

Glover in his monograph on electric auscultation traces the invention of the telephone to early French work and credits Boudet with one of the earliest medical applications (Glover 1925). Boudet presents a detailed review of the use of electricity in medicine in which he has several references to the amplification of body sounds (Boudet 1881a,b). He attributes to Dr Stein the first attempt to use the telephone to hear the sounds of the circulation, but it was very imperfect and unsuitable for examination of the heart. The practical application began with the development of the microphone which evolved from the telephone after it was invented in 1876. According to Boudet, Dr Richardson was the first to use a practical microphone in medicine around 1879, which he presented to the Medical Society of London. The use of the microphone in auscultation was subsequently studied in England, Belgium, France and many other countries. Boudet constructed a "microphone for transmission" (Figure 30) which he used to investigate the murmur in aortic insufficiency and its propagation to the crural (femoral) artery (Boudet 1882).

Albert Abrams introduced an electric instrument with a thumb slide and resistance units in 1899 (Abrams 1899). He later developed the stethophonometer which could be attached to a stethoscope to amplify the sounds (Abrams 1902).

Gottschalk introduced an electric stethoscope called the heartphone, in the early twentieth century. Gottschalk's instrument was "small enough to be carried in the pocket." The component parts were a transmitter, a receiver, a battery and a regulating controller. The transmitter case completely enclosed and protected the mechanism, which transmitted the sound unhampered to the receiver. The sounds were then passed on to the ears through soft rubber tubes protected by

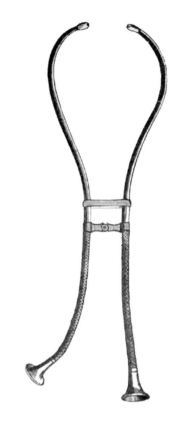

Figure 28b Alison's differential stethoscope

This illustration shows the assembled differential stethoscope (Hudson 1887).

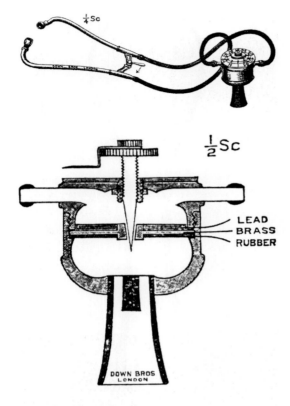

$\frac{1}{4}$ Sc

$\frac{1}{2}$ Sc

LEAD
BRASS
RUBBER

DOWN BROS
LONDON

Figure 29 The Bock stethoscope

Many catalogs show this as the Leyton Differential stethoscope but Leyton himself refers to it as Bock's in his article of 1916. Leyton in his article of 1918 does not name it, but uses the identical figure that he used in his 1916 article in which he clearly indicates that it is Bock's design.

A cross-section of the chest-piece illustrates how it worked: by turning the screw the opening between the chambers could be modified (Leyton 1918). Note the head-piece which has a lever mechanism to adjust the tension on the ears; this design was introduced by George Herschel (1891).

metal tubing. A sound regulating controller was placed on the cords between the transmitter and the receiver. C. C. Henry of New York published a strong endorsement of Mr Gottschalk in the *New York Medical Journal* (Henry 1918).

Another early amplified stethoscope was introduced by K. M. Turner who patented a modification of the dictograph transmitter "familiarly employed in ordinary secret and detective services." (US Patent #1,147,282). His device consisted of a telephonic transmitter, a receiver with ear tubes and a volume control and battery. This was invented in 1912 and patented in 1915.

A number of other electric stethoscopes were introduced in the next 25 years (A. B. Abbott, H. F. Dodge, F. E. Miller, J. Weinstein, C. A. Mason, US Patents #1,540,585, #1,686,504, #1,791,932, #1,976,707, #2,001,537). Similar attempts were made in England, France and Germany, but none achieved general use because the instruments usually were large and difficult to handle.

In 1935, an electrical stethoscope was placed in experimental use in Canada. The instrument magnified the sound of the human heart 100 times (CMJ, 1935).

The device was based on the telephone principle, with the heart doing the "talking." It was originally developed several years earlier by the Western Electric Company for a medical student whose poor hearing prevented his using the ordinary stethoscope (Figure 31). Its success aroused the interest of physicians having the same handicap and also of physicians who had to make examinations in noisy places. The detector was a modified telephone receiver which when placed on the chest amplified the sound (Figure A88). The sounds were transmitted over a short telephone cord to a tiny amplifier, which multiplied the signal strength by 10 times and then to a telephone receiver. The gain was about 60 decibels and the sensitivity was from 60 to 1500 Hz. A physician could hold the receiver directly to his ear, or attach it to the tube of his own stethoscope. A second physician could also listen. The whole unit was run by four flashlight cells and two plate batteries. The original device was not readily portable, but the later modified version (Western Electric 3A) was lighter and more easily moved about. It was 12½ by 8¾ by 4¾ inches and weighed 14 pounds. It also was equipped with some filters to modify the sound and a volume control. This portable stethoscope was a miniature of the large hospital type through which an entire auditorium of students could listen at the same time.

Amplified stethoscopes were largely abandoned for many years during the twentieth century, but in 1999 Hewlett-Packard introduced the Stethos fully electronic stethoscope. The Stethos has a bell, diaphragm and extended diaphragm and is cutting edge technology with built in microchip and a broad frequency response including frequencies below 10 Hz. It has volume control and memory features, and the whole unit is only slightly larger than an ordinary stethoscope. The amplification is 14 times that of an acoustical stethoscope. It comes in a 28-inch and a 40-inch length and the whole unit weighs 6.5 ounces for the 40-inch and 5.8 ounces for the 28-inch (see chapter 10).

Auscultatory percussion

A form of percussion which intimately coupled the two techniques and has been discussed throughout the text was "auscultory percussion." Alonzo Clark (1807–1887), who was born in Massachusetts, received his MD from the College of Physicians and Surgeons of New York in 1835 and worked with Drs G. P. Cammann and C. T. Mitchell to prove the value of auscultatory percussion by postmortem experiments. Clark also introduced a large funnel-shaped stethoscope similar to the one shown in Figure A9. He and Dr G. P. Cammann wrote: *A New Mode of Ascertaining the Dimensions, Form and Condition of Internal Organs by Percussion* in 1840. He became Professor of Pathology and Practical Medicine at the College of Physicians and Surgeons.

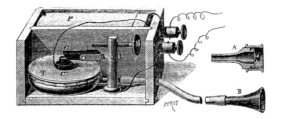

Figure 30 Boudet's "microphone à transmission"

Boudet developed this from a concept given to him by Dr Arsonval and had it fabricated by M. Gaiffe, a prominent Parisian medical electrical instrument company. The device worked with a battery. P is the battery, A is an alternative pectoral end with a button for localization of the sound. The volume is regulated by the steel screw M. The whole unit is in a small portable box. (Boudet 1882)

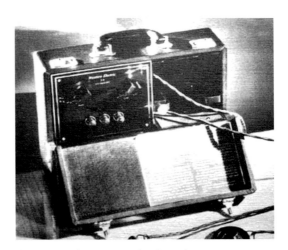

Figure 31 The Western Electric stethoscope

The various parts comprising the Western Electric design are shown for this "portable device." It obviously would not be very convenient to use in most circumstances. However it was well accepted at the time and was useful for teaching and for physicians with hearing problems. The stethoscope itself was almost of the usual size, but it was necessary to carry the box with the amplifying system.

They found that a stethoscope modified to fit between the ribs was the most satisfactory instrument to use (Cammann & Clark 1840). It was a solid cylinder of cedar, shaped in the direction of the wood fibers, 6 inches long, and 10 or 12 lines in diameter with a wedge-shaped pectoral end. Piorry was derisive of Cammann's invention, suggesting that he himself had first suggested it and that his technique was far superior. Stethoscopes designed to fit between the ribs were introduced also by McBride and by Heineman (Cammann 1886). Solid stethoscopes were used for many years for routine auscultation and were a source of continuing debate over their value (Blakiston 1848). Niemeyer was a strong advocate of their use (Sommerbrodt 1869) and used one made of fir. Sommerbrodt found that the perforated stethoscope transmitted finer sounds better than the solid one, but he did not apply it as firmly to the chest as others.

S. Fleet Speir (1838–1895), who graduated from the medical department of the University of the City of New York in 1860, was a surgeon at the Brooklyn City Hospital, New York. He devised the echoscope to intensify the sounds produced by percussion. It was composed of two tubes curved in such a way that their free ends could be adjusted to the ears of the observer. The other ends were connected with a trumpet-shaped sound receiver, which was supported, when in use, by a rest from the chin of the operator. This stethoscope was easily kept in position while the operator was percussing the chest of the patient (Speir 1870–1872). It could be used as a standard stethoscope by changing the chest-piece.

D. M. Cammann's modified binaural stethoscope (Cammann 1886) was intended for auscultatory percussion (Figure 21). It was closed at both ends and filled with water. The two tubes leading from the ears to the flexible portion of the stethoscope were of hard rubber. The chest-piece consisted of a rubber bulb surrounding the central tube, and was connected with a circular chamber in the chest-piece by a tubular opening. When the instrument was placed on the chest, the chamber was closed on all sides. By pressing upon the rubber bulb and then relaxing pressure, the air in the chamber was exhausted, and the instrument was held firmly against the chest by pressure of the external air in a manner similar to Paul's stethoscope. The central circular opening, which was the termination of the tube leading from the ears, was closed by a soft rubber diaphragm. The ear-pieces, made of hard rubber, were hollow and very thin. Cammann notes that the modification was useful only for auscultatory percussion. Unlike Alison (discussed later) who thought that the use of water improved the transmission of sound by the stethoscope, Cammann reports that vocal and respiratory sounds were not as well conveyed as with the ordinary stethoscope.

Denison's stethoscope had several bells which could be fitted on the end. The largest, 3 inches in diameter, was used for what he called "stethoscopic percussion." He carried this out by holding the large bell in front of the patients mouth and percussing forcibly over the suspected area. He notes: "An excavation connected with the bronchial tract is thus very nicely mapped out… Hence I make a point of this stethoscopic percussion." He listened for a "cavernous and cracked sound."

T. O'Kelly, of Chipping Norton, modified the binaural stethoscope to perform auscultatory percussion unassisted (O'Kelly 1894). It consisted of a metal rod 8 inches in length, and ⅕ inch in diameter. This was surmounted by a metal disc one inch in diameter which was covered by an India-rubber cushion for the forehead to rest on. This cushion resembled a ball and socket joint in that, when it was in contact with the auscultator's forehead, it allowed considerable movement of the head in any direction, without tilting up any portion of the chest-piece.

Louis Kolipinski, of Washington DC, devised an instrument which he named the auscultoplectrum. He combined the tubeophone (a form of ear trumpet) with a percussion hammer to create an instrument by which it would be possible to percuss and auscultate at the same time. The chest-piece consisted of an Otis urethroscope, with the obturator removed, heavily gold-plated and connected to 41 inches of red or black rubber tubing which was ⅕ inch in diameter and an ear-piece which was a small, acorn-shaped piece of hard rubber. The length of the whole instrument was 45 inches. Kolipinski carried his auscultoplectrum in a small bag in which he also carried two or three eight-ounce velvet corks. The cork served a pleximeter with its narrower end being applied to the body. The base of the cork was tapped with the plectrum (Kolipinski 1915).

James Cantlie, FRCS, used a tuning-fork as an aid to outlining with precision both the solid and hollow viscera. The principle involved in the use of the tuning-fork-stethoscope method is that when the stethoscope is placed over an organ, the note of the tuning-fork manifests by its loudness the limit of the organ under examination, and the moment the limits are passed the note becomes faint, distant or inaudible (Cantlie 1914). Although auscultatory percussion fell into disuse, it enjoyed great popularity around 1900 and numerous stethoscopes were produced to facilitate its use.

Other stethoscopes

S. Scott Alison, who invented the differential stethoscope, performed experiments on the propagation of sound with a variety of materials. He ascertained that water placed between the end of a hearing tube and an object such as a watch increased the sound conveyed to the ear (Alison 1859). The quantity of water could be only a fine film under the hearing tube, extensive enough to connect the entire circumference of the aperture with the source of the sound. Based on these observations Alison made a very thin waterproof India-rubber bag, about the size of a large watch and ⅓ inch thick, which could contain the water. He reported that the sounds of the body were

easily conveyed through the stethoscope when the water bag was placed between it and the body. One advantage of the "hydrophone," and probably the most important, was that it could fit exactly upon the part of the chest to which it was applied, however uneven and irregular the surface might be. Alison notes in his report that a water stethoscope had been invented earlier, but that he was unaware of the details. He may be referring to the stethoscope of Koenig which had a tube for injection of water into the chest-piece, and was dated at 1864 by Huard and Niaussat. They also mention a water stethoscope of Somerville of around 1859 (Huard & Niaussat 1982). According to Gerhardt, however (1890), Koenig's stethoscope consisted of a double rubber membrane with compressed air and a flexible rubber tube which lead to a wooden ear-piece. Alison obtained satisfactory results with the hydrophone using air-conducting stethoscopes such as Cammann's, but rigid wooden or metal stethoscopes apparently were not enhanced by its use. The ultimate use of water in the stethoscope is the "hydrophone" of D. H. Cammann which is discussed in the section on auscultatory percussion.

In 1892, Benjamin Ward Richardson of London examined a patient who appeared to have a stricture of the esophagus. Richardson tried the "water-gurgle" test to verify his diagnosis. This consisted of auscultating in the line of the esophagus anteriorly and posteriorly while the patient attempted to swallow fluid. A stricture was associated with a loud gurgling sound, followed by a sharp noise which resembled a passing current of fluid through a constricted passage. This was not conclusive, so he decided to pass an esophageal tube into the stomach of the patient. After the tube had reached the stomach it occurred to Richardson to auscultate through the esophageal tube:

> At once I sliced off a portion of the free end of
> the tube obliquely, slipped over this sliced end the
> terminal part of the double stethoscope, and made

in this fashion the exploring tube a continuous stethoscope. The effect of auscultating in this way was most interesting and satisfactory. I could hear soft friction of the tube against the walls of the oesophagus and was made quite sure that the friction was uniform throughout and that there was no special constriction or induration in any portion of the tube. When I passed the tube into the cavity of the stomach itself I obtained a sound new to me, like a gentle seething as of air or gas agitated in a thickish fluid and at times a gurgling sound of gas with another sound probably due to muscular contraction of the stomach itself... I withdrew the tube until the opening on the left side came in contact with that portion of the oesophagus that lies in immediate proximity with the heart... I counted the beats of the heart very deliberately from the inside of the thorax, seventy beats per minute, the sounds and the pause in proper order and the action perfectly regular.

...From these observations I have been led to the new departure in physical diagnosis in which I am anxious others should take part, and I have devoted some time to certain preliminary steps in its development. Briefly it is a means for auscultating on an extensive scale the organs of the body *from within the body*. (Richardson 1892)

Similar variations of this concept were introduced by Cohen (1893) Debenedetti (1934) and others.

Arthur S. W. Touroff, of Mt. Sinai Hospital in New York City, felt that a short flexible tape measure was a necessary item for the physician who attempted to achieve accuracy and precision in the field of physical diagnosis. His modified stethoscope had a very thin strip of white rubber, $\frac{1}{6}$ inch wide on one tube with calibrations $\frac{1}{6}$ inch apart. (Touroff 1932).

It was common for the stethoscope to be modified to be used as a reflex hammer (Figure A82). The variations described here represent only a small fraction of the countless variety of adaptations of the stethoscope to other uses.

9 Head-pieces and membranes

Headpieces

The suggestion that the ear-pieces should be so fashioned that they could be introduced into the auditory meatus was made early in the evolution of the stethoscope. This is seen in the stethoscope of Dr C. J. B. Williams of 1829 (Williams 1907), in which a trumpet-shaped chest-piece of mahogany was connected with "two bent lead pipes which could be adjusted to the ears," in principle, the modern binaural stethoscope. When in 1852 Cammann of New York added ivory knobs as ear-pieces, made each conducting tube in part flexible and in part rigid, and united the two rigid parts by a jointed bar and elastic band which kept the ear-pieces firmly in position, the binaural stethoscope acquired a comfortable and convenient form.

The evolution to the modern head-pieces of the type shown in Figure 30 was a relatively rapid development. Bowles in his 1894 patent shows head-pieces resembling Cammann's, and in 1901 has the modern type. Denison, and Bartlett and Knight, used a tube with a complex adjustable spring arrangement, although Barlett and Knight's were constructed of lighter metal tubes closer to the modern form. Davis introduced two types of stethoscope which were very close in form to the simpler head-piece. No one individual can claim full credit for this development. Many variations were introduced to try to provide more function-ality to this intrinsic part of the stethoscope. For many years after good quality head-pieces were available, physicians continued to use the flexible rubber tubing with an ear-piece which was stuck into each ear.

Irwin Palmer (1881) applied a circular box spring at the hinge of the head-piece of a Cammann-like stethoscope for the purpose of using the head-piece as a caliber as well, and to provide measurements such as the relative expanding power of the two sides of the chest in lung disease. He attached a dial plate at the hinge which registered the divergence of the metal arms.

The 1887 Lynch and Company catalog illus-trates a stethoscope with a head-piece which is very close to the modern form with two metal arms and a flat spring which it lists as the "clinical model."

Herschell of London felt that the weak point of the binaural stethoscope was the spring. If it were strong enough to keep the instrument in position, the pressure hurt the ears, and if it were weak enough to be comfortable to the user, it was too weak to keep the instrument in place. Conse-quently, Herschell removed the spring and substi-tuted a clamp at the joint (Herschell 1891) (Figure 29). When the lever was in one position the hinge of the stethoscope was loose. The instrument could then be adjusted to the proper pressure on the ears of the user. The lever was then moved to the other position, tightening the hinge and holding the stethoscope in position. It could then be removed without touching the lever.

A practical modification of the design that dominated stethoscope head-pieces for the next century was introduced and patented by O. H. Sheppard in July 1896 (US Patent #563,421). He introduced a swivel joint at the center point of the spring with the type head-piece shown in Figure A37. The joint made it possible to fold the head-piece so that it would fit more readily in the pocket for carrying (Figure 32).

The length of the tubing connecting the chest-piece to the head-piece also evolved, and in

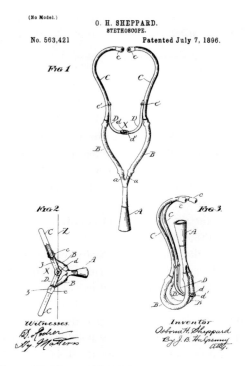

O. H. SHEPPARD.
STETHOSCOPE.

No. 563,421   Patented July 7, 1896.

Fig 1

Fig 2   *Fig 3*

Witnesses

Inventor
Osborn H. Sheppard
By J. B. Halpenny
atty.

Figure 32 Sheppard headpiece

From Sheppard's patent of 1896. By this time the head
piece was basically of a modern form. Sheppard as well as
several others introduced the concept of a joint to facilitate folding the stethoscope for easy portability. The
major innovation from Cammann's head piece is the
flat spring to maintain tension on the ears which was
introduced earlier.

1907 J. Langley formally suggested that a tube
which bifurcates as close to the chest piece as
possible would be more practical than models in
which there were two tubes all of the way down
to the pectoral end (Langley 1907).

Stethoscope membrane

Landouzy mentions experimenting with placing a
membrane over the tubing of his stethoscope. He
noted that when a thin membrane of parchment
was applied to either end of a metal instrument
the sound was augmented, but in his final recommendations he suggests using one only for multiple observers and placing it on the aural end of
the extra tubes (Landouzy 1841). It has been
reported that part of Marsh's patent of 1851 was
the suggested use of a membrane over the chest
end (Davis 1981; Editorial 1855). However the
actual document from the US Patent Office does
not give any indication of this, and there is no
membrane in the accompanying drawing. (Marsh
1851).

In 1859 Alison reported on his water stethoscope (the "hydrophone"). This was in reality a
membrane stethoscope as well (Alison 1859).
Alison notes that even a thin film of water works
in his stethoscope, and discusses the nature of the
membrane. The water was separated from the
tube by "some thin moveable or vibrating body,
such as thin India-ruber, gutta-percha or other
membrane … a thin membrane offers no sensible
impediment." Alison had probably discovered the
advantage of a membrane, but he does not discuss
the use of a membrane without the water although
he does comment in passing that a membrane
alone will augment sound.

Hogeboom (1866) reported

> In using the stethoscope a certain degree of pres-
> sure is requisite in order to have the sounds well
> conveyed. The greatest condensation of sound lies
> under the circular edge of the instrument and
> adjacent to it, both exteriorly and interiorly. By

making compression over the entire disk we obtain a greater quantity of sound from those parts lying immediately beneath the center of the stethoscope. This can be effected by stretching across the pectoral extremity of the stethoscope a membranous substance containing sufficient firmness and elasticity combined to compress the tissues and transmit sonorous vibrations. A piece of beef's or pig's bladder answers the purpose admirably. ... The membrane can be applied to any stethoscope and I think will be found to reduce the "roaring."

Boudet in France introduced a membrane inserted in a bell with a button to localize sound, around 1880. His device consisted of two chest-pieces (resonance boxes) each tuned differently and connected through a single tube, each with a localizing button on a membrane. The concept was to use the end that provided the best clarity of sound. It had flexible ear tubes (Figure A84). He also experimented with amplification (Boudet 1881b).

Another modification which was similar to the membrane was the addition of a rubber ring fitted to the bell of the stethoscope, In this case the ring on the bell provided a better fit to the chest and protection to the patient, but did not materially affect the sound. It was suggested by James Murray in 1889 and reported in the *Lancet* (Bishop 1980).

In 1911, while serving as a house officer at the Boston Floating Hospital, George Clifford King started using a baby's nipple over a Snofton stethoscope from which the hard rubber bell had been removed. He found the combination very successful in listening to the chests of thin and emaciated babies. The rubber allowed closer application of the stethoscope to the chest, and eliminated outside noises. The nipple could be easily and economically changed as soon as the rubber had lost its tone (King 1931).

John B. Donaldson of Ohio modified the stethoscope by fitting a rubber diaphragm over the bell. He suggested that a more durable diaphragm might be made of vulcanized rubber, celluloid or metal with a retaining coiled spring of wire situated above the diaphragm on the bell. This spring held the diaphragm firmly in place (Donaldson 1919).

J. D. Pollard patented a unique design in 1920 in which the membrane was attached to the bell like a drum with screws which could be used to tighten it (US Patent #1,329,430) (Figure A52).

Numerous other inventors suggested the use of the diaphragm (Figures A54–A56; A64–A66), the most notable of whom was Bianchi. However it was the Bowles design which achieved popularity and has persisted to the present time.

10 Current practice

Modern stethoscopes

Among the incredible number of stethoscope designs introduced during the nineteenth and early twentieth century only a few survive. The most remarkable aspect is that between 1926 and modern times the design changes have been minimal and today we are still using the same basic stethoscope that was used in 1925. Perhaps the single exception is the Stethos electronic stethoscope which is discussed under the section on amplification (Figure 33). Although the Littmann (1961) was introduced later, it was based on the preceding designs of Bowles and Sprague. Its main innovation has been in the improvement of the materials available for its manufacture (stainless steel and tygon) and refinement to a point where models weighing only 3 ounces are available. 3M markets eleven models of the Littmann, of all colors and styles. They range in weight from 3 to 6½ ounces and in length from 22 inches to 28 inches with a 40 inch teaching model. The very wide variety available attests to the fact that there is no perfect model for everyone. Even the Bowles model is still being sold with a chest-piece which is very close to the original. Modified Bowles chest-pieces are available which combine the Bowles diaphragm with the Ford bell and have a lever to switch from one to the other. The head-pieces in all of these are the simple style of the original Bowles. The Rappaport–Sprague stethoscope is also readily available and is advertised as "the standard by which all acoustic stethoscopes are judged."

Numerous other versions are marketed, of course, but the message is clear that the most important innovations in the stethoscope were

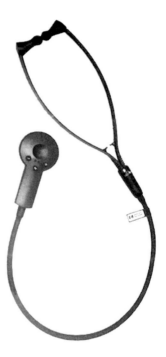

Figure 33 Hewlett Packard (Agilent) Stethos stethoscope
A modern electronic stethoscope is being marketed by Hewlett Packard as well as others. The modern miniaturization of electronics has made this approach practical (Courtesy of Agilent Technologies). The electronics are completely self-contained in the stethoscope itself.

largely accomplished by 1930, and this provides the justification for choosing to concentrate the contents of this monograph on the period preceding that date. It is of interest that a similar developmental evolution applies to the sphygmomanometer. Techniques for blood pressure recording and auscultation were essentially perfected by 1930. Major innovations did not occur until the last decade when miniaturized electronics made significant new approaches possible. Changes in diagnostic technology as well are beginning to have a dramatic effect on these approaches to physical diagnosis. The physical evolution toward the form of the modern stethoscope is summarized in Table 3.

Table 3 Major events in the evolution of the modern stethoscope before 1930

Date	Event
1816	Quire of newspaper
1816	Wooden cylinder
1828	Tapered cylinder with narrow stem, numerous modifications of size, shape, form. Ear-piece becomes concave, bell deeper
1841	Flexible monaural introduced evolves into various combinations
1851	Practical binaural introduced, tubing evolves to more reliable materials with greater flexibility
1894	Practical diaphragm introduced, evolves into Bowles type
1929	Combination chest-piece using bell and diaphragm

Competing modalities

Corvisart in his book on percussion (1808) wrote that, of all of the physical sciences, there is none so important as the interrogation of the senses in medical practice. Nothing cedes a place at the bedside of the patient to observation and experience; all theory is of no value without these faithful guides.

Concerns about physical diagnosis may be appreciated from sphygmography which during the later half of the nineteenth century remained a semi-quantitative method. Towards the end of nineteenth century the majority of physicians preferred to depend on palpation rather than the sphygmograph. They remained committed to physical diagnosis, which they had to learn after a long period of apprenticeship. A frequently quoted statement from the 1905 *British Medical Journal* deprecating the use of the sphygmograph reflects their concern: 'we pauperize our senses and weaken clinical acuity.' The author certainly would have been dismayed by the loss of skills in physical diagnosis that have accompanied modern technological developments.

In 1979, Andrews and Badger wrote, "Auscultation and percussion of the chest are still extremely valuable diagnostic tools in the hands of the skilled clinician, despite widespread reliance on chest roentgenograms and blood tests and the resulting atrophy of basic physical diagnosis techniques." (Andrews & Badger 1979)

The basis of medical diagnosis established by centuries of practice continues to be eroded. Politicians and medical economists lament the great cost of medicine, but do nothing to help students regain these skills which are being rapidly lost. Even worse, there are fewer and fewer practitioners to teach these skills. It is not uncommon for patients to have computed tomography scans or magnetic resonance imaging without ever having been examined. It is common for a patient to see an orthopedist with X-rays having been obtained before the first visit. There is no question that the development of imaging procedures including nuclear medicine, magnetic resonance imaging, computed tomography and ultrasound have given physicians a view of the working of the body in far greater detail than Hook or Harvey or Auenbrugger or Laennec could ever have imagined possible (Figure 34). But we have lost sight of the fact that most afflictions are not really that complicated to diagnose or treat. In a sense, the anxieties of many physicians about early diagnostic instruments have begun to come true. Although the stethoscope has greatly facilitated physical diagnosis, it is being put aside by devices which obviate the basic skills of history-taking, observation and examination.

Perhaps it is time to stop worrying about patenting our ideas, avoiding lawsuits with unnecessary tests and advertising to gain more patients. It is time to return to the practice of medicine as a profession rather than a business, and to provide better care to the patient.

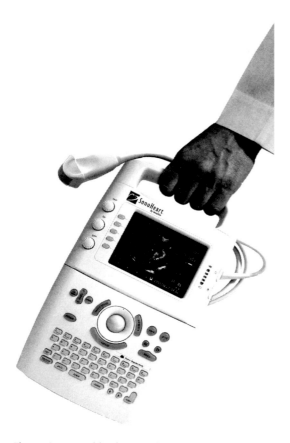

Figure 34 Portable ultrasound unit

The sonoheart, hand-carried echocardiography unit is shown. The entire unit weighs 5.4 lbs and provides a digital quality image for echocardiography. It is 13.3 in high, 7.6 in wide and 2.4 in deep. It can be used for 2D imaging, color Doppler and contains a cardiac calculation package (Courtesy of Sonosite Inc.).

References and suggested reading

Abrahams R. Stethoscopic examinations. *NY Med J* June 10 1911;93:1124–6

Abrams A. Measuring the intensity of the heart tones. *Med News* 1899;75:40–2

Abrams A. Studies in stethophonemetry. *NY Med J* Oct 18 1902;76:677–9

Aitken W. *Science and Practice of Medicine*, 4th edn. London: Griffin, 1866

Aitken W. *The Science and Practice of Medicine*. Philadelphia: Lindsay & Blakiston, 1868

Aitken W. *Science and Practice of Medicine*, 6th edn. London: Griffin, 1872

Alcock T. A biographical notice of the late Charles Thomas Haden. In *Practical Observations on the Management and Diseases of Children* by the late Charles Thomas Haden. London: Burgess and Hill, 1827

Alder N. A new form of straight monaural stethoscope. *Lancet*, Oct 23 1920;2:856

Alison SS. The employment of water in auscultation. *Med Tim Gaz* 1859 n.s.; 28, o.s., 40:7–9; 28–30 (July)

Alison SS. The physical examination of the chest in pulmonary consumption and its intercurrent diseases. Medical Times and Gazette 1859–1861; n.s.19:313–337, 406–421 n.s. 20:447

Andrews JL Jr, Badger TL. Lung sounds through the ages. *JAMA* 1979;241:2625–30

Andry F. *Manuel Practique de Percussion et d'Auscultation*. Paris: Baillière, 1844

Anon. A multiple stethoscope. *Lancet* 1904;1:731

Anon. A new binaural stethoscope. *Lancet* 1909;2:154

Anon. An addition to the binaural stethoscope. *Lond Med Record* 1881;9:219

Anon. Directions for the use of the stethoscope. *Lancet* 1826;10:667–70; 1827;11:312–4

Anon. Electrical Stethoscope. *Can Med Assoc J* March 1935;32:304–5

Anon. Flexible clinical stethoscope. *Med Tim Gaz* 1875;2:82

Atkinson WB, ed. *The Physicians and Surgeons of the United States*. Philadelphia: Charles Robson, 1878;788

Auenbrugger JL. *Inventum Novum ex Percussione Thoracis Humani ut Signo Abstrusos Interni Pectoris Morbos Detegendi* 1761;95

Aurness PA. Duplex stethoscope. *J Am Med Assoc* 1907;48:876

Baas JH. *Outlines of the History of Medicine and the Medical Profession*. New York: J.H. Vail & Co., 1889:1173

Bamberger J. Elin neues Stethoskop zur Bluldruckmessring nach Korotkow. *Deutche medizinische Wochensch* 1923;49:485–6

Barss WR, Eade WF, Fitzgerald EB. Stethoscopes. *Boston Med Surg J* 1926;195:116–21

Barth K. Rubber caps for phonendoscope. *Munchener med Wochensch* Jan 9 1931;78:61

Barth M, Roger H. *Traite pratique d'auscultation ou exposé méthodique des diverses applications de ce mode d'examen a l'état physiologique et morbide de l'économie suivi d'un précis de percussion*. Paris: P. Labe, 1850

Baruch HB. The Phonendoscope. New York: *Med Record* 1896;50:624–6

Batten RW. Binaural stethoscope. *Br Med J* 1887;2:1342

Bell J. Some general remarks on the use of the stethoscope. *NY Med Phys J* 1824;3: 269–81

Bennet H. On the comparative value of auscultation practised with and without the stethoscope. *Lancet* Jan 6 1868;1:461–6

Benoit EP. *Le Stethophone* (Part 1). Paris: Presse Medicale 1926;34:140

Bettany GT. *Eminent Doctors, Their Lives and Their Work*. London: J. Hogg, 1885ß

Bianchi A. Il Fonendoscopio; Nuovo strumento per l'indagine dei suoni interni. (The Phonendoscope; A new instrument for the investigation of internal sounds.) *Policlinico, Roma, sez. Med.* 1894;1:179–80

Bianchi A. Del Fonendoscopio; e della sua applicazione practica in medicina. *Clinica Moderna* 1895;1:421–7

Bianchi A. *The Phonendoscope and Its Practical Application*, translated by AG Baker. Philadelphia: G. P. Pilling & Son, 1900

Bianchi A. Estudios de fonendoscopia. *La Semana Medica* Oct 22 1925;2:1052–5

Bing HI. Some remarks on stethoscopy. *Int Clini* Dec 1927;4:111–22

Bird G. Observations on advantages presented by the employment of a stethoscope with a flexible tube. *Lond Med Gaz* 1840–41; n.s. 1:440–442

Bishop PJ. Evolution of the stethoscope. *J R Soc Med* 1980;73:448–56

Blackwell TC. An improved stethoscope. *Br Med J* 1911;1:697, 1361

Blakiston P. Practical Observations on Certain Diseases of the Chest and on the Principles of Auscultation. Philadelphia: Leas and Blanchard, 1848

Bluth EI. James Hope and the acceptance of auscultation. *J Hist Med All Sci* 1970;25:202–10

Bock H. Ein Neues Stethoskop zur Messung der Subjektiven Starke der Herzklange. *Munch Med Wochensch* 1908;55:551–3

Bock H. Ueber die Verwendbarkeit des Differential Stethoskopes Nach Bock. *Berlin Klin Wochensch* 1909;46:544

Bock H. Differential stethoscope for the examination of the heart and lungs. *Mod Hosp* 1915; 4:449

Boston LN. Clinical advantages of the double stethoscope. *J Am Med Assoc* 1927;88:1796–7

Boudet Dr L'électricité. *Rev Med* 1881a;760–77

Boudet Dr L'électricité ses applications au diagnostic et au traitement des maladies. *Rev Med* 1881b;829–62

Bowditch HI. *The Young Stethoscopist or the Student's Aid to Auscultation*. New York: J. & H. G. Langley, 1846

Bowditch HI. Double self adjusting stethoscope, invented by Dr Cammann. *Am J Med Sc* 1854; n.s. 28:85

Bowles RCM. A new pattern of bowles' stethoscope. *Med Rec* 1904;66:719

Brown J. A new form of bi-aural stethoscope. *Lancet* 1877;1:335

Brown JG. *Medical Diagnosis; A Manual of Clinical Methods*. New York: E. B. Treat, 1888;147–64

Budd G. Observations on the Stethoscope. *Elec J Med* 1837;1:397–403

Cabot RC. *Physical Diagnosis of Diseases of the Chest*, 2nd edn. New York: William Wood and Co., 1903:86–92

Cabot RC. A multiple electrical stethoscope for teaching purposes. *J Am Med Assoc* 1923; 4,81:298–9

Cabot RC. Note on the multiple electrical stethoscope for teaching purposes. *Med Press Cir* 1923; n.s., 116:199–200

Cahan JM. Stethoscope hanger in coat. *Med J Rec* March 5 1930;131:268

Camac CNB. Laennec and his stethoscope. *Med News* May 20 1905;86:918–23

Cammann DM. An historical sketch of the stethoscope. *Am Climatol Assoc Trans* May 1885a; 170–4

Cammann DM. A modification of cammann's binaural stethoscope. *NY Med J* 1885b;41: 27–8

Cammann DM. An historical sketch of the stethoscope. *NY Med J* April 24 1886;43:465

Cammann DM. Remarks on auscultatory percussion, and on a new binaural hydrophone. *NY Med J* 1886;43:241–2

Cammann DM, Scott RJE. Stethoscopes. In *Reference Handbook of the Medical Sciences*. New York, 1917;8:642–4

Cammann GP, Clark A. A new mode of ascertaining the dimensions, form and condition of internal organs by percussion. *NY J Med Surg* Jan–July 1840;3:62–96

Cammann GP. Letter to the Editors. *NY J Med* Dec 2 1856

Cammann GP. The double self adjusting stethoscope. *NY J Med* 1857;139–40

Cantlie J. *Br Med J* 1914;Feb 21

Carrick GL. On the differential stethoscope and its values in the diagnosis of diseases of the lungs and heart. *Edin Med J* 1872–73;18:894–916

Casper VW. Description of new stethoscope which permits simultaneous auscultation by several persons. *Med Klin* Dec 21 1928;24:1991

Chevalier D. Modification proposée au stethoscope (Rap de M de Kergaradec). *Bull Acad Imp Med* 1861–62;27:403–5

Clark A. Obituary. *Med Record* 1887;32:414

Clark A. *Lectures on Diseases of the Heart*. New York: E. B. Treat, 1891:251

Clendening L. The centenary of the stethoscope. *J Missouri Med Assoc* 1920;17:9–12

Clutterback H. *Lectures on Blood Letting*. Philadelphia: Haswell, Barrington and Haswell, 1839

Cohen SS. An esophageal stethoscope, with remarks on intra-thoracic auscultation. *Med News* 1893;63:688–9

Collin V. *Des Diverses methodes d'exploration de la poitrine, et de leur application au diagnostic de ses maladies*. Paris: J. B. Baillière, 1824;1:116

Collin V. *Manual for the Use of the Stethoscope: A Short Treatise on the Different Methods of Investigating the Diseases of the Chest*, translated from the French by WN Ryland. Boston: Benjamin Perkins & Co., 1829

Combes RH. A new stethoscope. *Lancet* Dec 12 1885;2:1100

Comins NP. Flexible stethoscope. *Lancet* 1828–1829;2:685–7

Comins NP. New stethoscope. *Lond Med Gaz* 1829;4:427–30

Comins NP. Flexible stethoscope. *Lancet* 1829–30;1:49–50

Conner LA. On certain acoustic limitations of the stethoscope and their clinical importance. *NY Med J* 1907;86:56–9

Cornell EL. The head stethoscope. *Surg Clin Chicago* Oct 1919;3:1304–6

Corning JL. A memorial address on the late Dr James R. Leaming. *Med Record* 1893;43:196–9

Corper HJ. Centenary of the death of rené Theophile Hyacinthe Laennec; brief review of his work. *Colorado Med Aug* 1926;23:261–8

Corvisart JN. *Nouvelle methode pour reconnaître les maladies internes de la poitrine*. Paris: Migneret, 1808

Councell RW. Binaural stethoscope. *Br Med J* 1911;2:168

Cousins JW. On a new convertible stethoscope. *Br Med J* Jan 14 1882;1:45–6

Crummer L. *Clinical Features of Heart Disease*. New York: P. B. Hoeber, Inc., 1925;353

DaCosta JC. *Principles and Practice of Physical Diagnosis*, 3rd edn. Philadelphia: W. B. Saunders & Co., 1915

DaCosta JM. *Medical Diagnosis with Special Reference to Practical Medicine*. Philadelphia: J. B. Lippincott & Co., 1895

Dana JT. Use of the stethoscope in determining the presentation and position of the foetus in utero. *Boston Med Surg J* 1853;47:427–30

Davies AT. Laennec and the stethoscope. *Br Med J* 1908;1:840

Davies H. A double stethoscope. *Med Times Gazette* 1862;1:359

Davis AB. *Medicine and its Technology*. Westport CT: Greenwood Press, 1981

Debenedetti E. Estetoscopio esofagico. *La Semana Medica* Sept 27 1934;2:980–1

DeLee JB. Several every day obstetric problems. *Am J Obste* 1917;76:15–25

DeLee JB. New stethoscope especially for maternity cases. *Zentralblatt Gynakol* Oct 21 1922; 46:1688–9

DeMarco F. Stethoscope à double paroi pneumatique. *Presse Medicale* Part I, June 13 1928; 36:750

Denison C. An improved binaural stethoscope. *Med Record* April 4 1885;27:391

Denison C. The essentials of a good stethoscope. *Med Record* Oct 22 1892;41:494–5

Denison C. My latest improved binaural stethoscope. *Transactions of the Colorado State Medical Society* 1896;257–61

Depaul JAH. *Leçons de Clinique obstetricale*. Paris: V. Adrien Delahaye et Cie, 1872–1876

Dickinson RL. Phonendoscope. *Brooklyn Med J* 1897;11:137–45

Dickinson SW. Laennec's stethoscope. *Virginia Med Monthly* May 1920;47:70–2

Dobell H. *Coughs, Consumption and Diet in Disease*. Philadelphia: D. G. Brinton, 1877;19–36

Donaldson JB. A stethoscope of increased sensitiveness. *J Am Med Assoc* 1919;73:1303

Double FJ. *Semiologie général où traite des signes et de leur valeur dans les maladies*. Paris: Croullebois, 1817

DuBois EF. A small stethoscope bell. *US Naval Med Bull* 1918;12:75–6

Duffin J. *To See with a Better Eye, A Life of R. T. H. Laennec*. Princeton: Princeton University Press, 1998

Ebstein E. Einige Bemerkungen uber die Form des Stethoskops. *Berlin Klin Wochensch* July 7 1913;50:1262

Editorial. Self adjusting stethoscope of Dr Cammann. *NY Med Times* 1855;4:140–2

Edwards WA. A new binaural stethoscope. *Med News* Nov 7 1885;47:527–8

Elliotson J. *On the Recent Improvements in the Art of Distinguishing the Various Diseases of the Heart*. London: Longman, Rees, Orme, Brown and Green, 1830

Elmquist R. Cheap electric stethoscope for lecture hall. *Klin Wochensch* Dec 19 1931;10:2374

Evans W. A teaching stethoscope. *Lancet* Jan 19 1935;1:153

Falls FH. Use of vaginal stethoscope in early diagnosis of pregnancy. *Am J Obstet Gyne* March 1926;11:309–13

Falls FH, Hunter TA. An improved head stethoscope for the hearing and counting of fetal heart tones. *Am J Obstet Gynecol* Sept 1924;8:356–8

Falls FH, Rockwood AC. Use of microphonic stethoscope in demonstration of fetal heart tones. *J Am Med Assoc* 1923;No. 20, 81:1683–4

Faught FA. *Blood Pressure from the Clinical Standpoint*. Philadelphia & London: Saunders W. B. & Co., 1913;276

Finlayson J. *Clinical Diagnosis: A Handbook for Students and Practitioners of Medicine*. Philadelphia: H. C. Lea, 1891;440–2

Finot A. Francois-Joseph Double Inventeur de l'auscultation en 1817. *J Hist Sci Med* 1972;6:14–21

Fisher JD. Stethoscopic diagnosis of pregnancy. *Boston Med Surg J* 1831;3:97–106

Flint A. *A Practical Treatise on the Diagnosis, Pathology and Treatment of Diseases of the Heart*. Philadelphia: Blanchard & Lea, 1859

Flint A. The life and labors of Laennec. *New Orleans Med News* 1859–60;6:736–56

Flint A. Stethoscopes and their use. *Med Record* 1870;5:234–6

Flint A. *A Manual of Percussion and Auscultation*. Philadelphia: H. C. Lea, 1876

Flint A. *A Manual of Auscultation and Percussion*, 2nd edn. Philadelphia: H. C. Lea, 1880

Floersheim S. Practical arrangement of the stethoscope or phonendoscope for the examination of the heart sounds, murmurs and the heart in general. *California and Western Med* Oct 1924;22:531

Forbes J. *A Treatise on the Diseases of the Chest by R.T.H. Laennec*. London: T. and G. Underwood, 1821

Forbes J. Original cases, with dissections and observations, illustrating the use of the stethoscope and percussion in the diagnosis of the diseases of the chest: together with a translation of Auenbrugger's treatise and Corvisart's commentaries, etc. Book Review. *Lancet* Oct 30 1824;5:144–60; Nov 6 169–80

Forbes J. *A Treatise on the Diseases of the Chest, and on Mediate Auscultation by RTH Laennec.* New York: Samuel S. Wood and William Wood, 1838

Forbes J, Conolly J. *Analytical and Critical Reviews, The British and Foreign Medical Review.* London: Sherwood Gilbert and Piper, 1837

Foy G. The centenary of the discovery of the stethoscope. *Med Press* 1919; n.s. 108:311

Foy G. The discovery of the stethoscope. *Med Press and Circular* 1924; n.s. 118:235

Froschels E. Differential stethoscope. *Medizin Klinik* Aug 17 1934;30:1099–100

Frossard HJ. Un Stethoscope pour la localisation des epanchements pleuretiques. *Presse Medicale* Aug 16 1924;32:1385–6

Fuller HW. *On Diseases of the Lungs and Air.* H. C. Lea, Philadelphia 1867

Gairdner WT. *Clinical Medicine Observations Recorded at Bedside with Commentaries.* Edinburgh: Edmonston and Douglas, 1862;17:741

Gamble CJ. Multiple electrical stethoscope and electrical filters as aids to diagnosis. *J Am Med Assoc* 1924;1230–2

Gamble CJ, Replogle DE. A multiple electrical stethoscope for teaching. *J Am Med Assoc* Feb 2 1924;82:387–8

Garstang W. On an improved stethoscope. *Lancet* 1856;2:437

Gee SJ. *Auscultation and Percussion together with Other Methods of Physical Examination of the Chest,* 3rd edn. London: J. Walton 1870

Geigel R. Die Akustische Leistung von Communicationsrohren und Stethoskopen. *Archiv fur Pathologische Anatomie* 1895;140: 165–91

Geigel R. Ueber Communicationsrohren und Stethoskope. *Wiener klini Wochenschr* 1895; 8:261

Gerhardt C. *Lehrbuch der Auscultation und Percussion.* Tubingen: H. Laupp, 1866

Gerhardt C. *Lehrbuch der Auscultation und Percussion.* Tubingen: H. Laupp, 1890

Glover H. *L'Auscultation électrique en physiologie et en clinique.* Paris: Fumouze, 1925

Good JM. *The Study of Medicine.* New York: Harper & Brothers, 1836;2:51–5

Gordon B. A modification of the bell type of stethoscope. *J Lab Clin Med* Aug 1929;14: 1111

Gordon B. Description of a mon-aural diaphragm type of stethoscope with discussion of its special field of usefulness. *Am Heart J* Aug 1933;8:845–9

Granville AB. *Sudden Death.* London: John Churchill, 1854

Graves RJ, Stokes W. Dr. Hope on Auscultation. *Dublin J Med Sci* 1839;178–80

Gregory G. *Elements of the Theory and Practice of Physic.* Philadelphia: Towar & Hogan, 1829;1: 399–405

Griffiths FG. Commemoration of Laennec: his work on the heart and lungs: his invention of the stethoscope. *Med J Austral* Dec 11 1926; 13th year, No. 24, 2:796–9

Groedel D. Das Binaurale Stethoskop. *Berlin klin Wochensch* 1891;28:59–62

Guthrie JB. Modification of the Bowles stethoscope. *J Am Med Assoc* Sept 22 1923;81: 1013–4

Guttmann P. *A Handbook of Physical Diagnosis.* New York: W. Wood, & Co., 1880

Hagenbach A, Krethlow A, Bachtiger P. Physical tests of ear tubes for stethoscopes. *Schweizerische med Wochensch* Jan 21 1928;58:49–54

Haig HA. A new form of chest–piece for the binaural stethoscope. *Lancet* 1911;1:1088

Hall M. The Principles of Diagnosis. New York: D. Appleton & Co., 1835

Harris I. A stethoscopic chest-piece. *Lancet* April 27 1935;1:994

Hart S. Stethoscopy. *Popular Science Monthly* 1884–85;25:189–201

Hartlett EM. A head clamp stethoscope holder for the rapid and secure adaptation of the standard bell stethoscope to the head. *Surg Gynecol Obstet* 1924;38:411

Hartshorne H. *Essentials of the Principles and Practice of Medicine*, 5th edn. Philadelphia: H. C. Lea & Co., 1881;103–4

Harvey W. *The Anatomical Exercises of Dr William Harvey*. London: Richard Lowndes, 1673

Hasenfeld A. Mein Polyauscultator. *Deutshe med Wochensch* Aug 16 1929;55:1384–5

Haus CJ. *Die Auscultation in Bezug auf Schwangerschaft*. Wurzburg: Johann Stephen Richter, 1823

Hawthorne CO. The differential (double) stethoscope. *Irish J Med Sci* 7th series, Feb 1935; 49–53

Hayden AA. Auscultation and Percussion in the Diagnosis of Accessory Nasal Sinus Disease Preliminary Report. *J Am Med Assoc* Oct 23 1926;87:1390–2

Hayden T. *The Diseases of the Heart and of the Aorta*. Philadelphia: Lindsay & Blakiston, 1875; I and II.

Hecker. Das Deppelhorrohr. Berlin: *Deutche med Wochensch* 1903;29:834

Heermann. Ein Neues Doppel Horrohr. *Deutche med Wochensch* 1903;29:249

Heise FH. The Physics of Percussion and Auscultation of the Chest. *Med Record* 1916;90:191–4

Henry CC. The heartphone: a newly perfected electric stethoscope. *NY Med J* 1918;107:162

Henry FP. A Modification of the stethoscope. *Philadelphia Med Times* 1876;6:295

Herrick JB. In Defense of the stethoscope. *Ann Intern Med* Aug 1930–31;4:113–6

Herschell G. An Improvement in binaural stethoscopes. *Tr Med Soc* 1890–1891;14:439–40

Herschell G. An improved binaural stethoscope. *Lancet* March 14 1891;1:609

Higgins JA. A type of stethoscope receiving bowl for use in the teaching of medical students. *J Lab Clin Med* 1918–19;4:450–2

Hildebrand B. Mono-auricular rubber tube stethoscope. *Munchen med Wochensch* July 8 1927;74:1134

Hildebrandt W. Eine Neue Verbesserung des Stethoskopes. *Munchener Medizinische Wochenschrift* March 1904;51:523

Hilliard RH. On a new double stethoscope: the head spring stethoscope. *Br Med J* 1875;2:610

Hillis DS. Attachment for the stethoscope. *J Am Med Assoc* 1917;68:910

Hogeboom CL. On the application of a compressing membrane to the stethoscope. *NY Med J* 1866;3:287–90

Holden FC. A good illustration of the DeLee stethoscope. *Med Rec* 1917;92:1009

Holmes OW. *Boylston Prize Dissertations for the Years 1836 and 1837*. Boston: Little, Brown, 1837

Holmes OW. *Poems*. Boston: Ticknor and Fields, 1856

Hope J. *A Treatise on the Diseases of the Heart and Great Vessels, and on the Affections which May be Mistaken for Them*. Philadelphia: Haswell & Johnson, 1842;116–22

Hoskin J. A Multiple Electrical Stethoscope. *Lancet* 1925;2:1164–5

Huard P, Niaussat P. L'Evolution du Stethoscope. *Comptes Rendus du 106 Congrés National des Sociétés Savantes* Paris: Bibliotheque Nationale, 1982

Hudson ED. *A Manual of the Physical Diagnosis of Thoracic Diseases*. New York: W. Wood and Co., 1887:162

Huter V. Das Somatoskop. *Berlin klin Wochensch* 1877;14:160

Jagic N. Phonendoscope for Class Teaching. *Wiener med Wochensch* Jan 14 1928;78:82

Jagic N, Spengler G. Auscultation with Electrostethoscope. *Wiener klin Wochensch* June 30 1927;40:847

Jessop CM. The Finger-ended stethoscope. *Br Med J* April 5 1879;1:514

Johnston FD, Kline EM. An acoustical study of the stethoscope. *Arch Int Med* 1940;65:328–39

Kane EO. Wearing of branching stethoscope by surgeons and anesthetist during Operation. *Surg, Gynecol Obstet* Oct 1924;39:508

Keele KD. *The Evolution of Clinical Methods in Medicine*. Springfield. Ill: Charles C. Thomas, 1963

Kelly HA. *A Cyclopedia of American Medical Biography*. Philadelphia: W. B Saunders & Co., 1912;I and II

Kelly HA, Burrage WL. American Medical Biographies. Baltimore: Norman Remington Co., 1920

King GC. A simple stethoscope tip. *J Am Med Assoc* July 4 1931;97:24

Kintzing P. *The Signs of Internal Disease*. Chicago: Cleveland Press, 1906;23–6

Kirschstein. Stethoscope with detachable reserve parts for use in infectious cases. *Deutsche med wochensch* Dec 2 1927;53:2084–5

Knapp MI. A new and improved stethoscope. *Med Record* 1895;48:682–3

Knapp MI. An improved stethoscope. *Med Record* 1900;58:119

Knight FI. An addition to Cammann's double or binaural stethoscope, intended to regulate the amount of pressure on the ears. *Boston Med Surg J* 1869;80:221–2

Knopf SA. An improved stethoscope with an attachable plessimeter. *Med Record* 1897;51:646–7

Knopf SA. A new binaural stethoscope with armamentarium for complete physical examination. *J Am Med Assoc* 1898;30:27–8

Kolipinski L. The auscultoplectrum, a combined stethoscope and percussion hammer. *NY Med J* 1915;101:194–6

Koplik H. A new binaural stethoscope for the examination of infants and children. *Transactions of the American Pediatric Society* 1899;11:171–2

Kretzschmar. Ein Praktisches Arztliches Untersuchungsinstrument. *Munchen med Wochensch* May 1908;55:970

Kuhn A. Biphoscope. *Munchen Med Wochensch* March 20 1925;72:479

Kuhn A. History of stethoscope with double membrane. *Munchen Med Wochensch* July 3 1925;72:1113–4

Laennec RTH. De l'Auscultation mediate ou traite du diagnostic des maladies des poumons et du coeur. Paris: Brosson et Chaude, 1819

Laennec RTH. *A Treatise on the Diseases of the Chest*, translated by J. Forbes. Philadelphia: J. Webster, 1823;211–9

Laennec RTH. *Traite de l'auscultation mediate du diagnostic des maladies des poumons et du coeur.* Paris: Brosson et Chaude, 1826

Laennec RTH. *A Treatise on the Diseases of the Chest and on Mediate Auscultation*, Philadelphia: DeSilver, Thomas & Co., translated by J. L. Forbes from the 4th London edn. 1835

Laennec RTH. *Traite de l'auscultation mediate et des maladies des poumons et du coeur*, edited and augmented by M. Laennec and G. Andral. Brussels: Wahlen & Co., 1837

Lamb DS. The stethoscope: A history. *Washington Med Ann* 1910–1911; No. 3, 9:260–9

Landes G. Weitere Untersuchungen uber die Schallubertragung des Stethoskops. *Deutsches Arch klin Med* 1931;171:607–23

Landouzy H. Memoire sur les procédés acoustiques de l'auscultation et sur un nouveau mode de stethoscopie applicable aux etudes cliniques. *Gaz Med Paeia* 1841;9:305–11

Langley I. Improved stethoscope. *Br Med J* Dec 14 1907;2:1720

Leaming JR. *Contributions to the Study of the Heart and Lungs*. New York: E. B. Treat, 1887

Leared A. *Catalogue of Great Exhibition*. 1851;9:477

Leared A. On the self–adjusting double stethoscope. *Lancet* August 2 1856

Leared A. *On the Sounds Caused by the Circulation of the Blood*. London: John Churchill, 1861

Leared A. Dictionary of National Biography. 1892;32:326

Leff M. A Stethoscope for auscultating the fetal heart. *Am J Obstet Gynecol* July 1930;20:108–9

Leyton O. Differential stethoscopes. *Lancet* 1916;2:24

Leyton O. The differential stethoscope as an aid to the diagnosis of myocardial changes. *Practitioner* 1918;100:224–34

Littmann D. An approach to the ideal stethoscope. *JAMA* 1961;178:504–5

Loewenberg SA. *Diagnostic Methods and Interpretations in Internal Medicine.* Philadelphia: F. A. Davis & Co., 1929;271–4

Loomis AL. *Diseases of the Respiratory Organs, Heart and Kidneys.* New York: W. Wood & Co., 1876

Loomis AL. Lessons in Physical Diagnosis. New York: W. Wood & Co., 1893;289

Losse H. Alte Faelle neu gelesen: Pneumonie. *Schweiz Rundschau Med (Praxis) 80 Nr* 1991; 48:1352–6

Louis B. Lecture on the auscultation of the chest (from the *Presse Medicale*). *Med Gazette* 1837; 20:711–7

Lowenthal L. A modified rigid stethoscope. *Br Med J* 1918a;1:673

Lowenthal L. An improved mon-aural stethoscope. *Lancet* 1918b;2:110

Ludlow JL. A new flexible stethoscope. *Am J Med Sci* 1844; n.s. 7:509–10

Lynch & Co., *Catalogue of Druggists Sundries and Surgical Instruments.* London: Lynch & Co., 1887

Lyons RSD. On a double bell stethoscope. *QJM Sc* 1862;33:364–6

Lyons RSD. Observations on the motions and sounds of the human heart during life as witnessed in the case of M. Groux. *Atlantis, Catholic University of Ireland* 1858;1:451–75

Malet H. The physical difference between binaural and uniaural stethoscopes. *Br Med J* 1882;2:774–5

Manges M. The phonendoscope. *NY Med J* 1904

Manheimer G. A modified Bowles stethoscope. *Med Record* 1909;75:18

Marsh N. *Stethoscope.* US Patent No. 8591, December 16, 1851

Martini P. Die Schallubertragung des Stethoskops. *Zeitschrift Fur Biologie* 1920;71:117–36

Martini P. Die Schallubertragung des Stethoskops. *Zeitschruft Fur Biologie* 1920;76:221–6

Masserman JH. Two new instruments of physical diagnosis: A stethoscope and electric resonator. *California and Western Medicine* July 1931;35: 44–5

Medical and Surgical Appliances. The stethoscope (the revolving). *Med Ann* 1915:756–7

Meyer-Steineg TH, Sudhoff K. *Hippokrates und die hippokratische Medizin. Geschichte der Medizin,* 4th edn. Jena: Verlag Gustav Fischer, 1950;60

Middleton WS. The medical aspect of Robert Hooke. *Ann Med Hist* 1927;9:227–43

Miller JW. Another binaural stethoscope. *Br Med J* 1888;1:862

Minchin WC. A new stethoscope. *Med Press* 1921; n.s. 111:300

Minchin WC. A new stethoscope. *Lancet* 1921; 2:1010

Minchin WC. Stethoscope for recording blood pressure. *Lancet* Feb 6 1926;1:294

Mitchell AR. An improved stethoscope for stethoscope percussion. *Med Detroit* 1896;2: 372–3

Mitchell SW. The history of instruments of precision in medicine. *Med Record* 1878;14: 285–8

M'Keever T. On the information afforded by the stethoscope in detecting the presence of foetal life. *Lancet* 1832–1833;2:715–7

Morris S. The Advent and Development of the Binaural Stethoscope. *The Practitioner* Nov 1967; 199:674–80

Moss MN. Combination stethoscope. *J Am Med Assoc* June 28 1924;82:2118–2119

Muller F. Principles of percussion and auscultation. *Lancet* 1913;1:674–675

Mumey N. *An Iconographic Sketch of the Life of René Theophile Hyacinthe Laennec.* Denver: Privately printed, 1932

Musser JH. *A Practical Treatise on Medical Diagnosis for Students and Physicians.* Philadelphia: Lea & Febiger, 1913;818

Myers JA, Cady LH. René Theophile Hyacinthe Laennec, inventor of the stethoscope. *Minnesota Medicine* June 1927;10:370–6

Naegele HF. *Die geburtshülfliche Auscultation.* Mainz: Zabern, 1838

Naegele HF. *A Treatise on Obstetric Auscultation,* translated from the German by Charles West. London: Renshaw, 1839

Nagle DC. On the use of the stethoscope for the detection of twins in utero, the presentation, etc. *Lancet* 1830–31;1:232–4; 395–400;497–502

Nagle DC. Observations on the use of the stethoscope in the practice of midwifery. *Lancet* 1831–32;1:449–51

Newton RC. A sketch of the origin of auscultation and percussion and of the state of clinical medicine in the time of Auenbrugger and Laennec. *Med Record* Sept 5 1914;86:415–19

New York Medical Times, Self Adjusting Stethoscope. *NY J Med* 1855;14:472–4

Norris GW, Landis HRM. *Diseases of the Chest and the Principles of Physical Diagnosis*, 5th edn. Philadelphia: W. B. Saunders & Co., 1933

Oden CLA. A soft rubber tip for the bell type of stethoscope. *J Am Med Assoc* 1921;77:623

O'Kelly T. Binaural stethoscope for auscultatory percussion. *Br Med J* 1894;1:919

Olpp VPD. Zur Stimmgabel Stethoskop Methode. *Munchen Med Wochensch* July 1914;61:1674–6

Page RCM. *A Handbook of Physical Diagnosis of Diseases of the Organs of Respiration and Heart, and of Aortic Aneurism.* New York: J. H. Vail & Co., 1895

Palmer I. An addition to the binaural stethoscope. *Lond Med Record* 1881:219

Park R. *An Epitome of the History of Medicine.* Philadelphia: F. A. Davis & Co., 1898;362

Parker FD. New thoracic murmurs with two new instruments, the refractoscope and the partial stethoscope. *J Exp Med* 1918;28:607–22

Paul C. Presentation d'instrument. *Paris Acad Med Bull* May 1881a; n.s. 10:552

Paul C. Un Nouveau Modéle de stethoscope flexible. *Gazette des Hopitaux* May 1881b;54:412–3

Paul C. *Diagnosis and Treatment of Diseases of the Heart.* New York: W. Wood & Co., 1884

Paul C. *Diagnostic et traitment des maladies du coevr.* Paris: Asselin et Houzeau, 1887

Pearson FW. Laennec and Skoda. *Maryland Med J* May 1879;5:1–7

Pel PK. Welches Stethoskop soll der Arzt Gebrauchen. *Berlin klin Wochensch* 1889;26: 929–31

Pennock CW. Notice of a new flexible stethoscope. *Am J Med Sci* 1844;7:509–10

Philpots JR. A new stethoscope. *Br Med J* 1892; 1:562

Pickering. Pickering's Panarkes' stethoscope. *Br Med J* 1887;2:1342

Pilling Instruments and Equipment for Surgeons and Hospital, Philadelphia: George P. Pilling & Co., 1932

Pinard A. *Clinique Obstetricale* Paris: G. Steinheil, Harve, Lemale, 1899

Piorry PA. Nouvelle Mèthode de percussion du thorax. *Arch Gen Med* 1826;10:471–2

Piorry PA. *De la Percussion mediate et des signes obtenus a l'aide de ce nouveau moyen d'exploration dans les maladies des organes thoraciques et abdominaux* Paris: Chaude JS, JB Baillière, 1828

Piorry PA. *Traite de ples simōt risme et d'organographisme.* Paris: Delahayé, 1866

Pitta. Sur des Modifications apportées au stethoscope ordinaire, rap de M. Kergaradec. *Bull Acad Imp Med* 1858–59;24:1148–56

Pocock TW. Letter to the Editor. *Lond Med Gazette* 1838;2:741–3

Pollack H. Stethoskop-Erka. *Deutsche med Wochensch* Jan 6 1933;59:16

Pollock JE. Self adjusting double stethoscope. *Lancet* 1856;1:398–9

Potter JC. The biresonating stethoscope. *Br Med J* 1901;2:814–15

Pratt JH, Bushnell GE. *Physical Diagnosis of Diseases of the Chest.* Philadelphia: W. B. Saunders & Co., 1925;522

Prest EE. The stethoscope in the diagnosis of pulmonary tuberculosis. *Lancet* 1930;1:990

Raciborski A. *Manuel complet d' auscultation et de percussion ou application de l' acoustique au diagnostic des maladies.* Bruxelles: Société Belge de Librairie Hauman et Cie, 1839

Ramsay J. Bock's stethoscope as an aid to determining the efficiency of the myocardium. *Br Med J* 1916;2:521–2

Rappaport MB, Sprague HB. Physiologic and physical laws that govern auscultation, and their clinical application. *Am Heart J* 1941;21:257–318

Rappaport MB, Sprague HB. The effects of tubing bore on stethoscope efficiency. *Am Heart J* 1951;42:605–9

Reed C. Improved double stethoscope. *Lancet* 1874;2:550

Reid JK, Morris WO. An improved stethoscope. *Lancet* Sept 8 1928;2:506

Reiser SJ. Aspects of role of the stethoscope in the introduction of auscultation to Great Britain and the United States. London: *Proceedings XXIII International Congress of the History of Medicine,* 1974:832–40

Remarks on the comparative value of auscultation practice with and without the stethoscope. *Lancet* 1843–1844;1:464

Reynaud. Memoire sur quelques faits et aperçus nouveaux, relatifs a l'auscultation de la poitrine (Note on some new facts and glances at auscultation of the chest). *Jour Hebd De Med* 1829;4:563–72

Richardson BW. *An India Rubber Double Stethoscope.* London: Asclepiad, Longmans, Green & Co., 1884;1:162–3

Richardson BW. *The Introduction of the Stethoscope Into English Practice.* London: Asclepiad, Longmans, Green & Co., 1888;5:382–6

Richardson BW. *René Theophile Hyacinthe Laennec, M.D. and the Discovery of Mediate Auscultation by the Stethoscope.* London: Asclepiad, Longmans, Green & Co., 1888;5:241–68

Richardson BW. Intra-thoracic auscultation: a new departure in physical diagnosis. *Lancet* 1892;2:1037–9

Risse GB, Pierre A. Piorry (1794–1879), the French "Master of Percussion." *Chest* 1971;60:484–8

Robertson WGA. A multiple stethoscope. *Br Med J* 1903;2:88

Robinson V. Laennec and Auscultation. *Medical Review of Reviews* 1912;18;456–65

Rolleston H. *Cardio-vascular Disease since Harvey's Discovery.* Cambridge: Cambridge University Press, 1928

Rose WD. *Physical Diagnosis.* St. Louis: Mosby, 1927;159–61

Rosenblatt S. Aural Auscultation. *Illinois Med J* March 1926;49:258–9

Rouit LM. *Essai sur L'Auscultation dans le diagnostic des maladies de poitrine.* Paris: Dido Le Jeune, 1828

Salter H. On the Stethoscope. *Assoc Med J* 1863;1:105–8;133–5

Sansom AE. *Lectures on the Physical Diagnosis of Diseases of the Heart,* 2nd edn. London: Churchill, 1876

Sansom AE. *Manual of the Physical Diagnosis of Diseases of the Heart,* 3rd edn. Philadelphia: Blakiston, 1881

Sansom AE. On Percussion as a Means of Precise Diagnosis. *Liverpool Medico-Chirurgical Journal* January 1885

Sansom AE. *The Diagnosis of Diseases of the Heart and Thoracic Aorta.* London: Charles Griffin & Co., 1892

Sato A, Nukiyama H (Japan). Magnoscope, an electrical stethoscope. *Am J Dis Children* 1925;29:618–20

Schall M. Ein Stethoskop. *Med Wochensch* March 1912;38:514

Scheminzky F. Electric stethoscope with reenforcer and graphic registrator. *Wiener klin Wochensch* May 26 1927;40;695

Schmalz KG. *Versuch einer medizinisch-chirurgischen Diagnostik in Tabellen, oder Erkenntniss und Unterscheidung der innern und aeussern krankheiten, mittels Nebeneinanderstellung der aehnlichen Formen.* In der Arnoldischen Buchhandlung, Dresden und Leipzig, 1825, 4th ed

Self-Adjusting Stethoscope of GP Cammann, M.D., of New York. The New York Journal of Medicine and the Collateral Sciences, New York: Purple & Smith, 1855; n.s. No 3, 14:472–4

Senator H. Zur Kenntniss der Schallerscheinungen an den peripheren Arterien nebst Bemerkungen uber die Auscultation mit holiden und soliden Stethoscopen. *Berlin klin Wochensch* 1878;15:297–300

Sewall H. The Role of the stethoscope in physical diagnosis. *Am J Med Sci* 1913;145:234–8

Sheldon PB, Doe J. The Development of the stethoscope. *Bull NY Acad Med* 1935;11: 609–26

Sibson F. The flexible stethoscope. *Lon Med Gazette* 1841;28:911–12

Singer JJ. A new simple stethoscope. *J Am Med Assoc* 1914;63:482

Skoda J. *Perkussion und Auskultation*, 4th edn. Aufl., Wien, Seidel LW, 1850

Skoda J. *A Treatise on Auscultation and Percussion*, translated by W. O. Markham. London: Highly and Sone, 1853

Smith AH. The use of the differential stethoscope in the study of cardiac murmurs. *Med Record* 1895;48:121

Smith DC. Austin Flint and auscultation in America. *J Hist Med All Sci* 1978;33:129–49

Smith ETA. A new form of stethoscope. *Br Med J* 1884;1:909–10

Snelling TG. Improvement of Cammann's stethoscope. *Med Record* 1870–71;5:44

Sommerbrodt J. Ueber das von Dr P. Niemeyer empfohlene massive Stethoscop (Horholz). *Berlin klin Wochensch* 1869;6:246–7

Souligoux L. Du Diagnostic Medical et Chirurgical par les moyens physicques. Paris: J. B. Baillière et Fils, 1868

Speir SF. Aids for the diagnosis and treatment of certain diseases. *Med Record* 1870–72;6:175

Spencer WH. On a new form of stethoscope in its relations to the theory and practice of auscultation. *Br Med J* 1874;1:409–11

Spencer WH. Binaural stethoscope, combining in the same instrument a stethoscope for ordinary use and a binaural differential stethoscope. *Br Med J* 1886;1:25

Sprague HB. A new combined stethoscope chestpiece. *J Am Med Assoc* June 19 1926;86:1909

Stephani J. Presentation d'un Stethoscope bilateral Biauriculaire. *Presse Medicale* Jan 21 1933;41: 133–4

Stephani J. Description of biauricular bilateral stethoscope. *Schweiz med Wochensch* Jan 21 1933;63:73

Stethoscope (The Revolving). *The Medical Annual*, London: 1915;756–7

Stofft H. Laennec et Kerkeradec, un amitié fecunde: application a l'obstetrique de l'auscultation. *Revue du la decouverte*, numero special 22 Aout 1981;152–69

Stokes W. Review From the West. *Lancet* 1825;9: 471–5

Stokes W. *An Introduction to the Use of Stethoscope with its Application to the Diagnosis in Diseases of the Thoracic Viscera*. Edinburgl: Maclachlan & Stewart, 1825

Stokes W. An introduction to the use of the stethoscope, with its application to the diagnosis in diseases of the thoracic viscera, including the pathology of these various affections. *Lancet* 1825–26;9:471–5

Stokes W. *A Treatise on the Diagnosis and Treatment of Diseases of the Chest*. Philadelphia: Barrington & Haswell, 1844

Stokes W. *The Diseases of the Heart and the Aorta*. Dublin: Hodges & Smith, 1854

Stokes W, Bell J. *Lectures on the Theory and Practice of Physic*. Philadelphia: Barrington & Haswell, 1842

Stroud W. On Mediate Auscultation. *Lond Med Gaz* 1841–1842; o.s. 29; n.s. 1:6–9

Strudwick E. Remarks on the stethoscope, in relation to phthistis pulmonalis. *J Med Phys Sci* 1824;8:33–52

Syers HW. The decay of auscultation and the use of the binaural stethoscope. *Lancet* 1902;1:369–70

Thilenius. Stethoskop Hygiene. *Deutsche med Wochensch* March 23 1928;54:477

Tobler W. Comparative physical tests of stethoscopes. *Schweiz med Wochensch* Sept 11 1926; 56:873–7

Tobler W. Comparative auscultatory tests of stethoscopes. *Schweiz med Wochensch* 1926; 56:973–5

Tobler W. Comparative physical tests of stethoscopes (Abstr.) *J Am Med Assoc* Nov 27 1926; 87:1870

Tobler W. Sound conductivity of rigid and flexible stethoscopes. *Schweiz med Wochensch* Oct 4 1930;60:933–41

Tomasinelli G. Stetoscopio lineari, una modificazione del comune stetoscopio de Laennec. *Riforma Med Napoli* 1918;34:165–8

Touroff ASW. Combined tape measure and stethoscope tube. *Am J Med Sci* 1932; n.s. 184: 213–5

Treis J. Eine Bandmanschette zum Membranstethoskop zur Blutdrckmessung nach Karotkow. *Deutche med Wochensch* 1922;48:1485–6

Turman CM. A vaginal stethoscope for use in locating a placenta in the lower uterine segment. *Am J Obstet Gynecol* June 1934;27:919–21

Valentine RK. An improved binaural stethoscope and improved soft rubber bell. *Med Record* 1895;47:30–1

Veale H. The medical officer's stethoscope. *Br Med J* Jan 17 1880;1:94

Voltolini R. Ein Besonderes Stethoskop. *Berlin klin Wochensch* 1875;12:205–7

Voltolini R. Nachtragliche Bemerkungen Zu Meinem Stethskop. *Berlin klin Wochensch* 1876;13:343–4

Wail VS. Appareils pourl' auscultation collective dans la clinique infantile. *Archives de Médecine des Enfants* 1935;38:33–6

Waldenburg L. Stethoskop, Hammer und Plessimeter in einem Stuck. *Berlin klin Wochensch* 1870;7:580–1

Wallgren A. Das Stethoskop als Massstab. Berlin: Beitrage Zur Klinik Der Tuberkulose, Verlag Von Julius Springer, 1922; 51

Walsh AS. New attachments for the phonendoscope. *Med Record* 1898;53:755

Walshe WH. *A Practical Treatise on the diseases of the Heart and Great Vessels including the Principles of Physical Diagnosis*. Philadelphia: Blanchard and Lea, 1862

Watson T. *Lectures on the Principles and Practice of Physic*. Philadelphia: Blanchard, 1852

Wechsler BB. Improved stethoscope for obstetricians. *J Am Med Assoc* Jan 16 1932;98:218

Weiss J. *John Weiss & Son: A Catalogue of Surgical instruments, Apparatus, Appliances, etc.* London: Rickerby, 1863

Welch WH. Memorial for Austin Flint at the New York County Medical Association. *Gaillard's Med Jrl* 1886;42:585–9

Wetherill HE. An Improved Form of Stethoscope. *Am J Med Sci* 1903;126:884–7

Whittaker JT. The history of auscultation. *Med Record* 1879;16:411–4

Whittaker. Disarticulating stethoscope. *Lancet* 1881;1:994

Wilcox RW. An improved stethoscope. *NY Med J* 1894;60:58–9

Wilks S. Abstract of evolution of the stethoscope. *Lancet* Nov 25 1882;2:882–3

Wilks S. Evolution of the stethoscope. *Popular Science Monthly* 1882–83;22:488–91

Wilks S, Bettany GT. *Biographical History of Guy's Hospital*. London: Ward, 1892;508

Williams CJB. On the construction and application of instruments used in auscultation. *Lond Med Gaz* Dec 16 1842;401–4

Williams CJB. Stethoscope. *Cyclopedia of Pract Med* 1845;4:237–9

Williams CJB. On the acoustic principles and construction of stethoscopes and ear trumpets. *Lancet* Nov 8 1873;2:664–6

Williams CJB. *Memoirs of Life and Work*. London: Smith, Elder & Co., 1884

Williams CT. A Lecture on Laennec and the evolution of the stethoscope. *Br Med J* 1907; 2:6–8

Willius FA, Keys TE. Cardiac Clinics; *A Collection of Classic Works on the Heart and Circulation with Comprehensive Biographic Accounts of the Authors*. St. Louis: Mosby, 1941;321–82

Wilson FN, Wishart SW. On the importance of the auscultatory signs of cardiac disease and the value of the electric stethoscope. *Ann Clin Med* (charts), July 1926;5:78–90

Wilson JC. A Handbook of Medical Diagnosis, 4th edn. Philadelphia and London: J. B. Lippincott, 1915:1473

Wintrich MA. *Handbuch der Speciellen Pathologie und Therapie: Krankheiten der Respirationsorgane* Erlangen: Ferdinand Enke, 1854

Witkowski G-J. *Histoire des Accouchments*. Paris: G. Steinheil, 1889

Wollaston WH. On the duration of muscular action. *Philos Trans R Soc Lon* 1810;2–5

Wood WB. Pulmonary tuberculosis in general practice. *Lancet* 1930;2:726–30

Woods EF. A new stethoscope. *J Am Med Assoc* 1906;47:1377

Young RA. The stethoscope: past and present. *Lancet* 1930;2:883–8

Young RA. The stethoscope: past and present. *Tr Med Soc* 1931;54:1–22

Appendix

The instruments illustrated here are from a collection which began about twenty years ago. In some instances very similar devices are included to show some of the modifications or options available. Commentary on historical significance and the evolution of the stethoscope is contained in the main body of the text. The purpose of this section is to allow the reader to see the wide variety of approaches that have been proposed for auscultation over the years and to bring a sense of reality to the words by showing real objects.

The organization of the section follows the general approach within the main text. Many of the stethoscopes are named after people because of minor changes in the head-piece or in the chest-piece. In some instances it is likely that the manufacturer chose to apply the name of some prominent physician to an instrument which he or she may have had little to do with designing. As noted in the commentary by Denison in the text, many manufacturers produced inferior versions of stethoscopes for the marketplace. In some catalogs the purchaser is offered a choice of a grade 1 or grade 2 instrument depending on how much he or she is willing to spend. For instance Sharp and Smith's Perfected Cammann's Stethoscope No. 1 cost $2.20 While No. 2 which was quite similar cost $1.85 (Sharp and Smith 1889).

Proper identification of the exact material of which a stethoscope is fabricated can be very difficult. The descriptions are a guide to the composition of the version illustrated. Many catalogs offer instruments in a broad choice of materials, especially the monaural stethoscopes. The Kny-Scheerer catalog of 1912 lists monaural stethoscopes made of cedar with or without ivory, hard rubber, aluminum with or without a celluloid ear-piece, and some which are simply described as metal. An article in the *Lancet* of 1826 states that walnut was the wood most frequently used at that time, with some cedar, ash or maple.

It should not be inferred that the inclusion of a stethoscope in the appendix means that it is of great historical significance. Some were, others are simply interesting in showing the wide variety that was produced. An incredible number of stethoscope designs were manufactured, most of no great consequence. Some idea of the popularity of a device can be gleaned from its listing in catalogs. Stethoscopes such as the Bazzi-Bianchi were very popular for a number of years after their introduction and are shown in almost every catalog of the period. Others simply cannot be found anywhere. The historic significance is best inferred from the discussion in the text rather than from the presence or absence of an illustration (which simply may mean I have not been able to obtain an example for my collection).

Another important point is the naming of the instruments. Some are unequivocal because they are unique. Others are so similar that it is extremely difficult to be sure which one is in hand. An example is the naming of monaural stethoscopes (which is more difficult since they differ less than binaural) by a German company. The *Kirchner and Wilhelm Diagnostic Instrument Catalogue* of about 1910 lists 150 varieties of monaural stethoscope. Among the names given are Winter, which resembles a Pinard (although Pinard's is listed as well), Kussmaul, Traube, which is a generally accepted name, Freerichs, Seitz, Leiter Muller and many other types named after

German physicians, reminiscent of the English calling the Cammann's a Leared. A Bazzi–Bianchi is called a micro–membrane stethoscope.

Finally there is the date. Patent dates are extremely valuable because they indicate the earliest time the device could have been manufactured. I have tried to assign dates which give a reasonable idea of when a particular stethoscope was likely to have been used and the period from which the example is derived. Many of the instruments may have been used significantly earlier than indicated and others later. I have grouped them in chronological order using the age I estimate for the example. Patent dates are given if noted on the instrument.

The catalog numbers shown refer to the numbering in the main collection which includes a broad range of medical instruments.

RIGID MONAURAL STETHOSCOPES

Figure A1

Catalog # 284

1830 Piorry stethoscope

(See page 19)

The instrument is shown with the extension piece attached. There is a 7" long oak stem which is 0.65" in diameter through most of its length but tapers to a 1.65" bell at the last 1.25" of its length. The end is fitted with a threaded ivory ring onto which a pleximeter of ivory 1.6"d screws. The 2" ear-piece can be screwed over it for convenient carrying. In addition there is a 5.25" wooden tube with ivory fittings at each end that are threaded to extend the length as shown in the illustration. See also Figure A4 for a later model and detail.

References: Laennec 1838; Piorry 1828; Piorry 1866

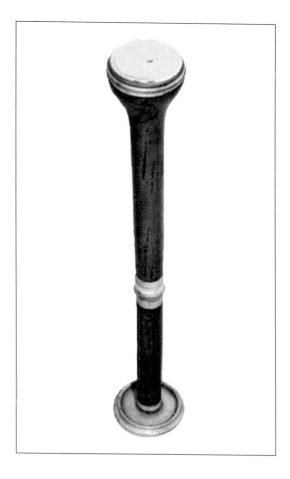

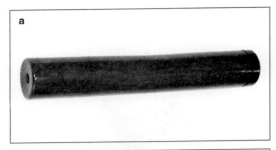

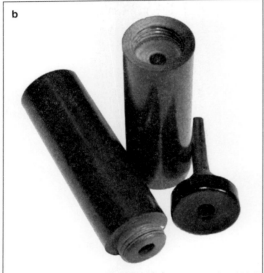

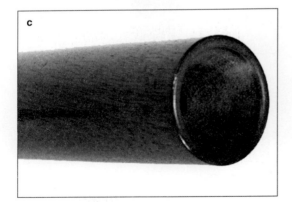

Figure A2
Catalog # 285
1830 Laennec's stethoscope
(See page 12)

This follows the design of the model published in 1819. It is 8.5″ long by 1.25″ and made of walnut. It is shorter than the original Laennec design and unscrews to form two 4″ long pieces. The bell end is formed by removing the cone-shaped insert which has a brass tube to hold it in place. The major change from original design is the shorter length. a: assembled, b: all parts separated, c: cone end without obturator for lung auscultation.
References: Davis 1981:98; Laennec 1837; Laennec 1838

Figure A3

Catalog # 544

1830 Modified Laennec stethoscope

(See page 28)

This version, which resembles the one that has been attributed to Haden is 5.8" long, 1"d, and made of walnut with an ivory ear-piece, 1.8"d, turned with rings. There is an ivory washer at 5". The remainder is an extension with a rounded end and with an insert that forms the usual hollowed out end of the Laennec. There is a brass tube to hold this piece on. Major modifications are the diameter that is slightly reduced, end is rounded and the stethoscope is basically one short piece instead of two. a: assembled, b: the obturator end, c: the obturator.

References: Laennec 1838; Laennec 1837; Lyons 1978:510

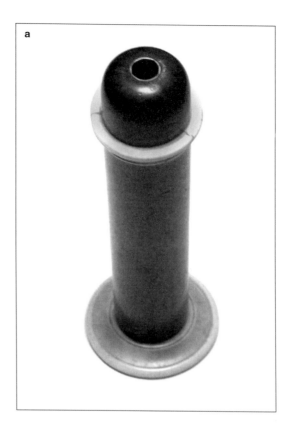

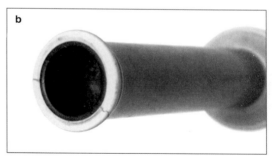

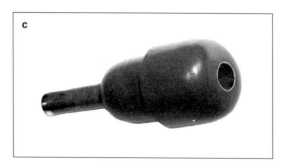

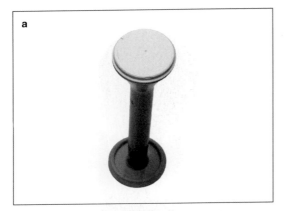

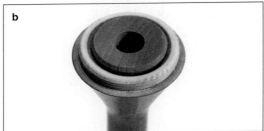

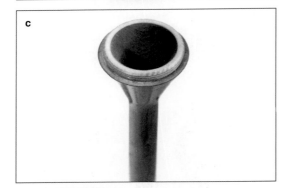

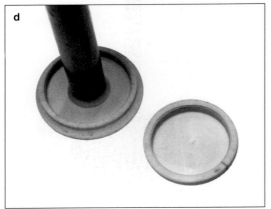

Figure A4

Catalog # 283

1835 Piorry stethoscope

(See page 20) (See also Figure A1)

The 6.25" long oak stem is 0.65" in diameter through most of its length but tapers to a 1.65" bell at the last 1.25" of its length. There is a hollow wooden plug which fits into the bell to reduce its caliber. The end is fitted with a threaded ivory ring onto which a pleximeter of ivory 1.6"d screws and the 2" earpiece can be screwed over it for convenient carrying.

a: with pleximeter on chest end, b: chest end with obturator, c: obturator removed, d: the pleximeter.

References: Laennec 1838; Piorry 1828; Piorry 1866

Figure A5

Catalog # 474

1835 stethoscope, early transitional from Laennec

(See page 32)

This very rare model is 5.75" long with the end in place. The end is a 1.5"d cone with a 3" brass rod which fits into the body of the stethoscope. It can be removed in the same manner shown in Figure A2. The ear-piece is 1.5"d with a 0.31"d hole throughout. It is made of cedar or other light wood. There is a line turned around the bell end for decoration. Stained light brown. The shape of this stethoscope resembles Billing's.

References: Laennec 1838; Laennec 1837; Wilbur 1987:21

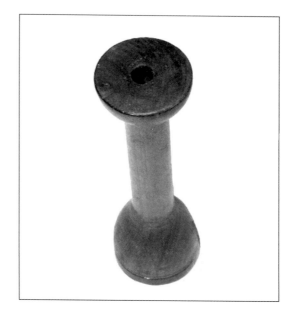

Figure A6

Catalog # 109

1850 Walsh's stethoscope

(See page 32)

A very commonly used design that is 7" long with a 2.5" ear-piece. It is made of fir with the ear-piece that unscrews of black natural plastic. It resembles Burrow's, or Fergusson's and in fact numerous others with only minor difference. It is distinctive for a somewhat greater length than usual.

References: Down 1889:412; Maw 1891; Tiemann 1879:81

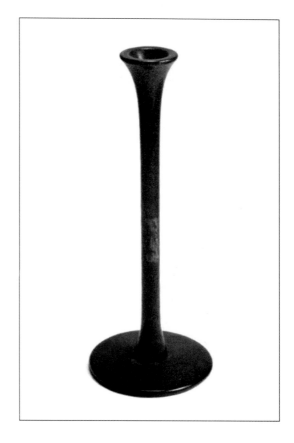

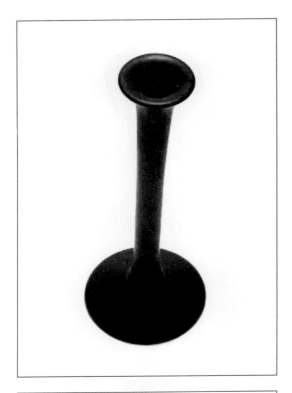

Figure A7

Catalog # 254

1860 simple stethoscope

(See page 32)

Another very common type that is 6.25" long with a 2.38" ear-piece and a 1.19" bell. It is a black simple monaural stethoscope. The ear-piece is a dark brown and may be made of a natural plastic or hard rubber, the shaft appears to be wood.

References: Sharp and Smith,1895:526

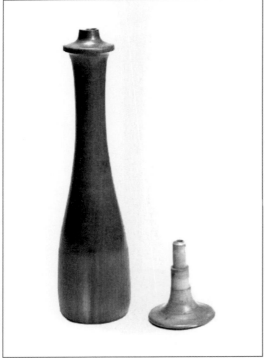

Figure A8

Catalog # 286

1860 cedar stethoscope

(See page 32)

This is a common model in early catalogs although it is rarely found today. It is clearly transitional in form and has the less popular ear-piece. It is 6.65" long with a broad taper to form a bell 1.5" in diameter. The ear-piece is of the plug type and is carved from the same piece of wood. The piece narrows to about 0.65" at its narrowest and is widest at the bell end. The ear-piece is 0.75" in diameter and 0.5" high There is a 1.5" wooden insert which is 2" long and fits into the bell to markedly reduce the diameter of the tube. The obturator is shown alongside the stethoscope in the figure. This is a very different form of obturater than originally described by Laennec.

References: Tiemann, George 1879:81; Wilbur 1987:23

Figure A9

Catalogue # 920

1865 Clark's stethoscope

(See page 32)

This is a very heavy and long instrument which is 9.5"
long with 2.38" ear-piece. The stem is 0.5" at the connection to the ear-piece and tapers gradually to a 2.13"
opening at the chest end. Made of a heavy wood, perhaps ash, with a dark stain. There are some delicate decorative turnings at each end. It is unusual for its length,
weight and the amount of decoration.

References: Maw and Thompson 1891:191

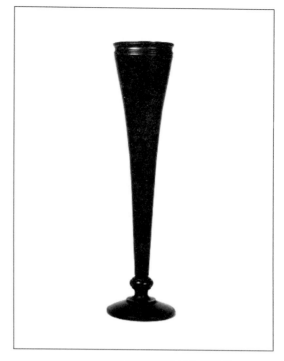

Figure A10

Catalog # 229

1880 Cedar stethoscope

(See page 32)

The same form as A8 but a more expensive design with
an ivory ear-piece. It is 6.25" long with broad taper to
form a bell 1.5" in diameter. The ear-piece is of the plug
type and is made of ivory. The piece narrows to about
0.5" at its narrowest and is widest at the bell end, the ear-
piece is 0.75" in diameter and 0.5" high.

References: Tiemann, George 1879:81; Wilbur 1987:23

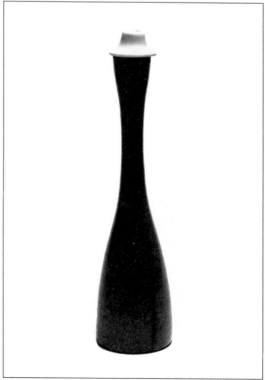

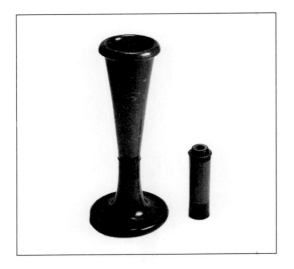

Figure A11

Catalog # 294

1860 three-piece monaural stethoscope

(See page 32)

Very unusual stethoscope which can be made into two lengths from the three-piece stem which screws together. It is 7.25" long when the center piece is attached, with a 2.25"d ear-piece that has a 0.5" vulcanite rim. The chest-piece is 1.5"d. The wood is ash, painted black at each of the two joints. The small joining piece is 2" long and can be clearly seen in the figure. When the center piece is not used as shown in the figure it resembles an obstetric stethoscope in form.

References: Jetter and Scheerer 1910:129

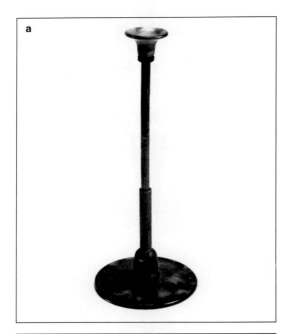

a

Figure A12

Catalog # 126

1880 folding stethoscope

(See page 32)

Unusual tortoiseshell monaural stethoscope. The 2.5"d ear-piece and the 0.75"d chest-piece are made of tor-toiseshell. The two are connected by a brass rod, the whole 6.25" in length. Unusual is the spring mechanism where if the ear and chest ends are pulled apart, the brass rod unlocks from the ear-piece and it can be folded down through a slot for carrying in the pocket. a: extended for use, b: folded for carrying.

References: Jetter and Scheerer 1910:129

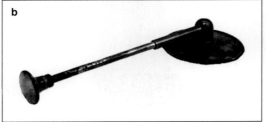

b

Figure A13

Catalog # 173

1880 folding stethoscope

(See page 32)

Another folding stethoscope that is 7" long and made of nickel plated brass. The ear-piece has a connector to the tube with a notch which permits it to be folded flat. It appears to be a folding version of Quain's.

References: Jetter and Scheerer 1910:129

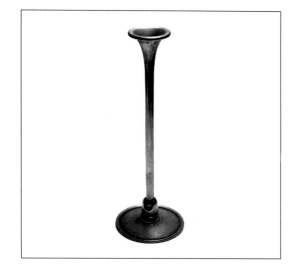

Figure A14

Catalog # 140

1880 Quains' stethoscope

(See page 32)

This was one of the more popular metal models. It is 7" long, made of brass, and divides in half by unscrewing. Then the top half (chest-piece) can be placed over the bottom half (ear-piece) and screwed in place for carrying. a: ready for use, b: for carrying.

References: Jetter and Scheerer 1910:129

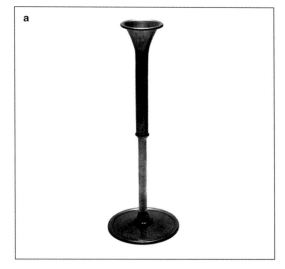

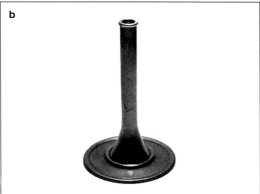

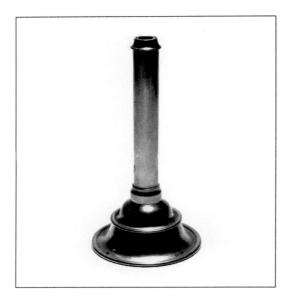

Figure A15

Catalog # 292

1880 Traube's stethoscope

Manufacturer: Kny-Scheerer, New York

(See page 33)

Another popular metal version is 6.63" long with 1.88" ear-piece and 1.19" chest-piece. The wide tube is 0.31" and the narrow tube is 0.25". The chest-piece can be inserted over the ear-piece for convenient carrying. It is made of white metal. Same concept as Quain's shown above. It is shown ready for transport.

References: Jetter and Scheerer 1910:127; Kny-Scheerer 1912:1024

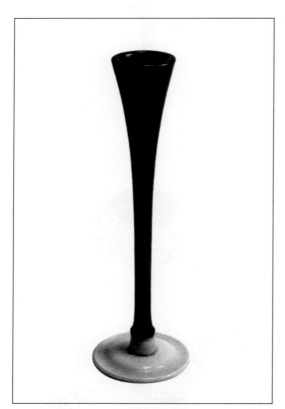

Figure A16

Catalog # 233

1880 cedar ivory mounted stethoscope

(See page 32)

This elegant model has a 6.75" cedar tube which tapers from about 0.5" to 1.2" at end to form a bell with a smooth taper. The ear-piece is ivory and is 2" in diameter, it screws onto a 0.5" ivory end on the wooden stem.

References: Hernstein 1881:114; Tiemann, George 1889:5

Figure A17

Catalog # 047

1880 Barclay's stethoscope

(See page 33)

Made of cedar 6.5" in height, stained brown, with an ear-piece 2" and a bell 1". This is of the simplest form.

References: Tiemann, George 1889:5

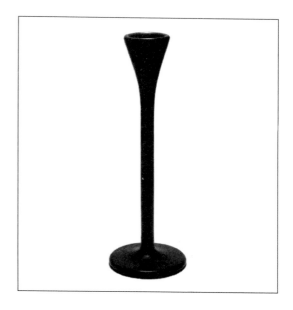

Figure A18

Catalog # 071

1890 Robert's stethoscope

(See page 32)

This portable stethoscope is made of black gutta-percha. It is composed of two pieces; the ear-piece has a hole to contain the tube for convenient carrying. It is 6.25" long. The Arnold catalog refers to a similar one as Roberts; in the Maw catalog it is listed as Maw's.

a: assembled, b: ready for carrying

References: Arnold 1904:519; Maw and Thompson 1891:191

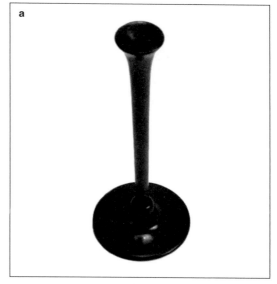

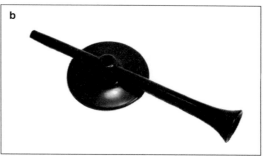

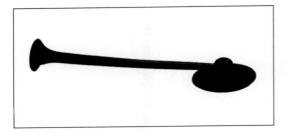

Figure A19
Catalog # 220
1890 Lichtheim's stethoscope
(See page 32)

A good example of national differences in naming stetho-scopes. This is 6.5" with a 2" ear-piece. The stem can be removed and inserted in the base through two holes. It is made of a composition material, apparently a thermo-plastic or hard rubber. It differs from Robert's in that the stem only fits into the hole at the end.
References: Arnold 1904:519; Jetter and Scheerer 1910:129; Maw and Thompson 1891:191

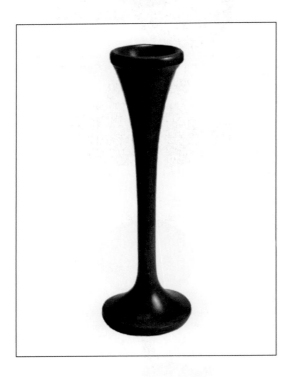

Figure A20
Catalog # 298
1890 Hughes' stethoscope
(See page 32)

This is 7" long with a 1.75" bell and a 2.25" ear-piece. It is made of cedar stained brown. The ear-piece is cupped as is the bell, with each tapering into the stem which is 0.38"d at its narrowest.
References: Arnold 1904:519; Down 1889:414; Jetter and Scheerer 1910:128

Figure A21

Catalog # 297

1890 Portable stethoscope

(See page 32)

Another portable model, this is 7" long with a 2.3" resin or hard rubber ear-piece which has a rectangular mount for the tube with two holes. The nickel-plated tube unscrews into two pieces that can be fitted into the base for carrying. The bell is 0.88"d and the same composition as the ear-piece. The tube is 0.25"d.

a: assembled, b: for carrying, c: the base.

References: Jetter and Scheerer 1910:131; Kny-Scheerer 1912:1024

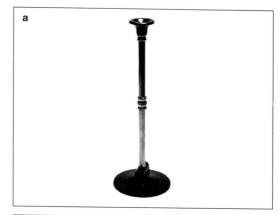

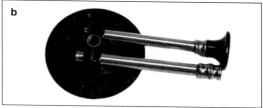

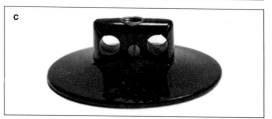

Figure A22

Catalog # 296

1890 English pattern stethoscope

(See page 32)

Several versions had this name, this one has a 6.75" nickel plated stem with letters EBS etched near the ear-piece which is made of hard rubber and is 2.44"d. The bell is 1.16" with a 0.16" center hole; The Arnold catalogue refers to a very similar design as Burrow's (see A6).

References: Arnold 1904:519; Jetter and Scheerer, 1910:128

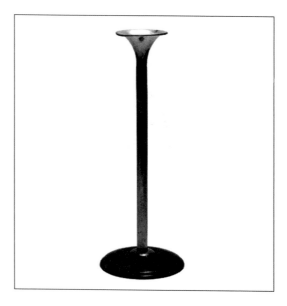

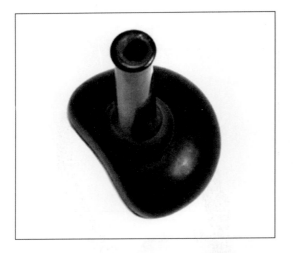

Figure A23
Catalog # 295
1900 stethoscope
(See page 32)

An unusually shaped stethoscope made of black hard rubber. It is 7.5" long with an ear-piece shaped crudely like an ear 2 x 2.75". The chest-piece is 1" with a 0.5"d and 0.38" perforation. Tube unscrews at middle to fit over ear-piece tube and make it suitable to carry in pocket. Shown closed with the chest end resting on the ear-piece and the connection viewed on end.
References: Jetter and Scheerer 1910:131

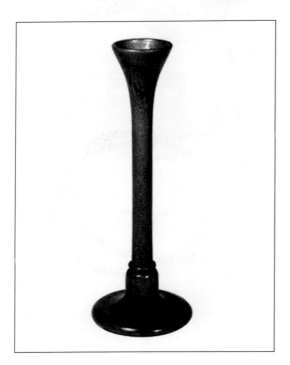

Figure A24
Catalog # 919
1920 monaural stethoscope
(See page 32)

A late monaural stethoscope that is 7" long with 2.5"d ear-piece and 1.38"d chest end The stem is 0.5" in diameter. It is made of pine with light tan stain. This was given out by a French pharmaceutical firm in 1920 as a gift to practicing physicians. It is noteworthy because of the late date at which the monaural version was still being used in spite of marked advances in binaural design.

FLEXIBLE MONAURAL STETHOSCOPES

Figure A25

Catalog # 430

1870 Golding Bird's stethoscope

(See page 35)

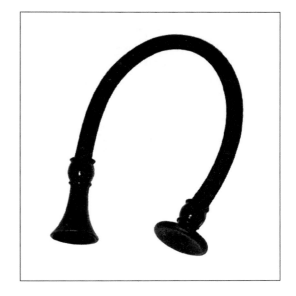

This nicely turned example is made of a 21" rubberized woven cloth tube with a wooden ear-piece at one end 2.25"d and a bell of wood at the other 3.5" x 1.88"d with black finish. The wood was lacquered but it is nearly worn off. The woven tube is 5/8" in diameter. This is a typical example of the popular flexible monaural stethoscopes.

References: Arnold 1904:521; Down 1900:872–873; Down 1889:412

Figure A26

Catalog # 428

1905 flexible monaural stethoscope

(See page 36)

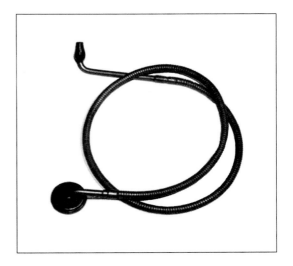

Another approach to the flexible monaural has a 36" flexible metal tube and a 1.25" diaphragm with a Bakelite membrane and a right angle connection (Bowles type) to the 5/16" metal tube. The other end is an ear-piece of gutta-percha which is 1/2"d and 0.75"l. This type of earpiece was used on the Stroud version of the flexible monaural. The entire tube probably was covered originally with cloth but is worn down to the bare brass.

References: Arnold 1904:521

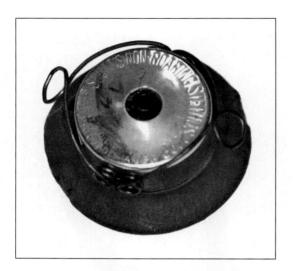

Figure A27

Catalog # 869

1901 Scott's non-roaring stethoscope

Manufacturer: Scott, Adelia, USA

(See page 38)

The head only is shown. It is 2"d x 0.75" with a rubber rim and bell-like opening. There is a metal spring on the sides and the top is embossed as shown above. There is an outlet for the connector to the ear-piece. A glass bell of smaller diameter to localize sound slips under the rubber on the chest surface. The spring is to facilitate connection to a belt to hold the stethoscope in place. The tubing to connect to the ear is missing, but it was designed to be used with a metal ear tube in one ear and a rubber earplug in the other. They were connected by an elastic cord so that the earplug would shut out sound from the ear which was not being used.

(US Patent # 676,999).

BINAURAL STETHOSCOPES WITH RIGID TUBES

Figure A28

Catalog # 310

1860 Cammann's stethoscope and pleximeter

Manufacturer: Codman and Shurtleff, Boston

(See Page 45)

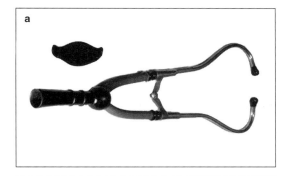
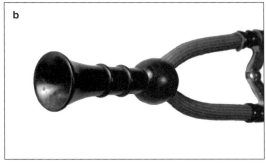

This early binaural is contained in a 9.63" x 3.25" x 2" brown wooden box with sliding lid. The stethoscope has a 4" x 0.88"d ebony bell. The last 2" screws off and can be replaced with a 1.38" x 1.38" flared bell The tubing is woven cloth over gum elastic. The 2.25" x 1.25" ebony pleximeter is signed Codman and Shurtleff. There is also a 1" x 1.88" bell which has a threaded tip with remnants of rubber — it may be Ware's modification. The rubber band which maintained the tension on the ear-pieces is missing. a: the stethoscope with the pleximeter, b: the larger bell chest-piece.

References: Hernstein 1881:114; Sharp and Smith 1889:524; Tiemann, George 1879:82

Figure A29

Catalog # 212

1880 Cammann's stethoscope

Manufacturer: Tiemann, New York

(See page 45)

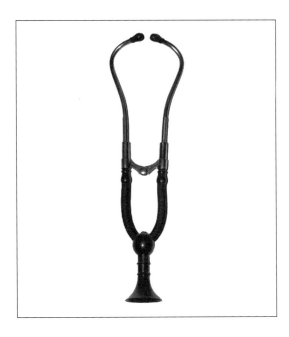

A 15" long binaural with woven tubes connecting 4" ebony chest-piece to the head-piece. Rubber band to maintain tension on ear-piece missing. Ear-pieces are ebony. The dating on this and A28 are approximations. The wooden box that A28 was contained in suggests an older date. Note that the head-pieces were the first step toward the development of the modern form that resulted mainly from the replacement of the joint with a spring.

References: Davis 1981:102; Tiemann, George 1879:82; Tiemann 1889:6

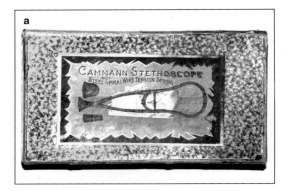

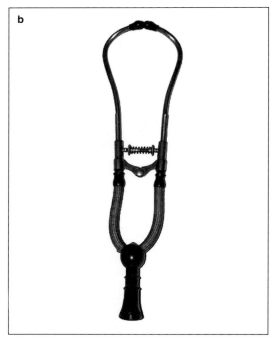

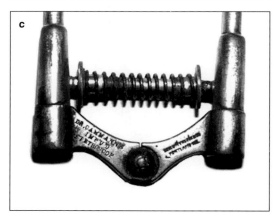

Figure A30

Catalog # 311

1880 Cammann's stethoscope with steel spiral wire tension spring

Manufacturer: Schlottenbeck and Co., Portland, Maine

(See page 45)

A very pretty 8" x 4.5" x 1.5" box with a picture of the stethoscope and label as above. It contains a stethoscope of the type pictured. The stethoscope has a 3" long x 1.63" ebony bell, woven tubing, ivory ear-pieces and a spring to adjust the ear-piece tension instead of a rubber band. The earliest version of Cammann's also had a spring but it was a simple loop and there was a rubber band as well. It is stamped "Dr Cammann's improved stethoscope". a: the closed box, b: the stethoscope, c: the spring mechanism.

References: Hernstein 1881:114; Reynders, John 1884: 231; Sharp and Smith 1889:524

Figure A31

Catalog # 426

1880 Cammann's spring improved stethoscope

Manufacturer: Tiemann, New York

(See page 45)

Almost identical to A30 this is a 15" long binaural with woven tubes connecting a 4" ebony chest-piece. Tension on head-piece is maintained by a spring device. Ear-pieces are also ebony. The hinge is marked Dr Cammann's Stethoscope, Tiemann & Co.

References: Davis 1981:102; Tiemann, George 1879:82; Tiemann, George 1889:6

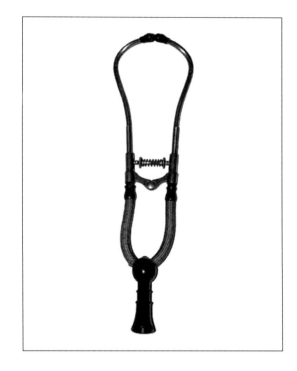

Figure A32

Catalog # 007

1890 Davis (modified Cammann's) stethoscope

(See page 53)

This is 14" long with woven rubberized tubes and a bell connected to a metal piece which in turn connects to the woven tubes. The bell is of ebony. It differs from Cammann because the ear-pieces are connected by a flat spring instead of a hinged joint and there is a metal connector for the bell. Snofton's also is quite similar. The head-piece has now more or less achieved the modern form.

References: Truax, Greene 1893:968

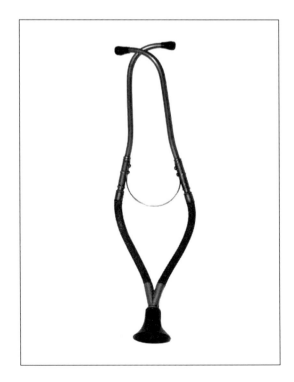

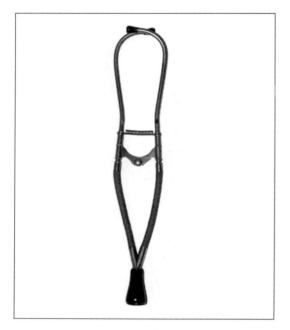

Figure A33

Catalog # 427

1890 Lynch's stethoscope

(See page 53)

A 15" long binaural with woven rubberized tubes connecting a 4" ebony chest-piece to the head-piece. Tension on the head-piece is maintained by a simple spiral spring. The ear-pieces are also ebony. The bell is narrow, (2" x 1") and is connected to the woven tubes by 1" metal tubing. It combines features of Cammann's (A31) and of Davis' (A32).

References: Davis 1981:102; Tiemann, George 1879:82

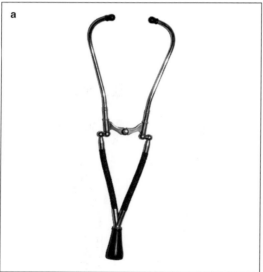

Figure A34

Catalog # 347

1890 Lynch's folding stethoscope

(See page 53)

This is another hybrid with features of Cammann and of the Lynch in A33. It is a 14.75" long binaural stethoscope with woven rubberized tubing connecting the head-piece to a 2" x 1" composition bell. The tubing connects at a hinge which allows the stethoscope to be folded in half. The rubber band to maintain pressure on the ear-pieces is missing as would be expected after this amount of time. a: open, b: folded.

References: Truax, Greene 1893:968

Figure A35

Catalog # 394

1895 Dennison's stethoscope

(See page 51)

A unique design which is 14" long with the intrinsic small pediatric bell that forms part of the connector to the tubing. There are also two interchangeable bells, 3"d and 1.63"d. There is a hard rubber joint for the two tubes and the bell and woven tubing which connects the head-piece. The head-piece is also hard rubber and there is an adjustable spring with a screw tension device. The spring mechanism was introduced by Knight. The special characteristics of this form are the tapering tubes providing a gradual reduction in caliber to the ear-pieces, the very smooth hard rubber and the design of the tubing which is discussed in the text.

References: Sharp and Smith 1889:527; Sharp and Smith 1895:527

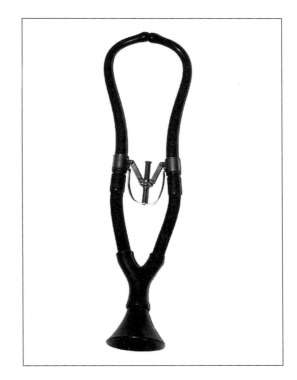

Figure A36

Catalog # 395

1895 Binaural stethoscope

Manufacturer: Down Bros, London

(See page 62)

A brass head-piece that has probably lost its nickel plating, with screw-on ivory ear-pieces. The connectors to the head-piece and the bell are bulbous; the bell is brass also with a screw-on hard rubber end to apply to the chest and is marked Down. The hard rubber end unscrews to leave a smaller bell which is intended for use with children. There were probably a variety of screw-on bells which were offered.

References: Down 1889:417; Down 1900:880; Down 1906:1142

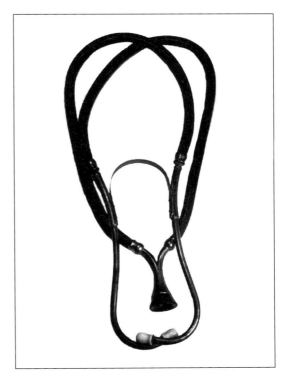

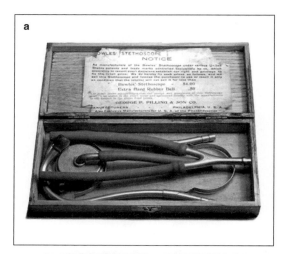

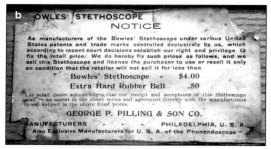

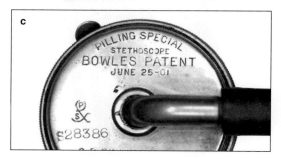

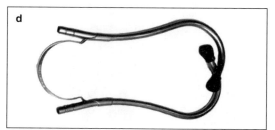

Figure A37

Catalog # 301

1901 Bowles stethoscope

Manufacturer: GP Pilling and Son Philadelphia, Pa

(See page 54)

A 7.5" x 3.38" x 1.25" oak box contains the directions and the price in the label on the top lid plus a Pilling special Bowles stethoscope patent date 6/25/01 in the box itself. The serial number is S28386. There is a protective metal plate over the hard rubber diaphragm which is 1.75"d It reads "this cover to be taken off before using stethoscope". Standard head-piece. This is the beginning of the modern binaural stethoscope. Note the option on the label to purchase a bell as well, recognizing the need for both forms for proper auscultation. a: in the box, b: the label, c: the patent information, d: the head-piece. References: Lentz, Charles 1914:302; Mueller 1908:14; Pilling 1932

Figure A38

Catalog # 855

1901 Bowles stethoscope

Manufacturer: GP Pilling and Son, Philadelphia, Pa

(See page 54)

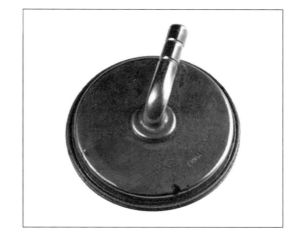

Another Pilling special Bowles stethoscope patent date 6/25/01. The hard rubber diaphragm is 2"d and there is a single connector to the rubber tubing. Standard head-piece. As noted in the text the Bowles chest-piece came in a variety of sizes.

References: Lentz 1914:302; Mueller 1908:14; Pilling 1932

Figure A39

Catalog # 856

1901 Bowles stethoscope

Manufacturer: GP Pilling and Son, Philadelphia, Pa

(See page 54)

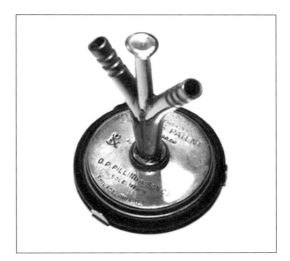

A different version of the Bowles stethoscope, patent date 6/25/01. There is a protective metal plate over the hard rubber diaphragm which is 1.75"d. It reads "this cover to be taken off before using stethoscope". Standard head-piece. This model has a metal connector at right angles to the head which divides in two and which has an arm in the middle for the examiner to hold the head in place.

References: Lentz 1914:302; Mueller 1908:14; Pilling 1932

Figure A40

Catalog # 857

1901 Bowles stethoscope

Manufacturer: GP Pilling and Son, Philadelphia, Pa

(See page 54)

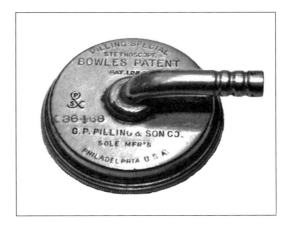

There is a protective metal plate similar to the example above in A39 on this head-piece. The hard rubber diaphragm is 1.75"d. There is a 1.13" raised circular portion to the head around the connector which is a single arm.

References: Lentz 1914:302; Mueller 1908:14; Pilling 1932

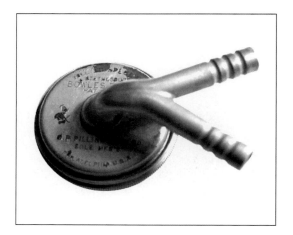

Figure A41

Catalog # 878

1901 stethoscope, Bowles

Manufacturer: GP Pilling and Son, Philadelphia, Pa

(See page 54)

Still another version of the Pilling special Bowles stethoscope. The hard rubber diaphragm is 1.25"d. A single connector leads to a V to connect to rubber tubing.

References: Pilling 1932; Mueller 1908:14; Lentz 1914:302

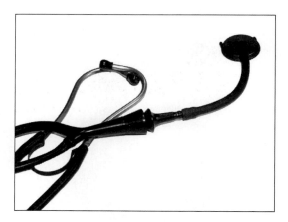

Figure A42

Catalog # 818

1905 Bowles stethoscope with Albion Ford chest-piece

(See page 54)

This instrument demonstrates the awareness of the need for a diaphragm and a bell for different sounds, but a crude solution to the problem. A 3" x 1" bell connects with rubber tubing to a standard binaural metal head-piece with ebony ear-pieces. The bell is made of hardened rubber with metal tubes to connect to the rubber tubing. In addition to the basic instrument there are two additional hard rubber bells which can be screwed into the end, one for pediatric use and the other with a smaller central hole. The main bell is for use with the diaphragm adapter, A43. The stethoscope is shown with the adapter in place.

References: Pilling 1932:152

Figure A43

Catalog # 815

1905 Bowles stethoscope (converts a bell to a diaphragm)

Manufacturer: GP Pilling and Son Philadelphia, Pa

(See page 54)

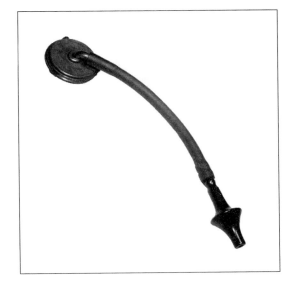

The stethoscope adapter shown in use in A42 consists of a Bowles patent Pilling special chest-piece which has a 1.5″ circular diaphragm and a metal protective plate. The tube bends immediately on exiting the detector and attaches to a rubber tube at the end of which is an ebony 3″ adapter that tapers to enter the rubber tube and again to the end piece which can plug into a bell. The whole unit is 9″ long. This is occasionally mistaken for a flexible monaural.

References: Pilling 1932:158,153

Figure A44

Catalog # 867

1905 Whitelaw stethoscope head

Manufacturer: Whitelaw

(See page 62)

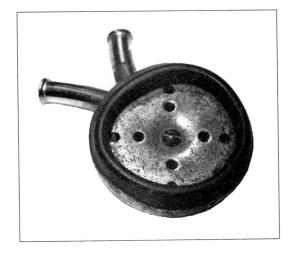

An interesting 1.5″ circular head, the rim of which is circled by a rubber ring. The unit has a metal chest-piece which is perforated with about 8 holes. The arms exit from the top and are slightly curved. There is a pointer on the top of the head which can be rotated to increase or decrease the number of holes open to the chest-piece thereby modifying the sound intensity.

Figure A45

Catalog # 871

1905 Stethoscope head

(See page 62)

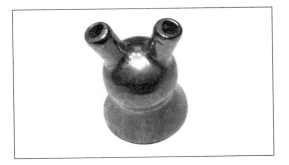

A 1.5″ x 1.5″ bell shaped like Snofton, but it is a single piece of metal with no screw-on end.

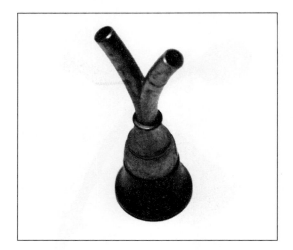

Figure A46

Catalog # 866

1910 Snofton stethoscope

(See page 62)

Typical 1.75" x 1" cone-shaped bell, the portion that applies to the chest is made of hard rubber and is inter-changeable with screw-threaded ends. The cone termi-nates in two arms that serve as attachments for the rubber tubing to the head-piece. Nickel plated body.

References: Pilling 1932

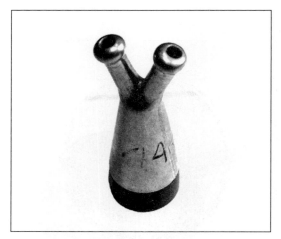

Figure A47

Catalog # 879

1910 stethoscope head

(See page 62)

A 1.75" x 1" cone-shaped bell; the portion that applies to the chest is made of hard rubber and is interchangeable with screw-threaded ends. The cone terminates in two arms which serve as attachments for the rubber tubing to the ear-piece. The body is made of a light metal, perhaps aluminum. Differs from other models in that the end is truly a bell rather than bell shaped with a central hole.

References: Jetter and Scheerer 1910:135; Pilling 1932

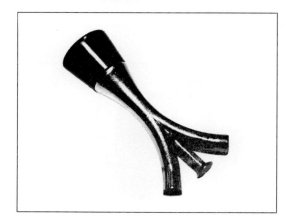

Figure A48

Catalog # 821

1920 Down stethoscope with finger rest

(See page 62)

A nickel-plated stethoscope bell with thermoplastic end. There are tubes to connect to two rubber tubes and a rod between them with a round end to use for pressure from the finger.

References: Pilling 1932:158

Figure A49

Catalog # 822

1920 Ford stethoscope

(See page 62)

The 3.75″ long stethoscope bell with hard rubber end is similar in shape to the Ford design. There are tubes to connect two rubber tubes.

References: Pilling 1932:158

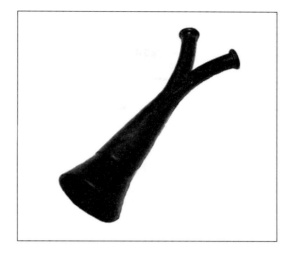

Figure A50

Catalog # 873

1912 Fosgate stethoscope

(See page 62)

A diaphragm-type head with each metal connector for the tubing protruding from top of the head separately. Similar to Figure A64 except that there is a metal fitting with a smaller bell over the diaphragm. The bell part is 1″d and is elevated 0.5″ in the center. A localizing button could be attached to the elevated portion, otherwise it was used as shown with a Bakelite diaphragm behind the bell portion. US Patent # 1,015,163

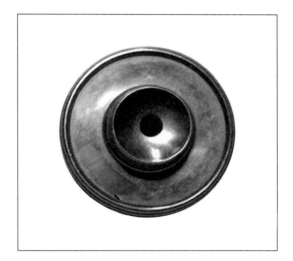

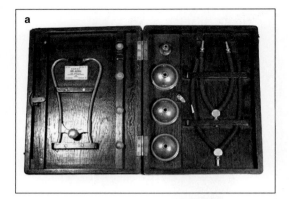

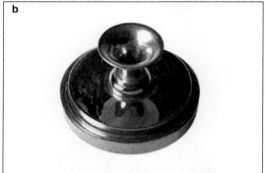

Figure A51

Catalog # 304

1920 Capac, binaural stethoscope

Manufacturer: Capac Co. Ltd., London

(See page 58)

A 13" x 9.5" x 2.5" brown stained oak box contains the head-piece that is adjusted with a central screw, four chest-pieces and parts of two sets of tubing. A 6" x 12" cover contains holders for the tubing and lifts out of the empty compartment. Three heavy bell-shaped diaphragm chest-pieces 2.5" by 1.25". There is one bell 1" x 1" which screws into the center of one of the three to provide a sound localizer. Two of the chest-pieces have a narrow hole which may fit a missing piece. a: the open box, b: with the bell extension screwed in place. Note resemblance to Fosgate (A50).

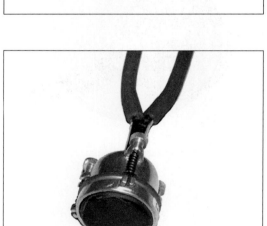

Figure A52

Catalog # 303

1920 Dr Pollards' stethoscope

(See page 77)

A very interesting aluminum- or nickel-plated stethoscope. The bell is a 1.5" x 1.5" cylinder which is covered by a leather membrane. There are three screws attached to a 0.25" rim that holds the membrane and can adjust the tension. The top leads to a 1.5" y tube which connects to two rubber tubes and a standard head-piece. US Patent # 1,329,430

Figure A53

Catalog # 446

1920 phonophore stethoscope

Manufacturer: Maw, London

(See page 62)

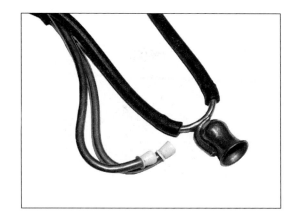

A 1"d x 1.75" bell shaped chest-piece with cone inset and U-shaped metal tube connected to C-shaped tube attached to bell. Rubber tubing connects to U and then to the usual metal binaural head-pieces with ivory ear plugs. The head-pieces can be folded like Sheppard's model and the tubing is 18" long and is the heavy 0.5" diameter black rubber of the period.

References: Maw 1913:359; Maw 1925:344

Figure A54

Catalog # 877

1924 Fleischer stethoscope

Manufacturer: Becton Dickenson and Co., Rutherford, NJ

(See page 56)

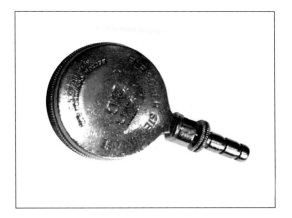

This 1.5" Bakelite diaphragm type head has a Luer Loc type connector to a tube which is shown connected without the rubber tubing. Like most of the stethoscope heads this was available in many sizes, a 2" one is also in the collection. The metal head is heavier than the Bowles chest-piece and the hole for transmission of the sound is on a rim rather that on the top.

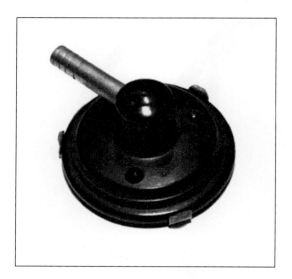

Figure A55
Catalog # 817
1930 Klagges' stethoscope
Manufacturer: CH Klagges
(See page 76)

This 1.75" circular chest-piece is made of hard rubber or Bakelite with a metal plate, both with C. H. Klagges inscribed on it. There is a metal tube that attaches at a right angle to the protruberance on the top of the diaphragm head.
References: Pilling 1932:152

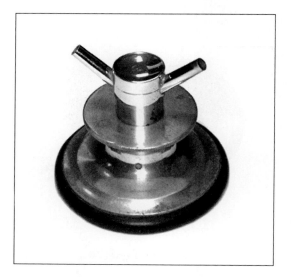

Figure A56
Catalog # 238
1930 Prof J. Minot endophone stethoscope
Manufacturer: Spengler Co., Paris
(See page 76)

This is a 2.75" bell that is 2.5" high. The piece applied to the chest is rimmed with rubber and there is a 0.75" circular piece which can be depressed resulting in the extrusion of a smaller 1" adapter into the lumen that can be used to localize the sound. The whole is contained in a box which is paper-covered with a standard set of tubing and head-piece.

BINAURAL STETHOSCOPES
WITH FLEXIBLE TUBES

Most of the manufacturers offered a choice of flexible tubing or rigid head-pieces to physicians when purchasing stethoscope heads. Many of the models below were used either way according to the preference of the physician.

Figure A57

Catalog # 429

1890 Sharp and Smiths' perfected Cammann (Korndoffer's) stethoscope

(See page 50)

This 16.5" long stethoscope has three interchangeable bells. There is a hard rubber joint for the two tubes and the bell and rubberized woven tubing which connects the head-piece. The ear-piece is also hard rubber. The tubing is 13" long and the two tubes are connected by a spring wire rather than by metal brackets. This appears in several versions in various catalogs. This model adheres most closely to Cammann's style except for the flexible tube ear-pieces. It is cited in the Otis Clapp catalogue as Korndoffer's stethoscope. a: the stethoscope, b: the extra chest-pieces. References: Clapp 1889:111; Sharp and Smith 1895:527; Sharp and Smith 1889:525

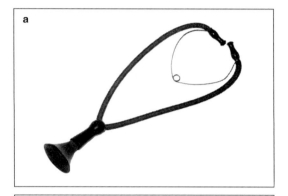

a

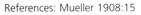

b

Figure A58

Catalog # 148

1890 Amplifone stethoscope

(See page 58)

A very interesting 2.5" circular diaphragm made of white metal and hard rubber. A small probe extends from the center of the piece and two side arms are also present to facilitate holding it in place. It connects to soft rubber tubing as shown. This resembles the Bazzi-Bianchi stethoscope in some respects. The patent date on the back reads Mar 29 1887. However I have been unable to locate the actual patent. The probe is detachable; it is for localizing internal sounds. Without the probe the device resembles A50 and A64.

References: Mueller 1908:15

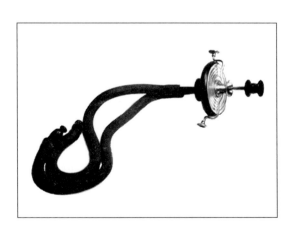

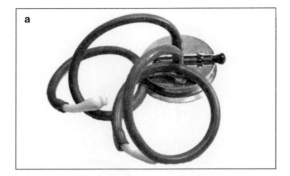

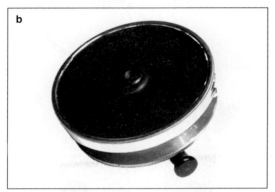

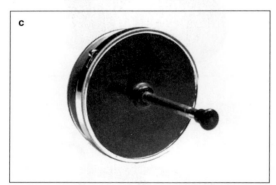

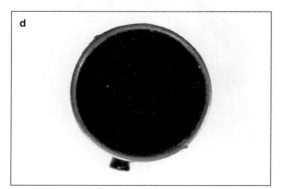

Figure A59
Catalog # 184
1895 stethoscope, Bazzi-Bianchi
Manufacturer: Gimber, London
(See page 59)

A very important and commonly encountered 2.4" x 0.75" diaphragm-type stethoscope. This may have been the first stethoscope with the modern diaphragm design. The head has a second diaphragm attachment with a detachable 2" long rod ending in a hard rubber tip that can be used to localize sound by percussion. The tubes are rubber and connect to bone or ivory ear-pieces. a: with ear tubes, b: the chest side with the place to attach the sound localizer, c: the localizer in place, d: the regular diaphragm which is exposed by removing the sound localizer diaphragm.
References: Arnold 1904:514; Pilling 1932:154; Wulfing-Luer 1904:19

Figure A60

Catalog # 920

1895 stethoscope, Bazzi-Bianchi

(See page 59)

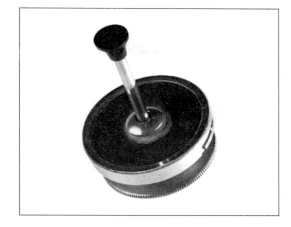

This example is noteworthy for its small size. It has a 1.63" diaphragm. It is the same as A59 but a very small version for use in children The diaphragm has a second attachment with a 1.75" long rod ending in a hard rubber tip that can be used to localize sound. The tubes (which are not shown) are rubber replacements and connect to ebony ear-pieces.

Figure A61

Catalog # 853'

1900 Oertel's stethoscope

Manufacturer: Waarenhaus Wein

(See page 62)

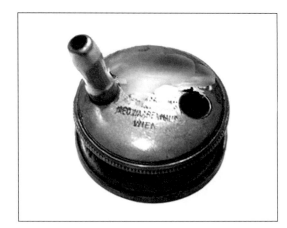

There is a 1" diaphragm head with an unusual 0.75" high notched shape. The rubber tubing is attached to two rods from the top, one rod is shown and the tubing missing. It differs from Figure A62 in that the diaphragm is white and the top curved instead of flat. Oertel was better known for his differential stethoscope.

References: Howarth-Ballard 1905:1026

Figure A62

Catalog # 852

1900 Oertel's stethoscope

(See page 62)

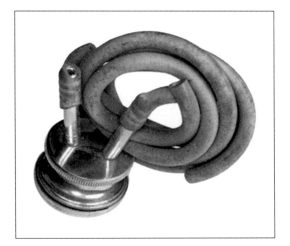

Another version of Oertel's with a 1" diaphragm head with 0.75" high notched shape. The notch was probably used to wrap the tubing when not in use, like the Bazzi-Bianchi. The diaphragm has a protective cover of metal. The rubber tubing is attached to two rods from the top. Some rubber remains. Very similar to the previous version (A61).

References: Howarth-Ballard 1905:1026

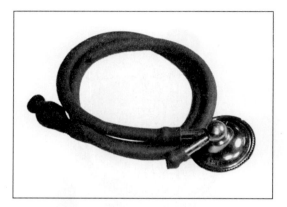

Figure A63

Catalog # 863

1900 Pulaski stethoscope

(See page 62)

A 1" diaphragm with metal cover. There are V-shaped connectors to the tubing. One ear-piece remains. The connectors fit into a dome on the back of the head. The back and the cover are both embossed.

a

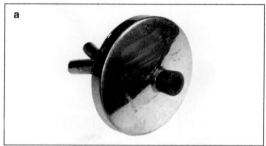

Figure A64

Catalog # 874

1900 Stethoscope

Manufacturer: Sharp and Smith

(See page 62)

This has a 2.25" diaphragm with V connector arising from the top. There is a metal plate which can be removed or used to cover the thermoplastic diaphragm and has a 0.5" x 0.5" circular elevation to localize sounds. Resembles Teske's head but the concept of a connector to localize sound was very commonly used in many designs. See Figure A50. The Bazzi-Bianchi design was the most popular. a: localizer attached, b: the regular diaphragm.

References: The Surgical Manufacturing Co. 1920:400

b

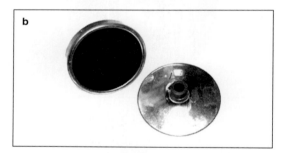

Figure A65

Catalog # 851

1901 Dr Kehler's improved stethoscope

Manufacturer: Becton Dickinson and Co, Rutherford, NJ

(See page 62)

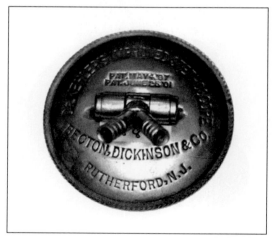

A 2" diaphragm head with engraving on the metal part as above plus patent dates of May 4 1897 and June 25 1901. It is unique in that the V-shaped connectors to the rubber tubing are attached to the head with a swivel device so that the angle at which they are held can vary as needed.

References: Hartz 1922:13

Figure A66

Catalog # 859

1901 Pilling Kehler's stethoscope

Manufacturer: Pilling, Philadelphia

(See page 62)

A 2" diaphragm head with engraving on metal part as above plus patent dates of May 4 1897 and June 25 1901. A raised 0.5" portion on the back serves as a connector to hold the two arms for the rubber tubing that are parallel to the surface in a V shape. There is a protective metal plate. Although both are attributed to Kehler, this is quite different from A65.

References: Hartz 1922:13; Mueller 1908:14

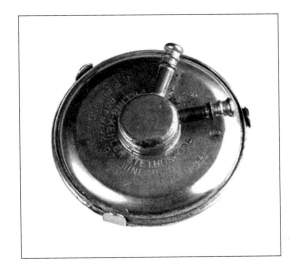

Figure A67

Catalog # 875

1905 Paul's pneumonic stethoscope

(See page 37)

A 1.25"d bell with 1"d inside ring also in a bell shape. There are two connectors at the top which is 1.5" high and another which emerges from the side for the connection to a rubber bulb to remove the air and increase adherence to the chest through a vacuum created between the two bell ends. This form of stethoscope appears in many instrument catalogues of the era.

References: Howarth-Ballard 1905:1025; Kny-Scheerer 1912:1025

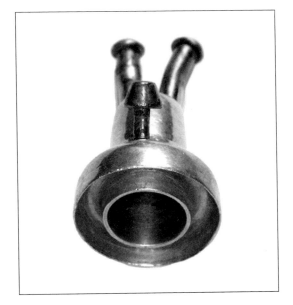

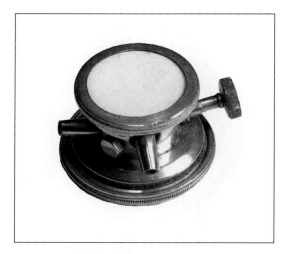

Figure A68
Catalog # 868
1905 Astatique stethoscope
Manufacturer: HJ Prossard, Paris
(See page 57)

A quite complex circular stethoscope head which is
1.75" x 1". There are thermoplastic membranes on each
side of the two heads, the smaller is 1.25". There are arms
for tubing which emerge from the sides and go in opposite directions. There is also a control button on the side.
This is similar to the Huston Akuophone and Carstens
Duplex. The button was used to determine which
diaphragm could transmit the sound. This was almost
identical to Fuch's Patent of 1910 (US Patent # 965,174).
References: Hartz 1922; Huston 1917:23

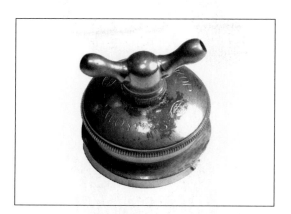

Figure A69
Catalog # 870
1905 Dr Woyla's echoskop stethoscope
(See page 58)

This 1.5" circular chest-piece is embossed as above with
connectors for tubing emerging from the top. A cover for
the bottom must have fitted on small pins protruding
from side but it is missing. It most likely was an attachment for localizing sound.

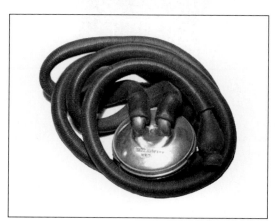

Figure A70
Catalog # 848
1906 C. M. Root stethoscope
Manufacturer: Penn
(See page 58)

A 1.25" diaphragm-type stethoscope with patent date
May 22 1906. It has two separate metal tubes to connect
rubber tubing which is present with hard rubber ear-
pieces. The diaphragm is covered with a protective metal
piece. Similar to the Bowles. US Patent # 821,315.
References: Mueller 1908:14

Figure A71

Catalog # 872

1906 stethoscope

(See page 58)

A larger 2″ diaphragm-type head with each metal connector for the tubing protruding from top of head separately. Similar to the Root stethoscope above (A70).

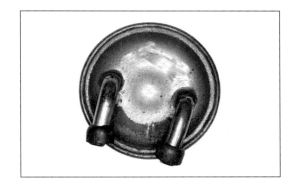

Figure A72

Catalog # 847

1915 Reid and Morris improved stethoscope

(See page 58)

A 1.2″ hard rubber bell-type unit with two tubes attached at the head to a V-shaped piece. One tube remains, quite hardened, and it has the original hard rubber ear-piece.

References: Down 1935:1417

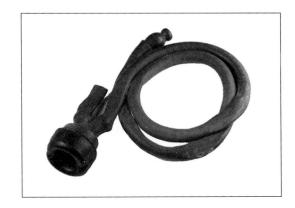

Figure A73

Catalog # 854

1926 Minchin stethoscope

Manufacturer: P Harris and Co. Ltd

(See page 55)

Dome-shaped stethoscope embossed RGD No. 6788E and manufacturer on top. It is a 1.25″d, diaphragm type. The dome-shaped head ends in two arms which serve as connectors for the rubber tubing. The advantage claimed for this unusual design was that it could be inserted under the patient's clothing. The diaphragm was unscrewed to use it as a bell. It was available with either a single or double connector. A trapezoidal shape of similar purpose was patented by Bowles much earlier.

References: Down 1935:1422; *The Surgical Manufac* 1920:400

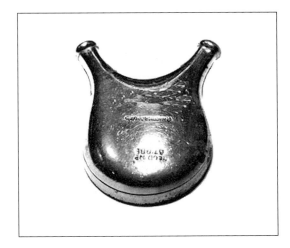

SPECIALTY STETHOSCOPES INCLUDING OBSTETRICS

Obstetrical

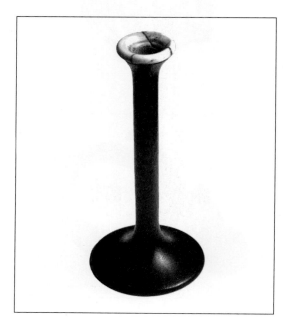

Figure A74

Catalog # 917

1850 obstetric stethoscope

(See page 65)

This very short stethoscope is 4.25" long with a 2" slightly concave ear-piece. The chest end is tipped with an ivory ring. The tube is 0.38" d. It is stained a dark brown and is notable for its short length indicating that it was used either for obstetric or pediatric applications, or both. References: Down 1889:414; Wilbur 1987:23; Witkowski 1889

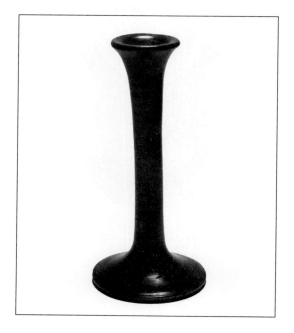

Figure A75

Catalog # 287

1860 DePaul stethoscope

(See page 65)

Another very short design which is 4.75" long with a thick tube that tapers at the end to form a bell 1.2" in diameter. The ear-piece is 2.25" in diameter and is carved from the same piece of wood. The piece narrows to about 0.65" at its narrowest. Notable for its short length. The chest end is not as broad as is usually noted in obstetrical stethoscopes and this one like A74 may have been used also in pediatrics. References: Down 1889:414; Wilbur 1987:23; Witkowski 1889

Figure A76
Catalog # 898
1860 Pajot stethoscope
(See page 65)

This 4.75" long instrument with a thick tube that tapers at the end to form a bell 1.5" in diameter is more like the common obstetrical design. The ear-piece is 2.25" in diameter and is carved from the same piece of wood. The piece narrows to about 0.5" at its narrowest. Notable for its short length.
References: Down 1889:414; Wilbur 1987:23; Witkowski 1889

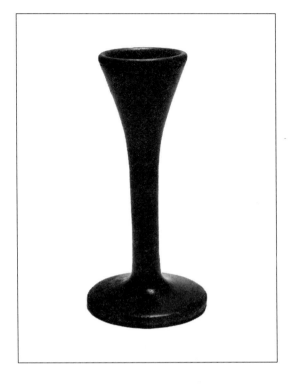

Figure A77
Catalog # 039
1895 Pinard stethoscope
Manufacturer: Down Bros, London
(See page 65)

This is the most commonly encountered obstetric stethoscope and it is 5.75" long and made of pewter. The earpiece is 2.38" and the bell end flares to 2". This is a typical example of the adaptation of the monaural stethoscope that occurred for obstetric use. There is no documentation that Pinard had anything to do with its invention.

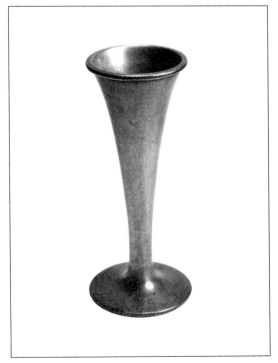

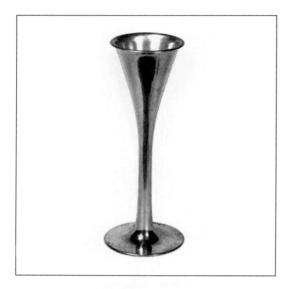

Figure A78

Catalog # 918

1910 Pinard's stethoscope

Manufacturer: Simian

(See page 65)

Another example which is 6″ long with 2″ trumpet shaped chest end 2.25″d and is made of white metal.

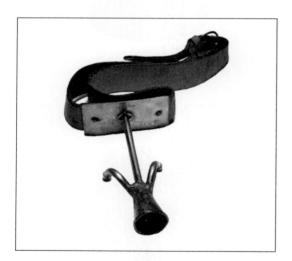

Figure A79

Catalog # 845

1920 Dr Lee-Hillis' fetal stethoscope

Manufacturer: Sharp and Smith

(See page 66)

A 5″ metal stethoscope of the bell type with two outlets to attach rubber tubing. The tube connecting to the bell is riveted to a plate which is in turn riveted to a leather head strap. This facilitated easy application to the abdomen in the pregnant woman, leaving the hands free. It was used well into the 20th century.

References: Down 1935:1415; Mueller 1938:439

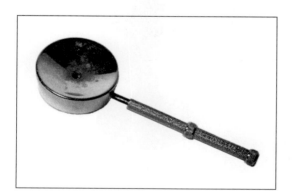

Figure A80

Catalog # 860

1950 Leff fetal stethoscope

Manufacturer: Klarr

(See page 66)

This is a very heavy 3″ weighted chrome-plated head with 5″ arm. It was made to rest on the abdomen by its own weight to permit monitoring fetal heart sounds.

References: Wilbur 1987:25

Figure A81

Catalog # 302

1980 Pinard stethoscope

(See page 65)

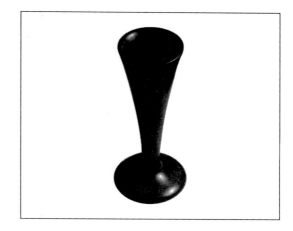

Monaural stethoscope of fetal design. The ear-piece is 2.25"d with 5.63" long tube tapering from 0.5" to a 1.94" bell. This was purchased new in a surgical supply shop in Manhattan in 1989 and illustrates well the difficulty in dating instruments as well as the duration of use of monaural stethoscopes which were particularly popular in obstetrics.

Other

Figure A82

Catalog # 293

1880 Burrows' combination reflex hammer stethoscope

(See page 73)

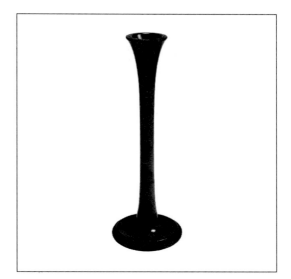

A 7" long, brown-stained pine stethoscope with vulcanite ear-piece 2.25" which has a rubber ring around it for use as a reflex hammer. The stem is 0.44"d.

References: Arnold 1904:517; Tiemann 1889:5

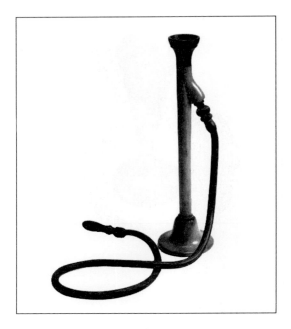

Figure A83
Catalog # 225
1903 Hecker's stethoscope
(See page 40)

A 7.5" horn and boxwood stethoscope with a 2"d convex ear-piece. The chest-piece resembles a bell 1" in
diameter. There is a side tube carved out of the wood
above the bell leading to a rubber tube which connects
with a valve-like connection to the main tube and on the
end has a hard rubber ear-piece. This tube was placed in
the opposite ear for binaural use. This is one of several
models of dual purpose stethoscope which could be
monaural or binaural. It is frequently mistaken for a
teaching model, but the original report by Hecker makes
it quite clear that it was intended for binaural use.
References: Jetter and Scheerer 1910:133

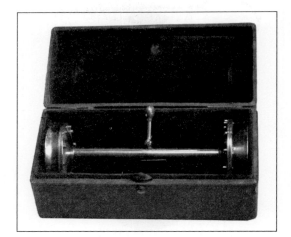

Figure A84
Catalog # 191
1883 Dr Boudet double stethoscope
Manufacturer: Ch. Verdin Paris
(See page 77)

A 6.5" x 3" x 2.63" black box is inscribed "Stethoscope
Double de Dr Boudet de Paris, construit par Ch. Verdin",
and is lined with purple velvet. It contains a 6" long nickel
plated double-ended stethoscope, one end 1.75" the
other 2.25" each with a hard rubber button protruding
from the membrane on the two bell heads and connected
by a 0.5" tube, the middle of which branches with a valve
and was connected to rubber tubing to the ears.
References: Verdin 1904:39

Figure A85

Catalog # 858

1924 Fleischer stethoscope

Manufacturer: Becton Dickenson and Co.

(See page 55)

A 1.5" Bakelite diaphragm-type head of the same basic design as in A54. There are metal loops on the sides for a cloth strap to pass through to allow attachment to the arm for the measurement of blood pressure. The Bakelite diaphragm is embossed J. Formichella.

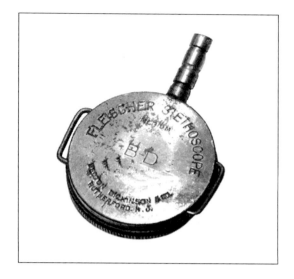

Figure A86

Catalog # 861

1924 Fleischer stethoscope

Manufacturer: Becton Dickenson and Co.

(See page 55)

A 1.5" Bakelite diaphragm-type head. Hard rubber or Bakelite construction. The Luer Loc type connector to the tubing can be seen. There are metal loops on the sides and a cloth strap passes through to allow attachment to the arm for blood pressure measurement, same concept as above except for construction material.

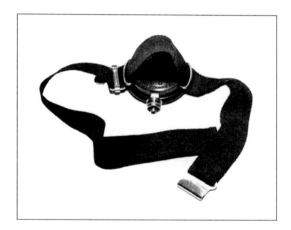

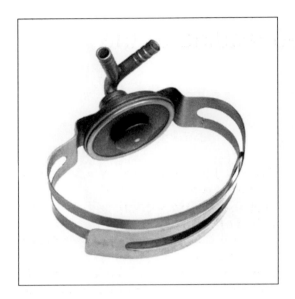

Figure A87
Catalog # 882
1930 Bracelet stethoscope
Manufacturer: Pilling, Pa
(See page 55)

A 1.5" diaphragm of Bowles type, reminiscent of his early patent before the button was dropped. The top has a screw protrusion and a metal bracelet screws in to the housing to allow attachment to the arm to hold it in place. The diaphragm is the type with a 0.5" button protruding to localize sound, for blood pressure measurement. The button was abandoned earlier to achieve the modern form but was useful for blood pressure measurement where it was helpful to localize the artery.
References: Allen and Hanburys 1930:1255; Down Bros 1935:1421; Hartz 1922

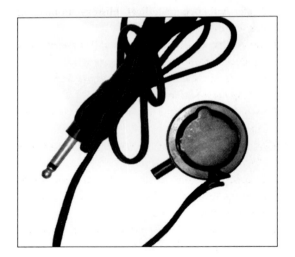

Figure A88
Catalog # 881
1920 Electric stethoscope
(See page 71)

A 1.25" circular diaphragm-type head with apparent microphone mechanism built in. There is a tube for connecting an ear-piece and also a wire emerges from the side with a coaxial plug-type connector. The amplifier section is lost and would have been fairly large.
References: Wilbur 1987:28

References and suggested reading to the appendix

Allen and Hanburys. *Surgical Instruments, Appliances and Hospital Equipment*. London, 1930

Arnold and Sons. *Catalogue of Surgical Instruments*. London, 1885

Arnold and Sons. *Instrument Catalogue*. London, 1895

Arnold and Sons. *Surgical Instruments and Appliances*. London, 1904

Aubry A. *Catalogue Illustré des instruments de chirurgie*. Paris, 1888

Bartlett JS. *The Physician's Pocket Synopsis*. Boston: Munroe and Francis, 1822

Bedini SA. *Early American Scientific Instruments and Their Makers*. Washington: Smithsonian Institution, 1964

Bennion E. *Antique Medical Instruments*. London: Sotheby Parke Bernet, 1979

Betz Co. *Catalogue*. 1907

Bianchi A. *The Phonendoscope and Its Practical Application*. Philadelphia: George P. Pilling and Son, 1900

Boulitte G. *Electrocardiographe de Boulitte*. Paris, 1922

Boulitte G. *Catalog*. Paris, 1923

Bowditch HI. *The Young Stethoscopist or The Student's Aid to Auscultation*. Samuel S. and William Wood, 1848

Burrows H. *Surgical Instruments and Appliances Used in Operations*. London: Faber and Faber, 1939

Catalogue of Surgical Instruments. San Francisco and New York: Norman Publishing and the Printers Devil, 1989

Charriere J. *Surgical Catalogue*. Paris, 1849

Charriere J. *Notice des instruments de chirurgie humaine et veterinaire*. Paris, 1862

Clapp, Otis and Sons. *Catalogue and Physicians Price Current*. Boston, 1889

Collin and Cie. *Catalogue général illustre d'instruments de chirurgie*. Paris, 1882

Dammann G. *Pictorial Encyclopedia of the Civil War: Medical Instruments*. Montana: Pictorial Histories Publishing Co., 1983

Davis A. *Medicine and Its Technology*. Westport: Greenwood Press, 1981

Davis A, Dreyfuss M. *The Finest Instruments Ever Made*. Arlington: Medical History Publishing Associates, 1986

Down Bros. *Catalogue of Surgical Instruments and Appliances*. London, 1889

Down Bros. *Catalogue of Surgical Instruments and Appliances*. London, 1900

Down Bros. *Catalogue of Surgical Instruments and Appliances*. London, 1906

Down Bros. *Catalogue of Surgical Instruments and Appliances*. London, 1935

Edmonson JM. *Nineteenth Century Surgical Instruments*. Cleveland: Cleveland Health Sciences Library, 1986

Evans and Wormull. *Illustrated Catalogue of Surgical Instruments*. London, 1893 473

Flint A. *A Manual of Percussion and Auscultation*. Philadelphia: Henry C. Lea, 1876

Flint A. *A Treatise on the Principles and Practice of Medicine*. Philadelphia: Henry C. Lea, 1878

Gardner J and Son. *Catalogue of Surgical Instruments and Appliances*. Edinburgh, 1913

Hamonic MP. *La Chirurgie et la médecine d'autrefois*. Paris: A. Maloine, 1900

Hartz JE. *Surgical Instruments*. JF Hartz, Detroit Michigan, 1922

Hay, Mackenzie J. *Graphic Methods in Heart Disease*. London: Oxford University Press, 1909

Hernstein AL. *Illustrated Catalogue of Surgical Instruments and Orthopaedic Appliances*. New York, 1881

Howarth-Ballard Drug Co. *Illustrated Catalogue of Surgical Instruments*. Utica, 1905

Huston B. *Catalogue of Huston Brothers Co*. Chicago, 1917

Inglis B. *A History of Medicine*. Cleveland: The World Publishing Co., 1965

Jetter and Scheerer Co. *General Catalogue*. South Germany, 1910

Kirchner and Wilhel Diagnostic Instrument Catalogue. Stuttgart, 1910

Kny-Scheerer Co. *X-Ray Apparatus*. New York, 1908

Kny-Scheerer Co. *Illustrated Catalogue of Surgical Instruments*. New York, 1912

Laennec RTH. *A Treatise on the Diseases of the Chest*. New York: Samuel S. and William Wood, 1838

Laennec RTH. *De l'Auscultation mediate, et des maladies des poumons et du coeur*. Brussels: Société Typographique Belge, 1837

Laennec RTH. *A Treatise on Mediate Auscultation with Notes and Additions of M. Mer*. London: Baillière, 1846

Lentz Charles and Sons. *Illustrated Catalogue and Price List of Surgical Instruments*. Philadelphia, 1900

Lentz Charles and Sons. *Surgical Instruments, Orthopedic Apparatus, etc*. Philadelphia, 1914

Luer, Surgical Catalog. 1867

Luer, Surgical Catalog. 1878

Lynch and Co. *A Catalogue of Druggists' Sundries*. 1887

Lyons A, Petrucelli J. *Medicine, An Illustrated History*. New York: Harry N. Abrams, 1978

Maison M. Arsenal Chirurgical. Lyons: Maison Mathieu, 1910

Matthews. *Surgical Instruments*. London, 1885

Maw and Thompson. *Surgeons' Instruments, Quarterly Price Current*. London, 1891

Maw S and Sons. *Surgical Instruments*. London, 1913

Maw S and Sons. *Maw's Catalogue of Surgeons' Instruments*. London, 1925

McKesson and Robbins. *Prices Current of Drugs and Druggists' Articles*. 1878

Mergier GE. *Technique instrumentale concernant les sciences medicales*. Paris: Octave Doin, 1891

Mills JF. *Encyclopedia of Antique Scientific Instruments*. London: Aurum Press, 1983

Mueller and Co. *Surgical Instruments*. Chicago, 1908

Mueller and Co. *Surgeons' Instruments Equipment Supplies*. Chicago, 1938

Mukhopadhyaya G. *The Surgical Instruments of the Hindus*. Calcutta: Calcutta University, 1913

Multhauf RP. *A Catalogue of Instruments and Models in the Possession of the America*. Philadelphia: The American Philosophical Society, 1961

Pilling GP and Son. *Pilling Made Surgical Instruments and Supplies*. Philadelphia, 1932

Piorry PA. *De la Percussion mediate*. Paris: J.S. Chaude J.B. Baillière, 1828

Piorry PA. *Traite de plessimetrisme et d'organographisme*. Paris: Adrien Delahaye, 1866

Reichert P. *The Reichert Collection*. New York: Burroughs Welcome and Co., 1942

Reynders J and Co. *Catalogue of Surgical Instruments*. New York, 1884

Robert and Collin. *Surgical Catalog*. 1867

Rouit LM. *Essai sur l'auscultation dans le diagnostic des maladies de poitrine*. Paris: Didot le jeune, 1828

Sansom AE. *Manual of the Physical Diagnosis of Diseases of the Heart*. London: Churchill, 1881

Sears Roeback and Co. *Surgical Instruments, Physicians and Hospital Supplies*. Chicago, 1904

Sharp and Smith. *Catalogue of Sharp and Smith Surgical Instruments*. Chicago, 1895

Sharp and Smith. *Surgical Instruments*. Chicago, 1889

The Surgical Manufacturing Co. *Catalogue of Surgical Instruments and Appliances*. Glasgow, 1920

Thompson CJS. *The History and Evolution of Surgical Instruments*. New York: Schuman's, 1942

Tiemann G and Co. *George Tiemann and Co*. New York, 1872

Tiemann G and Co. *The American Armamentarium Chirurgicum*. New York, 1879

Tiemann G and Co. *Catalogue of Surgical Instruments*. New York, 1889

Tiemann G and Co. *George Tiemann and Co*. New York, 1926

Truax C and Co. *Medical Supplies Surgical Instruments*. Chicago, 1890

Truax C and Co. *Mechanics of Surgery*. Chicago, 1899

Truax, Greene and Co. *Medical Supplies, Surgical Instruments*. Chicago, 1893

Velter A, Marie-Jose L. *Les Outils du corps*. Milan: Hier and Demain, 1974

Verdin C. *Catalogue des Instruments de Precision (Reproduction)*. Paris, 1904

Weed WA and Co. *Illustrated Yearbook*. 1872

Weiss J and Son. *Surgical Catalog*. 1831

Weiss J and Son. *Surgical Catalog*. 1889

Wilbur CK. *Antique Medical Instruments (Price Guide Included)*. PA: Schiffer Publishing Ltd., 1987

Witkowski GJ. *Histoire des Accouchments*. G. Steinheil, Paris 1889

Wulfing-Luer H. *Catalogue Général*. Paris, 1904

Index

teaching stethoscopes 63–65
Tomasinelli, G. 3
Touroff, Arthur S.W. 74
Turner, K.M. 70

vaginal stethoscope 66
Veale, H. 33

water stethoscopes 73, 76
Western Electric stethoscope 70–71
Whittaker, J.T. 33
Williams, C.J.B. 32–33, 34, 41, 75
Wintrich, M. Anton 19–21
Wollaston, William Hyde 12
Woods, Edmund F. 62

THE
DUKE'S
DESIGN

by
Margaret Westhaven

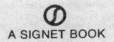

A SIGNET BOOK

SIGNET
Published by the Penguin Group
Penguin Books USA Inc., 375 Hudson Street,
New York, New York 10014, U.S.A.
Penguin Books Ltd, 27 Wrights Lane,
London W8 5TZ, England
Penguin Books Australia Ltd, Ringwood,
Victoria, Australia
Penguin Books Canada Ltd, 2801 John Street,
Markham, Ontario, Canada L3R 1B4
Penguin Books (N.Z.) Ltd, 182-190 Wairau Road,
Auckland 10, New Zealand

Penguin Books Ltd, Registered Offices:
Harmondsworth, Middlesex, England

First published by Signet, an imprint of New American Library, a division of
Penguin Books USA Inc.

First Printing, March, 1991
10 9 8 7 6 5 4 3 2 1

. . . you do me wrong . . . you do,
In such disdainful manner me to woo.

—*A Midsummer Night's Dream*

1

"VERY well," Matilda said. "I see no harm in it. And you're quite correct, your grace. I could use the money." Her voice was calm; she was counting on her training as an actress to hide how very much she did need funds and what a godsend this gentleman's proposition was.

The Duke of Arden turned upon the young woman the full power of his mischievous smile, that famous smile so often caricatured in the press. "You've made me very happy, my dear. And please, no need to be so formal. Do call me Duke."

Matilda choked back a nervous laugh. "If you wish . . . Duke."

The two were standing in a corner of the greenroom at the Royal George Theater. A rehearsal hall in the daytime, by night the greenroom became a social gathering place where actors and actresses might entertain friends and admirers.

It was understood that an actress who appeared here unattended was looking for more than homage from the many gentlemen of the *ton* who frequented all the greenrooms in London, quizzing glasses held aloft to ogle the newest faces on the market. Matilda, looking round at the brightly dressed female players and leering bucks in the crowd, knew that Arden and she appeared to be concluding the usual sort of bargain, and for just a moment, the thought depressed her.

It was not that she had a reputation to lose. Though she had never before ventured into the greenroom after the performance, nobody believed that Matilda Gra-

7

ham, actress, wasn't looking for a protector. She could
hardly pass down the corridor from the wings to her
dressing room without being mobbed by potential lovers. This evening she had been pounced upon the moment her slipper touched the carpet of the greenroom,
and she had experienced a moment of panic which she
hid under the frosty manner she always affected before
the rougher sex. Then, over the heads of the demanding males—all of whom were offering her anything
from diamonds to foreign travel if she would but grant
them the ultimate favor—a pair of sparkling dark eyes
met Matilda's.

"You received my note, Miss Graham," that deep,
rich voice had drawled, and the group of gentlemen
fell back as if by magic. And the Duke of Arden, left
alone with the lovely actress, proceeded to give to her
the facts of the "acting engagement" he had promised
her in a missive sent to her dressing room.

Now Matilda said, in a low voice suitable for their
odd conversation, "So we've agreed, then. One hundred pounds if I will let myself be found in the bed of
your old uncle. Is this a . . . a special occasion,
Duke?"

Arden grinned. "The old stick's birthday."

"And I am not to do anything but be found and run
out shrieking." Desperate for money, Matilda had resolved already to take part in the duke's prank. Still
she felt a need to repeat the terms, to reassure herself
and make the duke reiterate his promise that she would
not have to serve a possibly libidinous old uncle in
any capacity other than that of a practical joke.

"My life on it, Miss Graham. I will be waiting in
the cupboard to spring out and cry 'surprise.' "

The words rang with honesty as well as laughter,
and Matilda looked up into the eyes of Michael Beresford, Duke of Arden. His was a familiar figure; ever
since her arrival in London Matilda had known of the

famous Duke of Arden, the worst prankster in the *ton*. Indeed, even when she had lived in Oxford, items concerning this gentleman's practical jokes had appeared in the newspapers from time to time, and Matilda had always been secretly fascinated by the duke, for there was a side of her nature which appreciated atrocious pranks.

She supposed his handsome, aristocratic face and crisp dark curls helped ensure his notoriety. Not to mention a physique so tall and well-muscled that Matilda had caught her breath when she was finally, after weeks of seeing him only from behind the footlights, standing beside him. His evening clothes were everything that was elegant, from the tight-fitting satin breeches to the bicorne he carried under one muscular arm.

"When is this jest to take place?" she asked.

"Why, this very night," Arden said with a warm chuckle.

What wonderful brown eyes he had, and how happily they danced. Matilda often debated the reason why such a ruthless practical joker as the Duke of Arden could remain so popular. Now she knew. Obviously everyone he had ever played a prank upon needed nothing more than to look into those friendly ducal eyes. Forgiveness must follow, unless the victim of the joke had a heart of stone . . .

Matilda forced herself to snap to attention. She had been staring at him in fascination, and he was looking more amused than ever. "You mean I'm to go with you—now?" She thought quickly. "May I tell someone about this? Only one person, who might otherwise worry?"

The duke gave a start. As he understood it, this lovely young woman was as yet a citadel unstormed. Weeks of watching her performances from his first-tier box had made him admire her fire and spirit as

well as her beauty, and he had chosen her out of all
the actresses in London to play this joke on Uncle
precisely because he wished to know her better himself.
He hadn't counted on the encumbrance of a jealous
lover.

"Who is he, my dear?" he asked, hiding his disappointment. "Perhaps if I explain the circumstances
to the man myself. And assure him the whole thing's
innocent, don't you know. He might even go with us
in the carriage if he's the proprietary sort."

Matilda laughed and said that there was no gentleman; she always went home in a hackney with her old
aunt, who was waiting even now in the dressing room
and would fret if her niece didn't offer some explanation.

"Aunt." The duke nodded, trying to maintain his
seriousness in the face of this obvious bouncer. Fashionable actresses might possibly go home alone or with
a maid; but a superannuated aunt? Impossible. "And
do you wish me to speak with her?"

"Oh, no, sir," said Matilda at once, neatly confirm-
ing Arden's suspicions that, whoever was in the dressing room, it was no elderly female. "You would
overwhelm her, I'm afraid. Auntie is still quite coun-
trified, for all we've been in London six months. Let
me run back and tell her, then get my cloak. Do I
need . . . ought I to dress in character?"

"Have you a particularly enticing nightrail?" The
gentleman's lips twitched. Uncle would have an apo-
plexy.

"No," said Matilda a touch regretfully. "However,
Dulcie Moore might. We're nearly of a size; you must
know Miss Moore, she did Celia tonight. Shall I go
and ask her?" Matilda herself had done the part of
Rosalind, and Arden would be the first to agree that
she and Miss Moore had made the performance a
memorable one for any man with an eye.

Dulcie Moore was easy to locate in the press of people; the headdress of plumes she had donned after the play stood out even in the roomful of tall gentlemen. Dulcie, in common with most of the other actresses, put on full evening dress every night when the curtain came down. Matilda had done her best to follow that custom when she found she would need to make her first appearance in the greenroom to answer the duke's summons. She hoped none of the sometimes cattish females around her would mention that her low-necked gown of light-fawn tissue, scattered with brilliants, was out of the wardrobe rack.

The duke said, "If your friend would allow you to borrow a suitable, er, costume . . ." He watched Matilda's figure appreciatively as she made her way across the room. Her fellow actress Miss Moore *was* nearly of a size with Miss Graham. Perhaps it was Dulcie Moore's improbably guinea-gold hair, or her heavy use of paint, that made her figure seem coarse—not at all similar to Miss Graham's round, enticing shape.

Miss Graham broke through Dulcie's flanking admirers. The two young actresses put their heads together for a conspiratorial moment in an attractive pose which might have inspired an artist to paint them just so, the red head leaning toward the bright blond one. Matilda nodded in Arden's direction, and from across the room Dulcie Moore caught the duke's eye and gave him a broad wink. He winked back.

A short time later Miss Graham was by his side. "It's all arranged," she said. "Now, shall I meet you at your carriage? It will be outside the stage door, I presume?"

The duke detailed his arrangements and offered his arm. "Shall we be going, my dear?"

Matilda's expression was prim as she answered, "Do give me a few minutes' start of you, Duke. I still need to get my cloak and talk to Auntie. Besides, think how it would look if we left the room together.''

''About the same as it looks for us to be talking together, my dear young lady,'' Arden reminded her with a rueful shake of his head. ''At the carriage, then. Five minutes.'' He watched her out of the room, waited a beat or two, and then followed, enjoying the envious stares the other men were casting him. So they thought he'd stormed the citadel! Famous joke.

Matilda, who spent her days and nights cooped up in the theater or her lodging house in Bloomsbury, enjoyed the ride through the night in the duke's perfectly sprung carriage. They crossed the river at London Bridge and eventually left town behind, heading south. The chaise turned off the main road after the second toll to speed along hedge-lined lanes at what seemed to Matilda an extraordinary rate. The duke, in his seat across from her, was silent except for a quiet chuckle every once in a while. Much as Matilda wished to interrogate his grace on their destination, she was very much aware of her status as his employee. He might well call it impertinent if the woman he had hired asked too many questions.

The equipage slowed to enter a country town. The shadowy shapes of gabled buildings seemed to lean close when Matilda peered out of the coach window, and the horses were now clicking their way over cobbles. Soon the vehicle pulled up at what looked like the back entrance of a huge, hulking building, a house of a suitable size to belong to a duke's uncle.

''Shall I get into my nightgown?'' Matilda whispered.

''Splendid idea, Miss Graham. You don't wish me to observe you? A pity. Well, I'll descend and wait for you, carefully hiding my disappointment. Simply open the door when you've changed.''

Left alone inside the carriage, Matilda struggled with the tapes of the fawn evening gown and put herself into the mass of transparent pink ruffles lent her by Dulcie. The costume was hardly Matilda's best color, but she had not been hired as a fashion plate, she reasoned, and it *was* dark. Having stowed the evening gown in one corner of the seat, she retied her modest cloak around her neck and opened the carriage door.

"My dear!" the duke greeted her. "If I could see you I'm certain I'd have to congratulate you on how charming you look. Come this way, if you please. I've paid one of Uncle's servants to leave this back door unbarred, and I took the precaution of filching its key last time I visited." Arden couldn't hold back a soft chuckle; Uncle Theobald would be beside himself! It was time the old party was repaid for joining Arden's friends on the duke's own birthday. They had placed a live fox in his dressing room and, clad in full hunting regalia, stormed in on him in a body, preceded by a dozen hounds. Arden still had to laugh when he thought about it.

The door opened without a creak to disclose a lighted candle on a table in a small, shadowy vestibule. Obviously the servant had been well paid, thought Matilda. She followed the duke's solid form up a twisting maze of stairs, growing more nervous with each step.

Suddenly they were in a wide hall, well-lit by tapers. Rich red carpet, gleaming carved paneling, and stern portraits of churchmen danced before Matilda's eyes. And from behind one of the heavy oaken doors came the sound of masculine voices.

"Uncle was entertaining some learned men of his see tonight," the duke said, winking at Matilda. "Now, come along. His bedroom is on this floor."

Matilda had slipped off her shoes in nervous preparation for climbing into an old man's bed. To her embarrassment, Arden bent down at the same moment she did and captured her shoes before she had a chance to pick them up, causing their heads nearly to bump together.

"His see?" Matilda repeated. Taking off her shoes had surely distracted her; she couldn't have heard aright. She looked closer at the clerical portrait nearest her. "Who is your uncle, sir?"

"Why, the Bishop of Ardenminster. Didn't you know?" Arden spoke lightly. "This way, ma'am."

"You want me to humiliate a bishop?" the young woman hissed. "A man of the cloth?"

The duke looked down into her incredulous green eyes. "Oh, don't fret about his profession. I learned pranks at Uncle Theobald's knee. He isn't a stuffy fellow. And don't you agree that there is an extra fillip of humor to this joke, him being in orders?"

He said the last words to her back, for Matilda had turned on her heel and was retracing her steps on the dark staircase. She kept one hand on the stone wall and made it to the bottom, and the door, in safety.

Once outside the house—she supposed she ought to say palace—she had no choice but to return to the duke's carriage. She was miles from home and would fare poorly in these streets, dressed in a frilled nightgown. He had brought her to his own territory: Ardenminster, the cathedral town near the well-known ducal estates. She had no money and no acquaintance here and would have to rely on that horrid duke, her erstwhile employer, to take her home.

If the duke's coachman and grooms were surprised when the young lady who had so recently exited the carriage pulled open its door and hopped in, without the aid of steps, they gave no sign. Matilda slammed the door shut and sat down, hands pressed to her hot cheeks. She was ashamed of her lack of sophistication,

but there it was: she couldn't humiliate a bishop. One
hundred pounds, the proposed fee for this night's
work, had just slipped from her grasp.

Matilda had been raised in Oxford, where clergymen were plentiful. She tended to think of churchmen
as far above mere mortals in dignity and in kindness.
What would she have done without the vicar, to take
but one example, when Papa died and left her and
Aunt Poppy with only a mountain of debts?

Then there were the dozen or so earnest young men,
destined for the church, who had been among those
Papa had tutored over the years—

"I can't," whispered Matilda into the velvety darkness of the ducal carriage, punctuating her whirling
thoughts with the sound of her own voice. With a little
sigh of regret, she kissed the hundred pounds good-
bye and tried to think of something she might pawn.
There were other ways to get money. She had been
mad to break her strict rule about never dealing with
the gentlemen who watched her on the stage.

The door opened, and the Duke of Arden loomed
in the night. "Stage fright, my dear? Come, now,
there's yet time."

Matilda glared at him. "You still don't understand,
do you? Sir, if I'd known the . . . the butt of your joke
was a clergyman of any class, I wouldn't have agreed.
I imagined your uncle to be a degenerate old dandy,
perhaps, at any rate someone who would take the joke
in stride. Someone like . . ." She paused.

"Someone like myself, you would say?" Arden was
laughing as he climbed into the carriage and took the
seat opposite Matilda's. "I've assured you that my uncle is well up to the humiliation. He'd think it a famous
trick! No need to poker up—he really would. You're
resolved not to do it? Well, well. Who'd have thought
religious scruples would plague a girl of your profes-

sion? I'd have done better to ask your friend Dulcie, I expect.''

"I can't speak for Miss Moore," said Matilda in a hurt voice, seething at the disrespect for her profession implicit in his words, "and I can't claim the sort of religious feeling you kindly bestow upon me. It's simply that clergymen have always been exceptionally kind to me, and I just *can't—*''

"No need to distress yourself, Miss Graham." The duke heard the catch in Matilda's voice, and though he didn't understand the problem, he was quite willing to be the gentleman. He could always hire another girl for another evening; Uncle would keep. Had Miss Graham's first seducer been a curate, perhaps?

The ride back to town was accomplished in silence, Matilda sitting ramrod-straight on the lush velvet squabs, the duke lounging across from her, legs crossed. After what seemed to the nervous girl an eternity, the carriage rolled to a halt.

Arden assisted Matilda to descend. His post chaise immediately moved off and disappeared around a corner.

Matilda looked about her. "This isn't the theater, sir." They had agreed between them that he would deliver her back to the Royal George. There she might find a hackney easily, since job-coaches prowled the Covent Garden area until well into the morning hours.

"We're at my rooms. I thought you could change back into your proper clothes in comfort, and I'll see to it you're paid."

"Paid? But I didn't do anything but ruin your plans, Duke, and I can't accept payment."

"Be that as it may. Come up and get dressed again. I can't send you home in your nightdress, and it's deuced uncomfortable wiggling in and out of clothes in a carriage. Ought to know, I've done it once or twice."

Matilda took a deep breath, trying not to imagine in what connection the Duke of Arden might have changed his clothes in a carriage, and looked down at her flimsy costume and bare feet. Arden was holding out his arm quite as though they were about to promenade after a dance at a ball given by the fashionable set. Her little slippers were clutched in one of his hands; her evening gown hung over his arm. Matilda's eyes narrowed in suspicion. "You aren't going to give me my clothes, are you?"

"And let you change in the street? How uncomfortable that sounds when I have a warm room upstairs— a room that locks from the inside, if you're worried. My dear girl, don't you trust me at all?" returned Arden.

She wished she could see his face, but it was completely in shadow. "To be frank, no."

"I'm wounded, Miss Graham, deeply wounded."

"I doubt it."

"Well, my dear, I'm going in. If you would like to join me—and your clothes—come along."

Matilda frowned at the note of levity in his voice, but her practical nature, as well as her knowledge of what danger lurked in London by night, made her take Arden's arm.

She hadn't gone even a step toward the huge edifice before she remembered reading that Arden lived in that famous haven of masculinity, the Albany. He never used his huge family mansion in Cavendish Square. Matilda held her head high as the night porter, in a round hat and voluminous greatcoat, bowed low before her on seeing she was with the duke. Arden chuckled at the man's manner, flipping him a coin and guiding Matilda across a wide courtyard.

When Arden matter-of-factly directed her up a set of stairs, Matilda felt a tremor go through her: an odd and, to her logical mind, totally misplaced thrill of excitement. No respectable woman ever went up these steps after dark, and now she would change her clothes in the apartments of the foremost buck of the *ton*. She had Arden's word that nothing would happen to her, and she had no reason to think a duke of the realm would not be a man of honor. This was a rare adventure. How many young women got to see the inside of the Albany?

On the floor above the duke opened a door onto what looked, at first glance, like fairyland. Before Matilda's eyes was a very small rich room whose walls were entirely lined with leatherbound books. The gilt-trimmed bindings of the volumes glowed thanks to the candlelight and the flames of a cozy fire burning in a small grate. A door was ajar on the wall opposite the fireplace, giving a glimpse of what appeared to be a sumptuous sitting room beyond the enchanting miniature library.

Matilda barely glanced at the other appurtenances of the room. She hadn't seen so many books since the auction of Papa's library; it still made her shudder to think how even the rarest and most precious volumes had gone for a song. Somewhere in the back of her mind she wondered why a frivolous man like the Duke of Arden would have such a fine collection. As one in a dream, she stepped toward the books.

The door closed softly behind her.

The sound startled Matilda back to reality, and she noticed that a table before the fire was set for two.

"May I help you off with your cloak, my dear?" Arden's voice was affectionate, and his eyes as they looked Matilda up and down seemed to burn. "I told my man to prepare a cold supper and then gave him the night out."

"You did?" Matilda's voice was incredulous. Gazing into his mischievous face, she realized that he had been planning to bring her back here all along. Immediately she put on her ordinary armor: a cold, haughty expression and a forbidding stance.

The duke flung away Matilda's evening gown, and it landed on a sofa. He dropped her shoes onto the floor and reached her in two long strides. Then his arms were around her, and his smiling lips were descending on hers.

It had all happened so fast! Matilda gasped, struggled, and then, unaccountably relaxing for a moment within his incredibly strong, infinitely gentle embrace, she found herself returning the kiss. Except for the occasional peck onstage, this kiss was Matilda's first in her two-and-twenty years. It affected her as had no experience in her life before. Incoherent thoughts about collecting material for her craft danced through her mind, only to be replaced by dreams of a sunny summer day, herself in a field somewhere, dressed in white muslin, and this very man's arms holding her as closely as they were now. . . . She could almost feel the warm glow of the sun on her skin. Or was it the sun?

"Sir!" Matilda wrenched herself away. It took all her strength.

The duke's face swam above hers, the eyes heavy-lidded, the sensuous mouth set in puzzlement. "What's amiss, my sweet?"

"You actually planned this! You thought that after playing that prank on your uncle I'd come back here with you and . . . and stay. Now, don't deny it."

Arden's lips curved upward. "Deny the absolute truth? I'm not that sort of man."

"Neither are you the honorable sort," Matilda snapped. "You said I could change my clothes here. And you said you were hiring me only to play that joke, not to be your . . . your . . ."

"Mistress? I only hoped, Miss Graham. I didn't plan. My dear, I've been watching you for weeks now.

You're the loveliest thing to appear on the stage or off it in years. Naturally I want you. And I seem to recall a very recent kiss which would indicate that you want me.'' He moved forward.

Matilda stepped back as quickly. ''I never agreed to warm *your* bed, sir.''

''But wouldn't it be pleasant?'' The words were uttered so softly, with such caressing insinuation, that Matilda shuddered with something other than fear.

''No, it would not,'' she said levelly. In a sudden movement she sprang for the door.

He was too quick for her, catching her round the waist and pulling her close again. One large hand reached up to untie the strings of her gray cloak, which obligingly fell to the carpet, leaving Matilda exposed in all the questionable glory of transparent pink.

She looked down at herself. ''Plague take that Dulcie Moore. Does she call this a proper sort of outfit?''

''I doubt propriety is uppermost in her mind when she wears it,'' the duke pointed out with a warm laugh. His lips came down on Miss Graham's white neck. ''Pity Uncle couldn't see you in that,'' he muttered between kisses.

Once again Matilda pushed him away. ''Stop it, Duke! I'm leaving now, and you may find another woman for this little tryst you had the gall to arrange.''

''But, my dear girl, why? You're a beautiful actress; I'm a very well-set-up, and, forgive my lack of modesty, a very personable duke. What's to stop us from taking the combination to its logical conclusion?''

''Me,'' Matilda said. Pausing to grab the discarded evening gown, she headed for the door once more at a deliberate, stately pace.

Her very sureness dazzled Arden for a moment, but she hadn't reached the safety of the corridor before he moved to action again. Remembering her response to his caresses, he seized the young woman by the shoulders, turned her about matter-of-factly, and caught her in yet another searching, passionate kiss.

Matilda started to fight her way out of his embrace, but had second thoughts. The duke was maneuvering her toward the sofa, with who knew what lewd ambitions, and as she dragged herself with increasing reluctance from each kiss, she saw, out of the corner of her eye, a brandy decanter standing like a beacon on a small table to one side of the couch.

As he had intended, Arden sank to the sofa, his lady on top of him. His hands started in caressing her back.

Matilda stared down at him in disbelief at the liberties he was taking. Her face was pressed to his, and she tried to be unaffected by the closeness. Arden's hands were so obsessed in their wanderings that he had entirely loosened his hold on Matilda's arms.

It was now or never. Matilda thought virtuous thoughts. She had been incredibly stupid to come here, but she was not obliged to pay for her idiocy with her honor. She wouldn't be ruined on a whim by this light-minded seducer; not tonight, not ever!

One small white hand stole over Arden's head. He was too busy to notice.

Playing along with the duke was trying Matilda's nerves most sorely. Her breathing was ragged now, and she felt herself slipping away into some odd void where principles meant nothing and only passion held sway. At last her fingers closed around the neck of the decanter.

"My dear girl," Arden whispered. "I knew you'd come round."

Matilda brought the decanter down, with what she hoped was less than her full strength, on the duke's dark pate. Immediately his head rolled to one side.

Stopping only to reassure herself that her victim still breathed and to grab her cloak, Matilda shoved her feet into her slippers and ran from the room, down the stairs, and into the comparative safety of dawn-streaked London.

Not much later, the Duke of Arden struggled to a sitting position. What the devil! He put one hand to a head which seemed twice as heavy as any head should be. A lump was rising. The decanter, spilling brandy onto the Persian carpet at the duke's feet, told its own story. Arden was reassured to see that the vixen hadn't broken the heavy cut glass over his unfortunate crown; she did have some mercy.

The duke was smiling. "First round to you, Miss Graham," he said with a shaky laugh. "Here's to the play."

2

"**MICHAEL,**" said the duchess, a note of exasperation clear in her voice, "I know it's asking a great deal, but do be serious! How can I hold my head up this Season?"

"Why, the usual way, Mama," the Duke of Arden drawled. "Chin toward the sky and whatnot. How puzzling that you should want my advice on a matter of posture. I'd thought you were the expert there, for I remember a good deal of that sort of talk from you in years past."

A deep, rattling sigh escaped the Duchess of Arden. Her son was looking at her with a pleased expression. The plaguey boy did like his joke.

The duchess, a statuesque woman with a handsome, sharp face, looked born to the high position she held. In appearance she was more regal than any queen. Two wings of white sprang back from her temples and added a note of drama to her wealth of raven hair, serving as well as to make her recognizable at a glance throughout society. For the most part she enjoyed her notoriety.

She did not, however, enjoy her son's celebrity. The Duchess of Arden not only stood on her dignity but also had never been known to move off that imposing edifice. Her children had been bred up from birth to enhance the Arden name.

Michael, with his twinkling sense of humor and mania for atrocious puns, was not her favorite child. Quite often she gnashed her teeth over the unfortunate fact that he, of all her offspring, should be the one afflicted

23

by the most highly overactive sense of the ridiculous she had ever observed. He had not gotten it from her side of the family.

And Michael was the duke, the Duchess of Arden often reflected in surprise, for she did not quite believe it even after two years. As a duke, he ought to be dignified at all times, an example to the realm. His main claim to fame should *not* be the great number of occasions his name had appeared in the press as the instigator of some lurid practical joke.

There was no saving the situation, the duchess thought in resignation. The Duke of Arden was an eternal slap in the face to the family dignity.

"You must move home, Michael," she said, trying to invest her words with the ring of authority. If she could get him under her roof, as she had managed to do every Season so far by a judiciously administered dose of guilt, she would use her influence to curtail his most objectionable activities. (That her influence had never yet succeeded did not bother her one whit.) "How do you think it looks, you living at the Albany with me in town?"

Arden shrugged. He was determined that this Season, for once, he would *not* be forced into this mausoleum of a house. "I'll attend your parties, of course, Mama," he said as a conciliatory measure, though this prospect was almost as appealing as sitting through one of Uncle Theobald's sermons. "And I'll do the pretty, as usual, with all the spaniel-faced young hopefuls you can throw at me. But I need my privacy this year. I've work to do, don't you know."

"Work! You! No, I do not know," his mother retorted. "Thank heaven we have a respectable agent, or our lands could fall into the sea and you wouldn't notice. And isn't it way past time for your first speech in the House? And furthermore—"

Her son held up a hand in a vain effort to stanch the

duchess's flow of recriminations. There was nothing he could say to mollify her. He couldn't deny the charge of being a useless ornament of society, and he had no plans to change his ways.

In the two years since his father's death he had marveled at his mother's calm assumption that she was still the chatelaine of the Arden properties and the proper arbiter of the new duke's every action. Father having been quite under her thumb, she was used to a life of command. Arden supposed Mama would remain in office until he took a bride, and, considering that alternative, he could bear the duchess's constant yammering very well.

"Go to parties, dance with antidotes," he said over his mother's shrill words. "My final offer, Mama. Now, do excuse me. I have business." He rose, made his best bow over his mother's slender hand, and picked up a beribboned box he had brought into her salon with him, having preferred not to entrust it to what he knew was a deuced nosy pack of servants. "Thank you for the tea," he said over his shoulder.

The Duchess of Arden sighed. An after-dinner visit to drink tea, and the wretched boy doubtless thought she should fall all over herself with gratitude for the sunshine of his presence. And now, by his sleek evening clothes, one could assume he was going out to the opera or some such. And had he invited his very own mother? Well, the fact that he had not—and that he carried that strange box—indicated he was bent upon some mischief, as usual. He was insufferable!

His long-suffering mama's only consolation was that Michael would settle down once he was married to the Lady Davina Lowden. That match was a coup the duchess meant to bring off this very Season.

"Oh, Matilda," twittered the small old lady in rusty black. "Do look what came for you."

Matilda smiled affectionately at her great-aunt
Poppy, a lady of some seventy summers who had a
sweet, lined face and large blue eyes. The niece only
glanced at the huge white box, done up with red satin
ribbons, which reposed on the rickety dressing-room
table.

She didn't like exposing her innocent old auntie to
the seamy world of the London theater, but there
seemed to be no other solution. If Matilda were to
retain her respectability, she must have a duenna present with her in the theater at all times. And Aunt
Poppy, her only companion, was elected to the position by default.

Aunt Poppy had lived a very sheltered life. She
didn't seem to understand that the gifts Matilda sometimes received from eager gentlemen were not tokens
of esteem.

Matilda crossed to the table. Might as well get this
over quickly. She didn't even stop to loosen the laces
of a "Rosalind" outfit that didn't quite fit and had
been pinching her for two hours. She undid the red
ribbons and lifted the lid of the box.

Glittering up at her was the fawn tissue evening
gown.

Matilda had noticed that impossible duke leaning
over his box toward the stage this evening; indeed, on
more than one occasion she had been afraid he might
tumble out into the pit. She might have guessed that
he was staring, not in admiration, but in anticipation
of another joke.

Naturally she had been glad to see that the duke had
suffered no ill effects from being hit on the head. She
was extremely relieved, for not only did she wish him
the best of health, but as the day had worn on she had
been half-afraid that an officer of the law would come
to her door and haul her off to Newgate for assaulting
a peer of the realm.

And she was genuinely glad to get the dress back. When she'd discovered, the night before, that she had somehow left it in the duke's rooms in her haste to clear out of the place, she had been terrified that the wardrobe mistress would find the gown missing and remember who had had it last. Now Matilda could put it back with no one the wiser.

"Isn't this the same dress you were wearing last night?" Aunt Poppy queried, fingering the spangled material with interest.

"Yes, isn't it silly? I told you about that job I had to do last night. I was in another costume, and I accidentally left this dress behind." As she spoke, Matilda was lifting the folds of fragile material out of the box. She noticed that the dress was wrapped around something heavy.

A bottle of the finest French brandy! And fastened about the bottle with another red satin ribbon was a note for a hundred pounds.

"Why, how unusual," Aunt Poppy murmured.

Poor Aunt Poppy was more than a little dotty, a quality Matilda was sometimes grateful for.

"It is unusual, isn't it?" was all she had to say now, placing the brandy bottle in a conspicuous place on the table so they would remember to take it home. Brandy was a very practical gift, and Matilda decided on the spot to accept it.

The money, though. What was she to do about the money?

"Here is the hundred pounds, just as you said," Aunt Poppy was musing. She had taken the bill in her hands and was turning it over. Likely she had never seen such a thing before. "You performed the task well, then, child?"

"That's precisely the problem. I didn't," said Matilda. "Er . . . something occurred, and we weren't able to go to the engagement. I haven't earned this, and I expect my . . . my employer is only trying to be gallant. He knows we're poor, you see." Naturally Matilda didn't really ascribe such generous motives to the Duke of Arden. She more than suspected that he was simply being a tease.

"Well, so we are." Aunt Poppy nodded. "Poor. Very poor indeed, my dear. And if the gentleman, whoever he is, is disposed to be gallant, why not let him? I do so wish to go home soon."

Home was Oxford. Aunt Poppy had lived many years of her life there, and Matilda was a native of the place. When Matilda had brought her great-aunt to the metropolis she had promised the good lady they would stay for the minimum of time necessary to earn sufficient funds to keep them in their beloved university town.

Aunt Poppy would hopefully never know how poor they really were. Matilda had done a very foolish thing on first coming to London. Desperate to pay off her father's last debt and clear his name in Oxford, she had gotten herself into the hands of a City moneylender to the tune of one hundred pounds plus interest. She had been paying off the new debt in tiny installments, but unfortunately the moneylender chanced to go to the Royal George Theater one evening and discovered that his young lady debtor was an actress of some note. He had been pressing for larger payments ever since, assuming his lovely client had free access to the purses of countless gentlemen of the *beau monde*.

Matilda had pawned her mother's garnet earrings this very day, handed over the money to her creditor, and promised him more soon. He was staved off for the time being, but what a relief it would have been to cancel the debt.

Things were looking up even without the duke's money, Matilda reminded herself. She was no longer a newcomer to the theater company, and her new salary would allow her to put something toward the debt and at last begin to save for the return to Oxford.

She had already lectured herself on the folly of regretting the duke's money. Trust him to make her task harder. Was Matilda to return this banknote and see her goals recede by one hundred pounds? Was she to watch her dear aunt's lip tremble in chagrin, as it had the day their landlady raised the rent?

Well, Matilda had watched worse things than a trembling lip. The implications of keeping such a sum were too serious to be borne, for if the note were not returned, the duke would be justified in believing that Matilda had agreed to be his mistress.

"Auntie, we *must* give it back," she said, drawing the note from Aunt Poppy's fingers. She tucked it into her reticule, which was hanging from the back of the room's one ancient chair. There were no writing materials here; she would write the duke a note from home, enclosing the money. Unless . . .

Arden might possibly be in the greenroom tonight. If he indeed thought that Matilda's acceptance of his banknote meant acquiescence to his dark designs, he would surely be there.

Matilda grimly began to undo her costume. Her aunt, babbling slightly in her distress at the hundred pounds' fate, helped her to change.

"The pretty brown dress again?"

"Yes, Aunt Poppy, I'm going into the greenroom now, and I must be fine, you know."

"Into that dreadful room!" Aunt Poppy gave vent to predictions of doom should Matilda not have her wits about her. Auntie might be an innocent, but she had gleaned enough town bronze to realize what sorts of bargains were normally made in the notorious greenroom.

Matilda reassured the old lady and went on her way

through the backstage corridor, wishing as she walked along that she weren't so deep into this life of questionable morals.

The Duke of Arden was by no means the first lecherous nobleman to single out the voluptuous Miss Graham, and she was well-practiced in a cold refusal of a *carte blanche*. She did wish that she were as confident about depressing the Duke of Arden's pretensions as she had been with every other gentleman who had tried to seduce her.

Arden's case was different. He had not only kissed her; she had kissed *him*. She couldn't deny it, though she excused herself for the lapse. He was terribly attractive, and she had been watching him for weeks, indulging in schoolgirl dreams, even as he had admitted to observing her with his less innocent motives from the other side of the stage lights. It was only natural that she had lost her head for one brief moment and enjoyed herself in his arms.

How could she face him, though, with the proper icy reserve, when they both knew she had let herself go? Matilda was an honest girl. Yet she resolved, as she neared the greenroom, to be as distant and angry when returning the banknote as she would have been had she been completely innocent.

Matilda comforted herself with a stern reminder that this situation was her own fault for putting herself on the stage in the first place. Arden was simply one of the lumps in the bed she had made for herself—no, better not use that analogy, she chided herself as she stepped around a rolled-up backdrop and a huge coil of rope, drawing ever closer to the greenroom and the man she could feel awaited her there.

To act! It had seemed such a sensible plan when viewed from the grim spare room of the vicarage in Oxford.

Graham was a stage name. Matilda wished nothing

but honor to cling to the memory of her departed papa, and not for worlds would she bandy his respected surname about the boards. Though Aunt Poppy was her maternal great-aunt, Matilda insisted the old lady call herself "Graham" too, for the sake of privacy as well as simplicity.

On her father's death, when the pitiful state of his affairs was revealed, Matilda had clearly needed to find work. But as what?

Matilda had lost her mother at an early age, and her father hadn't hesitated to form the little girl in his image. He happened to be a learned classics tutor. Matilda's education, therefore, had fitted her for nothing so much as the life of a young men's preceptress. She had certainly picked up none of the feminine accomplishments so necessary to a modern governess. She could neither sing, nor play, nor sketch, nor had she ever longed to do so. The world of watercolors and fancy needlework was as mysterious to her as the land of the Eskimo—and as low on her list of places she wanted to explore.

The ladies of the parish assisted her in interviewing for several teaching positions, despite the fact that Greek, Latin, mathematics, and rhetoric were not considered indispensable to the education of those young ladies whose families could afford governesses.

Matilda was twenty-two, of quite a proper age to become a governess, but she looked sixteen. The combination of lush red-haired beauty, apparently excessive youth, and total ignorance of how a lady ought to be trained proved her undoing.

And though the kind vicar tried his best to aid her, a girl of her flamboyant looks was naturally unable to obtain a position as a tutor of young men.

Matilda searched through her scholarly past and realized that she did possess one frivolous skill. Her father had believed that young people should practice oratory by reciting the great works of Shakespeare and the Greek and Latin dramatists. His daughter had read and studied plays with him from an early age; and, what was more, she showed a decided bent for the art.

One day Matilda looked at herself in the mirror. Her red curls and full bosom seemed to shimmer back at her, defying her attempts to earn her living in a genteel way.

What choice did she have but to go on the stage?

She knew that by trying for such a position she would shock everyone in her native town; hence the change of name. And Aunt Poppy had had to go along, not only because there was nowhere in Oxford for the old lady to stay, but because Matilda was much too frightened to stray into the unknown world of London and playacting without some sort of companion.

Mr. Devlin, manager of the Royal George, the first minor theater Matilda tried once she arrived in London—she lacked the courage to go to Drury Lane or Covent Garden—was noted for preferring pulchritude to talent. He took a long look at Matilda and heard her read one scene. She later learned that, thanks to her looks, she probably would have been taken on had she been suffering from an acute constriction of the larynx.

Without a salary, only the customary board and lodging paid for her and, as a special mark of kindness, for her aunt, Matilda had begun her period of apprenticeship on the stage, acting at first in tiny roles, then graduating to minor speaking parts and finally to featured characters. She took to playacting naturally, as she had somehow known she would. The pose she maintained before Aunt Poppy, that acting was merely a necessary evil on the road to Oxford, became less honest by the day.

Now, six months later, Matilda could call herself a small success. Sundry plum roles went to her, for she, unlike most of her sister performers, could speak the lines with authority and move about without tripping over her own hem. And, the probationary period past, she was at last on her way to earning the dream which had brought her to London: the money to make her dear great-aunt's last days comfortable.

As the six months passed, another desire grew in Matilda, a wish she kept a dark secret from Aunt Poppy.

Matilda had discovered that more than financial need kept her on the stage. She loved to act, and she was good at it; the hours she spent lost in some play were more important to her than anything else. She couldn't bear the thought of giving up the stage for good; therefore, she would not. Though she still meant to go back to Oxford with her aunt as soon as they had enough money, she now intended to return to the theater someday, after Aunt Poppy had lived out her peaceful life in the company of a docile grandniece.

Many actresses found their greatest success after youth was past. Matilda would study her craft constantly. She would burst back upon the stage someday in a glory to equal that of Mrs. Siddons.

Matilda was thinking of this cherished secret as she pushed open the door to the greenroom. Blazing with light from a tawdry chandelier, the room seemed much less shabby by night than it did in the daytime, when every peeling place on the walls stood out. Now, if one but kept one's eyes half-shut, the crowds of people in evening dress made the greenroom seem to be the scene of an elegant rout party. The blend of exotic perfumes and masculine odors she had noticed the night before met Matilda's nose as the sound of shrill chattering assailed her ears.

As for her eyes, they were staring blankly into the handsome face towering above her. His grace of Arden had evidently been waiting just inside the door.

"Miss Graham! I was hoping you'd deign to honor us poor mortals tonight. Your performance was breathtaking as always, my dear." One hand reached up to his dark cropped curls, and he caressed the side of his head. "Absolutely stunning."

"How did you like the play?" Matilda asked.

He laughed in delight. Matilda noticed in irritation that at least a dozen knowing glances were shooting their way. In the minds of her fellow actresses and the bucks who attended them, she had already given herself to the duke. But the important thing was that she hadn't really done it, though she'd come uncomfortably close. There was no reason to become a loose woman simply because she'd been labeled one—and she had been so styled long before she had embroiled herself with the duke. Many respectable women graced the theatrical profession, and despite the drawback of her wanton looks, Matilda intended to be one of them.

"Duke," said Matilda, "give me your hand."

Arden's face seemed to light up like a candle. "Ah, cry pax, is it? I'm happy to do it, my dear. And then may we begin our friendship anew?"

He held out his gloved hand. Matilda shook it firmly, managing to transfer the tightly folded banknote from her palm to his without arousing any curiosity in the surrounding crowd.

He spoiled this subtlety by calmly taking the note and unfolding it. "Why, what is this?"

"It's your despicable money, you . . . you wicked libertine," Matilda snapped. Luckily she was an actress. While her words betrayed her anger, her face retained the blandest of social smiles. "How can you wave it about like that? Do put it in your pocket."

"Pardon me? Oh, the note." With a ribald chuckle, Arden obligingly folded the troublesome piece of paper and put it into the pocket of his corbeau-colored coat. "I'll keep it for you, if that's what you wish."

"It's not what I wish and you know it," Matilda said. "I want you to take it back. And in all fairness I must thank you for returning this gown. I would have had to pay for it if I'd lost it. And I'm grateful that you suffered no ill effects from . . . er, from last night."

Arden scrutinized the young woman, pleased that her last words had caused a blush to overspread her creamy skin. So she did desire him! Not that he had ever doubted it. The duke was a master of gauging women's reactions to his lovemaking, and this one had melted into his arms as though she were coming home.

Unfortunate that she'd also brained him with that decanter! Such coquetry would look like unwillingness to a lesser man.

"Oh." He raised his voice in response to her last remark. "I may be getting on in years, my dear, but never let it be said that I can't take even such a trial as you were pleased to offer me last night."

Necks swathed in highly starched cravats craned at the words, and there was an audible swish of silk as women also turned to stare at Arden and his companion in a sudden, unsettling silence.

Matilda struggled to maintain her air of queenly calm as her face, already rosy, turned scarlet with that speed which seems peculiar to redheads. Arden noted with interest that the flush stained even her lovely bosom.

Unfortunately, Matilda had a temper to match her hair. Her hand shot out. The Duke of Arden had never before received quite such a stinging slap. Matilda then stalked out of the room.

"Lovers' spat, Duke?" a raucous voice snickered from a nearby corner.

Arden, an idiotic smile bedecking his face, along with a fiery set of finger marks, turned toward the friend who had spoken. "Why, yes, my dear fellow. Quite the lovers' spat. I hadn't known she loved me quite that much."

3

"MY daughter, a duchess, my daughter, a duchess," said the Countess of Dauntry to herself. A short, round woman in fussy clothes, she sat in state among the chaperones in the gilded ballroom of Arden House in Cavendish Square.

These words were the charm Lady Dauntry always repeated when she was in the society of the duke's family. Despite their unassailable position in the *ton*, she had no fondness for the Ardens. She had loathed the old duke, thought the present duke a useless carouser, and detested the duchess. Eudocia had been a pompous stick long before she'd become a duchess, in fact ever since she and Lady Dauntry had been at school together.

But affection, or lack thereof, didn't alter the facts. Eudocia, Duchess of Arden, wanted only the best bloodlines for what she obviously considered her dynasty, and she had chosen as mate for her eldest son the Earl of Dauntry's only daughter, Davina, in whose rather prominent blue veins swirled most of the noblest blood in the kingdom.

The countess looked across the floor to where her daughter, the envy of all present, went down the dance with the Duke of Arden. A handsome devil, that one! No one could outshine him.

Chilly and well-bred, in a pale pink sarcenet gown chosen more for its high price than its attractions, Davina appeared, as usual, a cipher beside the magnificent duke. There was no doing much with Davina. The aristocratic bloodlines which the Duchess of Ar-

36

den so admired had evinced themselves, in Davina's case, by an excessive length of face and a nose which just missed the classic Grecian proportions by an inch or two. Lady Dauntry didn't trouble her mind over-much about her daughter's lack of personal beauties, though, for the girl's proposed marriage with the Duke of Arden would be a matter of business only.

If Arden wanted beauty, charm, and wit—and Davina, though intelligent enough, was tongue-tied in company—there were plenty of places he could get such things. The sordid dens where men, not except-ing Lord Dauntry, obtained companionship were le-gion. Lady Dauntry could not hold back a sneer, thinking of the fleshpots of London and the weakness of the male sex. In a determined mood, she continued with her internal chant: "My daughter, a duchess, my daughter, a duchess . . ."

Meanwhile Arden was smiling as he bowed over Lady Dauntry's daughter's hand. "Tell me, Lady Da-vina," he said, "does it ever bother you, the way our respective dams thrust us together for the good of En-gland?"

Lady Davina was examining the brilliant polished wood of the floor, her favorite pastime during dances. "It does become a little wearing," she returned. For an instant she looked up, and Arden thought he inter-cepted an honest gaze from large, clear blue eyes. She had shifted her attention back to her slippers before he could be certain. "You see, I don't like you either."

"My dear girl! I like you very well. How could it be otherwise, knowing the close connection between our families?" protested the duke. No need to men-tion that that close connection consisted of the matri-monial plotting of the two mothers and nothing else. "However, I am relieved that your fondness for *me* doesn't attain the heights of romantic fancy."

"Hardly that, Duke," Davina said.

Arden thought he detected a small smile; again, he couldn't be sure. It occurred to him that Davina, while not the woman of his dreams, did have her attractions.

"Well, my lady," he said, "it becomes clear that we ought to think on this problem. Our marriage would be a great waste of time, considering that neither one of us wishes it. Unless . . . can it be you're willing to bear with me in order to become a duchess?"

Davina looked at him in horror. "How can you say so, sir?" She paused, then added in her diffident way, "No one in my position, you see, could wish to do . . . that."

"Is that so?" Arden was surprised. According to his mother, not to mention the evidence of his own eyes, all young women of his class spent their waking hours scheming to attain that title which this lady professed to scorn.

Once more Davina directed her attention to the floor. She murmured, in so low a voice that his grace had to bend to hear her, "I ought to clarify that statement. I meant to say that I, personally, could never wish for the title of duchess. I've been taught from the cradle that I must strive with all my energies to become the Duchess of Arden. Do you blame me for not relishing the prospect?"

"Knowing your mother and my own," Arden said with a wise nod of his head, "I don't blame you at all. Well, my lady, this settles it. No matter how the storms of matchmaking toss us, we will not become man and wife."

"Oh, Duke!" Once more Davina favored him with the full power of her shining eyes as they came together in the dance. "Thank you."

"Think nothing of it." Arden's lips were twitching as he bowed to Lady Davina and turned aside to take his place in the line. If only all young ladies of marriageable age were as easy to please!

The Countess of Dauntry and the Duchess of Arden, from their different stations in the ballroom, sighed in happiness to see their children getting on so well. There they were, actually smiling as their hands met in time to the music. The duchess mentally dandled long-nosed grandchildren on her knee and traced their lineage back to the Conqueror. The countess merely envisioned Davina in coronet and purple robes of state. *Stand up straight, Davina,* hissed Lady Dauntry in her fancy, from the corner of an imaginary royal reception hall.

The dance ended, and Davina made her final curtsy. Then she allowed the duke to take her back to her mama. The couple's manners, as they walked across the ballroom floor, could only be described as friendly and intimate.

"Well, my child," said Lady Dauntry in eagerness as soon as they saw Arden's broad back, "what were you and the duke talking of so happily?"

"Nothing, Mama," Davina responded, frowning. She could hardly inform her mother that she and Arden had been discussing their mutual wish to avoid a marriage. A thought struck her. "We were merely talking of a joke he and some friends plan to play."

Lady Dauntry's eyes narrowed, but she caught herself before she made a snappish reference to the unbecoming levity of Arden and his intimate circle. "The dear duke," she said instead. "So playful, so charming."

Such a fribbet, Davina said to herself. She had given up arguing with Mama that Arden was not the man for her. How lucky that he seemed to feel the same! She had feared that the duke would go through with the marriage plot out of simple laziness, for a duke must marry someone. He might possibly even have shared his mother's absurd thoughts on old blood. Davina was

a secret student of physiology, and she thought her
family was much *too* old.

And though Davina had no confidence that she could
withstand the combined machinations of the Duchess
of Arden and her own mama, the duke would never
allow himself to be bullied and coerced into matrimony. It remained only to avoid being alone with him,
for Davina wouldn't put it past her mother to burst in
on any such *tête-à-tête* with cries of "compromise!"
to be followed shortly by the dissonant clanging of
wedding bells.

Davina did wish to marry, but she retained, at nineteen, a fancy that she would be better off wedded to a
man she could love and respect. Dreams of finding a
man who would be more her equal in looks also drifted
through Davina's mind in her most romantic moments.
She might be plain, but if the man of her dreams were
plain too, perhaps she wouldn't fade beside him. She
would simply disappear into the woodwork if she were
to marry the dashing Duke of Arden, for Davina considered that he outshone her mentally as well as phys-
ically. She did want to *exist* after her marriage.

Davina watched the duke's tall figure as he bowed
over the hand of another lady. In her gaze there was
something approaching fondness. How comfortable it
made her feel to have such a powerful ally as Arden
in her secret campaign not to become a duchess.

"Peterborough," the Duke of Arden was saying at
that moment, over his shoulder. "I'm going to ask you
and Waverman to help me in a little prank. We'll need
a great deal of pasteboard and some gilt paint."

The duke and Perry Peterborough were in the same
set of a quadrille. Their respective partners, nearly
identical damsels in white muslin gowns, rolled their
eyes and shrugged expressively behind the gentlemen's
backs.

"Gilt paint," said Lord Peterborough. "Pasteboard. What's it for?"

"An atrocious visual joke. Can you come by the stuff?"

"Easy as anything. Oh, your pardon, Miss Smythe."

"Miss Smytton," snapped his partner, tossing pale blond curls. "You've quite injured my foot, Lord Peterborough. Please return me to my mama. I have *no* desire to finish out this set."

Miss Smytton limped away. Either Peterborough had trodden hard on her toe, or she wished for a bit of drama.

"I say, ma'am." Peterborough, a large rawboned young man, hurried after the angry young lady, blundering between a pair of dancers. This left Arden, *his* partner, and the other two couples in the figure to bow to the air for a quarter of the remaining time. Thanks to Arden, it became an amusing jest to dance with the invisible couple, and his set ended the selection in high good humor.

After delivering his little blond partner, Miss What's-her-name, into the sheltering presence of her hatchet-faced dragon, Arden strolled about the richly appointed public rooms of Arden House, nodding to the occasional guest and feeling virtuous. He had danced with sundry young ladies, each one picked out by his mother. He had distinguished Lady Davina twice, and, what was more, he had finally gotten some indication that she thought as little of him as he did of her. Not that he didn't like the girl. If she could only keep from shrinking and shivering in his presence, he thought she might possess a creditable wit and even some personal attractions. But he would never marry her.

A shame for Lady Davina's second Season to be wasted in pursuit of his noble self, as her first had been. Her mother, with the lure of a dukedom to blind her, would never let Davina accept another.

There must be a way to set Lady Davina free of him, free to entertain other suitors and enjoy herself. Perhaps she would even perk up, look less wilted and hopeless, if she were cut loose from the web of expectations her mother and Arden's had entangled her in.

He could marry another . . . No, no need to go that far.

Arden furrowed his brow in deep thought. He and Lady Davina could kneel before their assembled relations and declare their mutual indifference . . .

"I say, Michael," spoke up two youthful voices in unison.

Arden started. "Boys! What the devil are you doing out of Cambridge? Didn't your tutor chain you up at night as he was told?"

Before the duke stood his youngest brothers, Lords Paul and Peter Beresford. "The fair-haired boys," Arden always called them in his mind. They were the only light-complexioned children in the family, besides being their mother's favorites. The twins had curling hair of dark blond, the family eyes of velvet brown, and tall, thin physiques which would perhaps fill out in time. They were eighteen.

They were dressed as they usually were, for effect, in identical foppish gear. Bright blue coats with extremely padded shoulders and large gleaming buttons; decorated brocade waistcoats, one yellow embroidered in purple, the other purple embroidered in yellow; cravats tied in an ornate and foolish style of their joint invention, which they had named "The Gemini Knot"; and pearl-colored breeches and stockings which fit their slim, strong legs like a second skin. Identical fobs and seals hung from opposite waistcoat pockets. The boys enjoyed the mirror-image ploy, which tended to make those who stared at them at first keep staring, in confusion.

"We've come down, Michael," said Paul.

"We weren't sent down, either," said Peter.

"We simply left."

"Mama says we're naughty, but welcome."

"Mama would," said the duke. He glared with what he hoped was parental disapprobation. Only before these boys did he play the Stern Duke. It was his duty, for they had lost their father much too young. At least, so his mother occasionally affirmed to excuse the twins' rampant truancy.

Arden was no stranger to pranks. Nor did he recall much fatherly advice from the last duke, who had been a remote and mostly absent figure in the lives of his sons. Even Mama hadn't appeared to miss her husband when he had died, rather suddenly, on a trip to London. (Rumor had it, in the bed of a courtesan, but the family never inquired too closely, fearing they would unearth the name of the respected peeress who had been old Arden's very good friend for several years.)

But whether Father had fulfilled his position as parent was not at issue here. Obviously a firm hand was needed with the twins. Unlike Arden, they hadn't grown up in an atmosphere of frozen nobility and stern tutelage. Their mother's last babies, they were the first to come to her attention. They had been spoiled from the cradle, and, as a result, were not inclined to think themselves less than perfect, nor their schooling anything but a waste of time.

At least they didn't go in for playing practical jokes. Arden would have been quite unable to take his young brothers to task for a failing he luxuriated in himself, and he was pleased to stand in an unassailable position to lecture them on their besetting sin. Dash it all, he might not be the most serious of young men today, but he had stuck it out at Harrow and at Cambridge until something more than a garish taste in clothes had sunk in.

"You'll go back tomorrow, *and* under the escort of my secretary," he said.

The boys still whined upon occasion.

"Deuce take it, Mama wants us here," Paul offered in that peculiarly irritating tone of voice, as Peter mewled out something which sounded profane.

"And Father's will stated you be educated at Cambridge, and so you shall be," Arden responded, implacable in his role of adoptive parent. "Let Mama dandle you in the long vacations, but during terms, stay put! Good Lord, you were always bolting out of Harrow too, and that was during Father's lifetime, so I don't know why she continues to excuse you as poor little orphans."

Peter and Paul both had the grace to blush while they gave each other sidelong glances.

"I know you feed her with that sort of talk too," Arden said with a long-suffering sigh he did not quite feel.

The twins looked up (they were half a head shorter than Arden), seeming to sense the lack of real rebuke in their elder brother's manner. "One day?" Paul asked plaintively.

"Well—"

"Perry Peterborough says you're planning a famous joke. Can't we help you on that and then go back?" asked Peter with great eagerness.

"Hmm." Arden paused to consider the request. Dandies were supposed to be indolent, and as budding dandies Lord Peter and Lord Paul were becoming more consciously languid with time, an irritating pose which Arden often longed to quash. Now, for once, they were practically jumping up and down in excitement. Their brother wondered if he shouldn't encourage them in this rare enthusiasm. And he could use them, as it happened.

One major flaw in his newest plan—the one involving the pasteboard and the gilt paint—was the need for a small and agile man to climb up high at one point in the scheme. The duke was a large man; Peterborough was even bigger; and Waverman, their other constant companion in joking, was round and ungainly. Peter and Paul were not small, but they were light and very wiry, with taut muscles trained by fencing.

"You may stay in town one day," said Arden. "And you may help me." His tone was that of royalty bestowing a boon. "And now," he added when the twins had thanked him, "seeing as you're here at a ball, make yourselves useful. Go over there and dance with Lady Davina Lowden."

"Nay," said Peter.

Paul brayed out the actual sound of a horse, neatly giving away the joke in case their aging brother had turned into a slow-top.

Arden groaned. He only enjoyed those atrocious puns which were executed by himself. Besides, in all fairness to Lady Davina, her equine qualities were highly exaggerated. "Do not, if you please, behave in such a way as to convince the world that you aren't gentlemen. Peter, the next dance," he said sternly. "Paul, the one after. That is, if the lady will consent to stand up with such infants."

The lads balked, but knowing that Michael had the power to send them packing on the instant, they were soon bowing in unison over the hand of an astonished Lady Davina. Arden, watching from across the room, smiled at her slack jaw and blank stare. Not far from Davina, he could see his mother beaming on her two gallant sons.

Arden turned his mind to the vastly more intriguing prospect of a certain actress. Matilda Graham was not a dancer, yet she had been pirouetting through his mind all the evening. He would go to see her now; would the play still be going on? A glance at his slim pocket watch informed him it would not. And he knew she had no part in the farce of the greenroom—unless, of course, she were summoned there by a special message.

He had a feeling she would no longer be enticed there by any message from him; and he didn't really blame her.

Miss Graham would have to wait until tomorrow night.

The duke decided that, all things considered, he would go on back to the Albany and read. No man would accuse him of not honoring his mother's ball to the best of his ability.

He began to hum in harmony with the Scottish reel now being danced to by a remarkably dull-looking set of people. Would Miss Graham yield to him soon? The vixen was driving him into a very pleasant state of frenzy.

4

MATILDA'S head emerged from the billowing white nightrobe. She suspected that Papa was at this very moment turning over in his grave.

Never in the history of the London theater, at least not since the days of boys in female roles, had a more unlikely Lady Macbeth trodden the boards. The reputation of the great Siddons seemed to taunt Matilda as she prepared to do her final scene in this plum role: the sleepwalking scene.

Luckily for Matilda's finer feelings, her idolized Mrs. Siddons had chosen to retire from the stage this year, in the wake of the Old Prince riots at the new Covent Garden. Siddons wasn't even in town, and Matilda hoped she would never hear of the very different interpretation a certain Miss Graham was giving to Lady Macbeth this season.

"I look like a dairymaid," she had protested to the manager when the question of casting this part came up.

"You know the lines already, and you're the only one can speak 'em without sounding like a ninny," Mr. Devlin retorted, and the decision was made. Mr. Frye, the company's lead actor, was a popular Macbeth, and Frye was insisting on a revival of the play. A Lady Macbeth had to be found, and quickly.

Matilda had learned a thing or two in her time on the stage, and she pretended to a little more reluctance in an effort to get more money. To her astonishment, it worked.

"You have red hair," one of the actors pointed out. "Lady Macbeth is supposed to be Scottish."

But Matilda shook her copper curls in doubt, fearing that a buxom, cheerful-looking Lady Macbeth bouncing around the stage would draw ridicule, not admiration.

For some reason unfathomable to Matilda, derision had not greeted her the other night when the play opened. She didn't realize it, but in this part she proved that she was, indeed, an actress. *Macbeth* had always been one of Matilda's favorite plays, fascinating in its tragic intensity, and her involvement showed.

Her lovely face turned set and cold in murderous intent, provoking at least one buck to wonder what he'd ever seen in her. Her green eyes blazed strangely, and her gestures, if not her appearance, were regal when she played Lady Macbeth as the queen. No, she wasn't Siddons by any means, but more than one theater buff said she made a perfect Lady Macbeth, if Lady Macbeth had been a rapacious child bride. And why should she not have been?

"Oh, don't you look nice," said Aunt Poppy as Matilda adjusted the nightgown. "Now, here is your candle, dear."

Nice? Matilda glanced down at herself. She was supposed to look deranged, but there was only so much that could be done with clothing. She had rumpled up her waves of red hair, and they hung down her back and over her breasts, which were adequately covered, for once in her stage career, by this virtual bale of cheap muslin chosen to resemble a medieval nightdress. This production of *Macbeth* was making a gesture to historically accurate costuming, a fact which had been made much of in the advertisements. Mr. Frye was appearing in a kilt as Macbeth and had caused a mild furor until theater buffs recalled that the great Macklin had performed the same role in Old Scottish costume over thirty years before.

Matilda pulled at her huge nightgown for one last time, accepted the candle, kissed Aunt Poppy on the forehead, and hurried on her way to the wings, leaving the old lady peacefully mending one of Matilda's costumes.

" 'Dagger I see before me,' " Matilda was murmuring as she marched along in her bare feet. Tonight Mr. Devlin had ordered her to lengthen her last scene by repeating part of Macbeth's soliloquy from Act II.

"That's a silly notion," Matilda had said frankly, thinking of her father's lectures on the purity of Shakespeare's poetry. She knew that the Bard's works were rarely left untouched for the popular market, but she still felt obliged to defend the great man.

"No such thing, m'dear. The crowd wants more of you, and we have to take the words from somewhere. We have it that you overhear Macbeth saying the piece. What more natural than repeating it in your mad sleepwalking? Er, I mean, Lady Macbeth's."

Was it only fancy, or did Devlin look a touch uncomfortable? Matilda wondered uneasily if one of her admirers—possibly even the Duke of Arden!—had bribed the company to lengthen her part. Well, she supposed there was no harm in it, and at least the extra lines were from the play. She wouldn't have put it past Devlin to make up new words for the occasion, and that she couldn't have borne.

Matilda was reflecting, as she reached the wings and heard the first lines of the Gentlewoman and the Doctor which preceded her own entrance, that one benefit of her encounters with the Duke of Arden was that other bucks of the *ton* had stopped pursuing her, presumably giving way to rank. For the past days, ever since she had lost her temper, delivered that slap to the duke's teasing face, and thus convinced every witness that she was his lover, not one bouquet or insistent note had been delivered to her dressing room, nor had her hackney coach been pursued down the streets after the performance. She hadn't been so comfortable since the first weeks of her London stay, before she had come into the fashion.

And since she was an actress anyway, what did it matter that her reputation was ruined? It was only the reputation of the fictional "Miss Graham," and, more important in Matilda's view, the rumors were not true.

It was probably the most convenient affair, from a balky virgin's point of view, in the history of the world. Matilda's greatest discomfort was her own unruly mind, for she had to admit to a little twinge of disappointment whenever she found the duke's box empty. Not only must she feel such a disagreeable emotion, she was wont to search the society columns of a newspaper filched from the porter until she could discover the reason for his absence. Even worse, on her first appearance this evening Matilda had been immeasurably pleased that the infuriating duke was once more leering down at her from his accustomed box to the right of the stage.

Someone standing near her struck a flint and lit her candle; Matilda took her usual two steps backward, then walked out onto a stage adorned by an illusionist backdrop of winding castle corridors. All thoughts of the duke fled, and Miss Graham the actress was deep in her role.

Her short scene was nearing its end; she had wrung her hands and rubbed in vain, trying to take off the imagined blood. Matilda inwardly shuddered and began her patched-on, supposedly raving version of Macbeth's earlier speech.

" 'Is this a dagger which I see before me, the handle toward my hand?' " Matilda's clear voice rang out, aquaver with maddened emotion as Lady Macbeth lived through her husband's earlier torment in her dreams. Those of the audience who were watching the performance were leaning forward, fascinated.

Something creaked, and Matilda, lost in the personality of Lady Macbeth, her eyes half-shut, didn't even notice the six-foot pasteboard dagger until it had been lowered all the way to the stage, directly in front of her.

After staring for one blank moment into a wall of gilt, Matilda glanced sharply upward. There, in the rafters, sat two elegantly dressed boys with light curls. They looked like nothing so much as leering, if skinny, cupids. Both young men were chuckling so much that they shook slightly on their unsteady perch.

There was no doubt in Matilda's mind as to who had perpetrated this. Instantly she knew whose coins had greased Mr. Devlin's palm and led to her additional lines this evening. Stepping majestically in front of the giant dagger—how thorough of the wretch to have it painted gold on both sides!—she threw one pained glance up to a certain box and was met by laughing brown eyes.

"Touché," Matilda muttered, looking into those eyes, and somehow she knew he understood her.

The duke and two other elegant gentlemen who sat beside him were clutching their sides in helpless laughter as Matilda resolutely went back to her role, to the admiration of the astonished Gentlewoman and Doctor. She raved out the rest of the Macbeth speech, casting her eyes only once above her head. The two curly-headed boys had disappeared.

She noticed through the haze of her stage manner that the Doctor's and the Gentlewoman's comments on Lady Macbeth's unhappy state of mind were uttered in slightly hysterical tones.

Her last speech! Matilda rushed through it, desperate to get off the stage. Then she noticed something

else as she urged an invisible Macbeth "to bed, to
bed, to bed": only a few members of the audience,
notably the raucous bucks and tulips in the pit, were
joining that shameless duke and his companions in
hearty laughter. Most of the spectators either blandly
surveyed the stage, or talked with others in that insouciant manner, typical of a theater crowd, which so in-
furiated Matilda ordinarily.

Either they thought the dagger was an ordinary stage
property or they hadn't even noticed it being lowered
at the crucial moment.

Matilda lost control and choked back giggles. One
or two people remarked that her shoulders were shaking as she made her somnambulant way offstage.

Putting the candle into the hands of the first person
she saw, Matilda ran back to her dressing room, alter-
nately laughing and wanting to cry. That man! How
dared he ruin her performance? She would have something to say to Mr. Devlin about this horrid prank,
though she had to admit that anyone, especially a
struggling theater manager, would have found it difficult to resist the commands of the Duke of Arden.

Despite all her better feelings of outrage, something
inside Matilda reached out to the duke and agreed that
this had, indeed, been a splendid if stupid joke, not
only on her, but on those idiotish theatergoers who
were so used to adulterated jumbles of Shakespeare,
not to mention the socializing which really brought
them to the play, that they hadn't even noticed that
giant paper dagger. Matilda had to stop outside her
dressing-room door and compose herself, for she was
still giggling wildly, and there were tears running down
her painted cheeks. No need to alarm Aunt Poppy.

As it happened, Aunt Poppy had already been startled out of her habitual state of calm. When Matilda
opened the door, it was onto a bright world of flowers.

"Matilda!" cried her aunt, appearing like a gray

deer through a thicket of roses. "Some duke sent all these."

Matilda nodded, and she had to wander around for a moment. Here was every sort of flower she had ever imagined. Early in the season as it was, most of the blooms must have come from hothouses. Hundreds of pounds were represented in the roses and lilies and lilacs and orchids which greeted the eye on every side, arranged on the floor in vases and baskets and adorning the few sticks of furniture. There were even several potted plants. Each bouquet had a card attached. Matilda looked at one.

"Your slave," was the two-word message on the back of the ducal calling card pinned on a silk ribbon to a dozen white roses. He wrote a strong scrawl.

"Fustian," sniffed Matilda, half to herself. "It's his slave he means *me* to be."

"Dear, what did you say?" Her aunt fluttered up. She had wreathed her gray hair with a garland of jonquils and was clutching a nosegay of violets, and she looked happier than Matilda had ever seen her.

"I said, at least you appreciate the duke's gifts, Auntie," Matilda improvised with a smile. "Do you know why he sent them?" She hoped she wouldn't have to detail the duke's black plan to her innocent old relation. Certainly Aunt couldn't be naive enough to think that this many flowers were an offering of anyone with a respectful purpose.

Nor was she. Aunt Poppy's face was thoughtful above the violets. "Well, I suppose it's an improper proposal. So many flowers, after all! But flowers aren't a thing you must return, so I say you're lucky, my dear. He could have sent diamonds, and then we shouldn't have had all these pretty blossoms for our very own."

"There is that," said Matilda, looking into her

aunt's bright countenance. No, she wouldn't send the flowers back.

The play would be nearly over, and Matilda had to run back for her curtain call, leaving Aunt Poppy to rove at will in the strange garden. Matilda's sympathy with the duke's joke disappeared and her temper blazed when she saw Arden's wide and knowing smile above his clapping hands. He was as sure of himself as though she'd shouted from behind the stage lights that she would be his this evening. And did he have to wave? She and the other cast members took their bows, Matilda wishing she knew of some way to teach the duke a lesson.

How could any man, however arrogant, think that his dreadful sense of humor and misplaced gifts of flowers would open all doors? There was no doubt in Matilda's mind that the duke had directed one of his renowned tasteless jokes at her as a very public form of lovemaking. He was determined to make Matilda his mistress; he might as well have written *that* on one of his cards, and Matilda was positive his assurance would have made her dig in her heels even if she, like most of the other actresses, were on the lookout for a rich protector.

It was merely her misfortune that her tormentor was a most attractive man, a man whose mind she understood in some strange way and whose kisses had been haunting her dreams ever since that disturbing night of their first meeting.

Back in the dressing room, Aunt Poppy was still humming about in the forest of flowers. Matilda shook her head in fond amusement, stripped off her costume, and put on the ancient cotton wrapper which was her only form of dishabille. She began to wander at her leisure, reading a card here and there.

"Darling, do not be bitter," said the card clipped to a miniature lemon tree.

"You have pierced my heart like a dagger," was the particularly unsubtle message attached to a spray of white orchids. Those lush flowers seemed embarrassingly lewd to Matilda, with their long tongues and heated, tropical look. She had never before seen an orchid, except in the illustrations in botany books.

"Several of the girls have stopped in to see the flowers," chatted Aunt Poppy, appearing behind the orchids with a pretty pot of heartsease in her hand. "By the way, this one says, 'Pansies, that's for thoughts.' How very literary of the dear duke."

"He is *not* the 'dear duke,' " Matilda said sharply. She was relieved that the other actresses had already made their visits. She wasn't on easy terms with more than a few of them, and they would all be dressing for the greenroom by now if not acting in the afterpiece, so she might expect no more curious callers. That was lucky, for she didn't think she could stand playing the innocent—or even the pleased mistress—before any sharp eyes tonight.

"Oh, I know that whoever he is, he must be a terrible libertine," said Aunt Poppy, setting down the pot and picking up another one, brimming with sweet william. "Still, so many flowers. And we do know, my sweet, that he is bound to get the wrong idea with you up on that stage for all the world to see."

"To be sure." Matilda glanced about. "I can't see the couch, Aunt. Is it still here? They didn't move it out to make room for these wretched things?" It would be tragic to lose her couch! And she somehow felt that more than one member of the company would be eager to deprive her of the ancient, moth-chewed thing. A sofa was an amenity not many people in the theater were lucky enough to possess.

So, for that matter, was a private dressing room. Matilda was well aware that she owed Aunt Poppy thanks for their little luxuries, for the old lady had

brought out the chivalry in more than one jaded actor.
Miss Graham's duenna was the pet of the company.

"The couch is right behind these lovely lilacs and
these tall lilies," Aunt Poppy informed her niece,
moving some vases about to uncover the disreputable
piece of furniture. "Do you want to lie down, my
love?"

"Yes. I . . . I have the headache," Matilda said. In
reality she wanted to stay put in this room until much
later, when the greenroom would be cleared and the
theater quiet. She couldn't face anyone quite yet.

And foremost on her list of people she couldn't face
was the Duke of Arden, who, some instinct told her,
would be waiting in the greenroom.

"Poor dear. Here, Matilda, you shall lie down with
your head in my lap, and I'll tell you a story."

Matilda was glad enough to obey. Aunt Poppy loved
to tell stories, and her reedlike voice, in combination
with the heavy floral scents pervading the room, would
soon drug Matilda into a much-needed sleep. She was
suddenly as weary as she had ever been in her life; the
aftermath, no doubt, of that trauma on stage.

"Once upon a time, there were five sisters," began
Aunt Poppy, stroking Matilda's forehead with a gentle
hand. "Each one more lovely than the last, and every
one as beautiful as a flower."

Matilda smiled. It was Aunt Poppy's favorite story.
She could almost see the famous Gainsborough portrait Aunt had told her about so many times. *A Garden
of Flowers,* it was called, and there the five sisters,
each named for a flower, sat or stood or played on
swings in a bower of leaves and birds and sunny summer sky. Matilda closed her eyes and, for an instant,
did see their pretty panniered dresses, their bright
faces, their powdered curls. What a shame the picture
had been lost.

Aunt Poppy's voice droned on. Matilda fell asleep,

thinking, not of flowers nor the pretty girls of fifty years gone by, but of a certain darkly handsome duke who seemed to have gotten into the garden, pushed the phantom sisters out, and now stood alone, taunting Matilda with his crooked, enchanting smile.

5

MATILDA struggled into consciousness. Something was trailing over her face. A spider? Horrors—not a mouse?

Her eyes opened wide. Rubbing at her face, she stared directly into the smiling countenance of the Duke of Arden, positioned about two inches from her own and oddly shadowed in the wavering light of the one candle which lit the little room.

"You've been kissing me," said Matilda in a tone of voice which might have been employed to tell him his trousers were undone. She couldn't hold back a sigh of relief that she had not felt some one of the crawling creatures with which this theater was fully staffed. "Where is my aunt?"

"Aunt?" Arden's glance was very tender. He reached out one hand and smoothed the young woman's hair back from her face, ignoring the fact that she immediately drew away. "Oh, yes, the aunt." He remembered now that Miss Graham had propounded the existence of that mythical person on the night of their meeting. "Er, she must have stepped out."

Matilda sat up, craning her neck to get a view over the masses of flowers. Aunt Poppy was nowhere to be seen. Arden had slipped in past the dragon.

"Thank you for the flowers," Matilda said grudgingly. She did her best to ignore the fact that this wonderfully handsome man was kneeling right at her feet.

"A mere nothing, my dear. I wish you'd allow me to give you much, much more," was the suave and smiling reply.

Looking down at her tightly folded hands, Matilda said, "Your wishes are nowhere near my own. I thought I'd made that clear."

"You have—and you haven't," Arden said. With an agile movement he rose to sit beside Matilda on the sofa. He put his arm around her waist, bent his head to hers, and kissed her ever so gently.

Matilda, caught off her guard, responded. And if that weren't shaming enough, she had no chance to shove him away with angry exclamations, for he released her very soon.

"You see? Your kisses are very friendly. Whatever is a man to think?" The duke was still smiling in that infuriating way of his. In an obvious pretense of propriety, he moved a safe distance away from Matilda and waited for her reply.

"I know what you think, and why you think it," Matilda said. "I'm an actress. Naturally you believe that I'm no better than I should be, and that if I haven't a protector now it's because I've been waiting for the most lucrative offer. But I assure you, sir, that simply isn't the case. I never went into the greenroom in my life, except to see you about that . . . that hundred pounds. And I'm sorry if I've given you cause to think your . . . your attentions would be welcome—" Matilda broke off with a nearly hysterical laugh. It struck her how similar her words were to those a young lady might use to turn down an offer of marriage. "Well, what do you expect if you *will* keep kissing me?" she finished crossly.

"Oh, no more than what I've gotten," the duke said airily. "The truth. From your own lips, as it were. I've been waiting for you in the greenroom for hours, my dear. Everyone in the theater has gone home, except for the rather surly old curmudgeon who guards the door and told me where I could find you. Won't you reward my patience, love—tonight?"

All at once he was beside Matilda again. His hands seemed to burn through the thin material of her wrapper; she couldn't quite remember what the world was like outside his broad chest and strong, sheltering arms. His face was descending again, and if he kissed her one more time, Matilda didn't know if she could trust herself. Extremely helpful was the knowledge that Aunt Poppy must be very nearby and would return at any moment, but even so, this was danger!

"No," said Matilda. One of her hands reached up to stop the duke's face in its progress, and she let out a helpless little whoop at the sight of his aristocratic nose peeking through her small white fingers.

The duke deftly removed her hand and encased it between his own, disturbing Matilda further. "And why not? You seem to be a bit touchy about appearances; here it is late enough that no one but the mice will see us leaving."

"I wish you wouldn't mention mice," said Matilda. "I thought you were . . . That is, they give me the shivers."

"Anything you wish. The word will never pass my lips again," Arden murmured, kissing her hand as he gave her a long, intense look. "Shall I help you dress, my sweet?"

"No." Matilda, not knowing how else to get away from those dancing dark eyes, wrenched her hand away, stood up, and turned her back. She stared into a bank of flowers. "I want you to leave, Duke. Now. I'm not . . . I couldn't possibly . . . Oh, I hate you!"

"Whatever your true opinion on the subject of my humble self, I can assure you hatred is not uppermost in your mind," the duke said. Matilda started as she heard him rise from the creaky sofa, and then she felt his hands on her shoulders and heard his next words whispered into her ear. "You keep resisting. Why? Is it the terms? I'll be as definite as you wish, and as generous. You mustn't forget this will be quite a coup for you. Think of it! A duke for your first protector. And I need you, my dear. I do wish you'd come with me now.''

"I suspect it is high time, Duke, that you learned your wishes won't open all doors. Why, you haven't even asked my pardon for that terrible joke you played this evening.''

He chuckled. "That was rather awful, wasn't it? I simply couldn't resist. And I had a spot of trouble, you know. The other night when I saw the play, I was sure Lady Macbeth was the one who did the dagger speech. Shows you that I was enraptured by your charms, and not paying attention. And when I was going through the play to find the exact scene when the boys should drop the dagger—those were my agile young brothers up there in the rafters . . . I saw you looking—I came to find out Macbeth says the dagger thing! And while I have every reason to believe your Mr. Frye has a fine sense of humor, he wasn't the one I wanted to—''

"Humiliate," supplied Matilda, stepping out of his arms and turning to face him once again. "Why, if more people had noticed, I would have been so very, very embarrassed . . .'' Her words trailed away, and she let a laugh escape her. The truth was, she hadn't been very embarrassed at all once she had seen that hardly anyone had remarked the prank. All those bland, bejeweled people on the other side of the footlights, so engrossed in their social activities that they didn't even notice the worst and most obvious joke in the world! Matilda clapped a hand over her mouth to stifle another giggle.

"It was amusing, wasn't it?" Arden stepped forward and reached out his arms again, but Matilda parried his advance and stepped behind a bank of gladioli.

"It was awful," she lied. "Now, get out, Duke, if

you please. And I do thank you for the flowers. A bit
excessive, perhaps, but I'll accept them as an apology
for what you put me through tonight. We actors like
to lose ourselves in the roles, you know. It was quite
upsetting to suddenly have a huge piece of pasteboard
appear in front of me.''

''My apologies, of course, ma'am,'' said the duke
with a smile that absolutely denied any such sentiments. ''And if you must know, I'd planned to have
the thing lowered in back of you. I know how actors
are. But my rapscallion brothers can never get anything the way it's supposed to be. Now, then. Am I
really to go? Wouldn't it be more pleasant to begin
now? Perhaps even here, in the midst of all these flowers. Though you're so lovely that you make all these
blooms pale by comparison.''

Matilda rolled her eyes. Here she was, tangled hair,
threadbare wrapper, and smudged paint, being told she
was lovely! Men would stick at nothing, then, when
bent upon seduction. How sickening. Her anger
mounted as she pictured the scene Aunt Poppy would
witness if Matilda were really to give herself to the
duke here in this room.

Surely Aunt would be returning any moment. The
duke must leave!

''Duke, my wish is that you go now,'' she said in
her clearest voice. ''You say you want to please me—''

''Coquette!'' The duke, his smile widening, bent
over the tall blooms that separated them and managed
to snatch Matilda's face between his hands. Briefly he
kissed her on the lips. Then he bowed, picked up his
hat from somewhere, and crossed the room. He paused
with his hand on the door. ''I do want to please you,
you know,'' he said with a last glance full of tender
meaning. Then he left he room.

Matilda pressed her hands to her cheeks. Why had

no one told her it would be so hard to remain a virtuous woman? It had been easy until now. All she had had to do was refuse to answer the many pleas which had been bombarding her since her first appearance on the stage. Nobody had been insistent; in the world of the theater, people seemed to accept that an actress would hold out for the best offer possible. The bucks and rakes understood this as well as Matilda's colleagues.

And now she had a handsome duke, not only filling her room with flowers but also making known to her for the first time a valid reason for whistling virtue down the wind.

The audacious thought sneaked its way into Matilda's consciousness. Being a fallen woman could be fun!

"Drat that man," Matilda said. And then she turned to smile, in the last light of the room's one guttering candle, as the door opened again and Aunt Poppy entered with a confused and too vivid account of her trip to the convenience.

When Matilda rose from her lumpy, chaste bed next morning, she was more than angry at his grace of Arden. She was furious. She hadn't seemed to get through to him at all in their encounter the night before. She had said no, she had told him to leave her, but somehow she still knew that, across town in the Albany, the Duke of Arden was sleeping late in the assurance that Matilda Graham, actress, would become his mistress. Not that this wasn't partly Matilda's fault. She had not been cold and rigid in his arms as any proper lady would have been when fighting off improper advances.

Matilda suspected she was really more angry at herself than at the duke. However, he made an excellent and deserving outlet for her rage.

Staggering across the room with heavy-lidded eyes—
Matilda was not a person who awoke with the birds,
eager to begin her day—she got out pen and ink and
one of the few pieces of hand-pressed paper she had
brought with her from Oxford. Sitting down under the
one window where the light was best, she wrote:

Your grace,
 Perhaps if you were to busy yourself in some worthy
 occupation you wouldn't feel the need to play stupid,
 irritating pranks on virtual strangers. I will never, ever
 become your mistress.

Respectfully,
 M. Graham

When Matilda read the letter over a bit later, after
her eyes had opened wider, the words struck her as
confused and lacking in style. She decided to send the
missive anyway. It expressed her opinions and wishes
clearly enough.

If she had known that the letter, when it arrived by
the two-penny post at Arden's residence, would have
the opposite effect from the one she intended, she
would have thrown it into the fire rather than send it.

"She cares," said the Duke of Arden, pressing the
letter to his heart in a melodramatic manner. "She
cares, Finley."

Mr. Finley nodded. The duke's thin, dry-looking
middle-aged secretary was an inheritance from Arden's father. "Very good, your grace." The man's ears
were still red from having opened by mistake a letter
from a female—and a female of easy virtue, from the
sound of it! Normally Finley laid aside all letters that
were highly scented or written in an obviously feminine hand. This one had been on plain paper and

penned in a scholarly script the secretary never would have identified as written by one of the fair sex.

Finley was somewhat embarrassed, also, to have read the letter-writer's suggestions to the duke, hints which so neatly summed up what he, Finley, had been thinking for years. His grace did need some active occupation other than practical jokes. His grace's father, for that matter, could have benefited from an occupation other than that of the latest crop of lightskirts.

"You see, my excellent Finley, my best of Finleys, why would she bother to write a cautionary letter to a man she didn't like?" The duke was taking his ease in his study, the same heavily paneled book-lined room he had ushered Miss Graham into not so many days before. He leaned back in his chair, drawing the letter back and forth in his fingers.

"Why, indeed, your grace." Finley stood at attention awaiting orders. His grace was waxing rhapsodic today, sure sign of an imminent practical joke. Finley was rarely used in any capacity in the preparation and finalizing of such amusements; his grace had his circle of friends for that. But Finley knew that, until said prank should have been played—as they always were, to his grace's satisfaction—there would be no dealing in matters of business.

Finley spent remarkably little time regaling his grace of Arden with estate matters. He was in closer communication with Mr. Slump, the man of business, and Mr. Fitzhubert, the land agent, than he was with the young man in whose name all these arrangements took place.

"Finley, sit down," said the Duke of Arden.

The secretary obeyed, choosing the hardest chair in the room to pull up near the ducal desk.

"If you could see her!" Arden said, his eyes going out of focus as he contemplated the charms of this newest conquest. "She's loveliness itself. Quite a fighter too."

Finley coughed and looked at the red Turkey carpet. He didn't care to know about his employer's quirks in the area of, er, congress.

"Last night I almost had her," the duke continued. "I daresay I would've, but her pride as an actress got in the way. It was the dagger, you see. I'll admit even I didn't picture it as being quite so big."

Finley nodded, not at all certain what his grace was saying, and not sure he wanted to know. He had not been in on the *Macbeth* plot and wondered uneasily if "dagger" was a new slang expression.

"And now," said Arden, "I feel the best thing to do is to let the young woman cool off, as it were, for a short time while I prepare everything for her reception. I'm sending you out today to rent a pretty house, Finley. In a fairly fashionable street; you know the sort of thing."

"I will confess I do, sir," said Finley. "Your late father made many such arrangements, if you'll forgive the reference."

"I do know of Father's peccadilloes. As it happens, I haven't yet had to set up a mistress from the ground up, so to speak. Always seem to hit upon the ones who have their own houses. I rely upon you, my most diligent Finley. When you have the house, it will need to be decorated in the first style. Come to me when you have the property in hand, and I'll take it from there."

The secretary stared. "Does your grace mean to take part in the decoration of the house? I would be happy to—as I always did for your father . . ."

"Ah, but this lady is special," the duke said. "I want to choose everything myself. And then there's the matter of her wardrobe . . . Do you know what I think, Finley?"

"Your grace?"

"This has all the appearance of an amusing diversion. Oh, and speaking of that, send round this note to Lord Peterborough, by a footman. Fred Farquhar, my old friend from Cambridge, has a wedding soon, you know. We'd hate to think of it coming off without one of our special little touches."

"Quite, your grace." And, his face wooden, Finley went off to do his master's bidding.

The Duke of Arden was left to meditate on Matilda's letter and to wish he had someone besides his cold fish of a secretary to confide in.

"M. Graham," indeed! Quite an inappropriate signature for the owner of a body that luscious, a face that enchanting.

How odd this little play was! Did she truly think that the Duke of Arden, who had been on the town for over ten years, would be taken in by the pose of innocence from a stage actress? She meant to dictate terms to him by pretending reluctance. Arden could think of no other excuse for her behavior.

She would find the terms mighty generous. And the duke didn't doubt that Miss Graham would be worth every penny he was about to spend in pursuit of her favors.

6

WHILE the Duke of Arden's plans for establishing Miss Graham were still in their infancy, his grace confined his romantic activities to showing up every night in his box at the Royal George to ogle his ladylove as she performed in her various roles. He could tell this drove her mad—that was obvious even through her considerable acting ability—but Arden felt he owed himself these treats. Barred for the moment from the joys of intimacy with the lovely lady, was he to forgo the mere sight of her?

And, in his favor, he wasn't lurking near her dressing room or haunting the greenroom in the hopes of seeing her. Even the sternest of women, the kind Matilda was pretending to be, wouldn't begrudge a poor besotted chap the pleasure of gazing on his love from afar.

Finley easily found a suitable house, in Half Moon Street, and on the duke's orders staffed it with servants. Then Arden began his own arrangements. Soon all would be ready! And Matilda, the duke was sure, would tumble into his arms once he had the proper trappings at her disposal.

Meanwhile the Season dragged on. The Countess of Dauntry and the Duchess of Arden continued their campaign for the duke's marriage, not really assisted, yet not quite hindered by the intended bride, Lady Davina Lowden. One day the duchess appeared in the drawing room of her prospective in-laws. She wore a decided air of triumph.

"My son has promised to drive me home from

here,'' she informed the countess. Her eyes had that predator's gleam which Lady Dauntry privately found unattractive.

"How delightful," said the countess, beaming. "Dear Davina should be down in an instant. Do you think . . . tell me, Eudocia, if we left them alone together, would the time be right for a declaration? You must know your son's mind.''

The duchess not only was totally ignorant of the workings of her eldest son's mind but also intended to remain so. He had a most whimsical and strange sort of brain. "Who better than his own mother?" she answered nevertheless. "We might as well try it. Davina is agreeable, of course?"

"Of course," muttered Davina's mother.

When Davina entered the room, it was to find two pairs of speculative, critical eyes riveted on her. She found herself sighing as she made her curtsy to the duchess.

"Run back upstairs, child," said Lady Dauntry at once, "and put on that new sprigged muslin with all the delightful flounces at the hem.''

"But, Mama, that's the stupidest-looking dress I own. I swear the modiste made some dreadful error. What's wrong with this one?" And Davina looked down at herself, finding no fault with her simple blue morning gown. It was her favorite, and boasted scalloped epaulets and long sheer white Mameluke sleeves caught in short puffs to the wrist. The neckline was high and ended in a pretty white ruff which did its best to soften Davina's narrow face.

The countess paused a moment before making an answer. The truth was, the sprigged muslin was low-necked and Davina had a neat figure. Lady Dauntry meant to trot out all the weapons at her, or her daughter's, disposal for the coming scene of courtship. But she could hardly talk of décolletage. "That dress has

a spot at the back," she lied. "I'm surprised your
maid would put you into it. I'll have to speak to her
very strongly. Now, go and change, there's a good girl.
We want you to be here when the duke stops by to
fetch his mother. I know he'll wish most particularly
to see you, dear."

Davina shrugged. She knew the dress she had on
was in perfect order. A spot, indeed! On the bright
side, perhaps if she appeared in the ridiculous muslin
costume the duke would find her even less attractive
than usual.

Upstairs in her room, Davina let her maid assist her
into the hated sprigged ensemble and warned the girl
not to pay any attention if the countess actually rep-
rimanded her for having let Davina wear the pristine
blue gown.

Davina dragged her feet on the way back, for she
was truly reluctant to appear in the drawing room, or
anywhere in company, in the frothy, low-necked dress
which suited her not at all. Lace and ribbons dripped
from every available surface and made Davina feel like
a particularly overdecorated piece of confectionery. As
for her bosom, it seemed to have swelled to twice its
normal size, the effect of the bodice's tight fit.

"Oh, how sweet," proclaimed the countess when
Davina entered the room for the second time. "Now,
go and arrange yourself under the Gainsborough.
Here—here's your embroidery. Do spread out your
skirts gracefully for once, Davina. There!"

Lady Dauntry followed her daughter over to the spot
in question and fussed about until Davina was in the
proper position. The duchess looked on and wondered
how any woman's taste in clothes could be as bad as
the countess's, and wondered further if Davina had
any more spirit than a stone. Ah, well, she would be
a perfect, malleable daughter-in-law.

The Duchess of Arden had no real intention of letting an opinionated or difficult young lady replace her. The duchess had plenty of life left, and it was imperative she spend it in her accustomed place as mistress of the Arden domains. Davina would suit to perfection.

"What a pretty picture you make, dear," Lady Dauntry said, clasping her hands in spurious admiration as she surveyed the sprigged-muslin skirts, the embroidery in the slim white hands, and last, Davina's scowling face.

The countess's eyes strayed to the painting above the striped silk sofa where Davina perched on display. The five beautiful faces of the storied Parmenter sisters stared back at her, rendered by Gainsborough at the peak of his career. *The Garden of Flowers*. One of the girls portrayed was Davina's grandmother, the last Countess of Dauntry. Why on earth hadn't the limpid beauty of that legendary Lady Rose Parmenter been transmitted to her granddaughter? Even a little would have helped.

Or—Lady Dauntry touched her own hair consciously—why hadn't Davina inherited her own, less brilliant loveliness? Belinda Dauntry had been the toast of London as a young matron. She remembered it quite well, though the Duchess of Arden, if queried on that point, would probably have recalled no such thing.

Lady Dauntry, with one of those lapses of logic common in such matters, thought it was quite Davina's own fault that she resembled her father almost to the last feature. And the earl was one of the least prepossessing men in England, a fact which was luckily offset by his ancient pedigree and more than ample fortune.

The countess gave a private nod to the duchess, went back to her chair, and poured both herself and the duchess another glass of canary wine from the small decanter at her elbow. She passed ratafia biscuits and comfit cakes. The two elder ladies began a conversation about the last night's rout party, excluding Davina as a matter of course.

Davina sighed and poked at her embroidery; she felt as little a part of things as the set piece at a banquet, and far less decorative. It was not that she wanted a ratafia biscuit, or even to join in that horrid society gossip she deplored. She merely wished . . . She didn't know what. To be away from her mama, for one thing.

The thought occurred to Davina that marriage would be a sure way to achieve that goal. Oh, if only she would meet the right man! Somehow she and her imagined knight would triumph over her mother's ambition and the Duchess of Arden's calm, cold insistence.

Thoughts of the right man seemed to bring the wrong one into the room. The butler flung wide the doors and the Duke of Arden, a spring in his step and a smile on his handsome face, was bowing over the countess's eagerly outstretched hand.

"Oh, my dear duke," twittered Davina's mama.

Davina tried to hold back a hoot of laughter at her mother's silliness, but was only half-successful. The choked snort brought the duke's eyes to her corner.

Having placed a kiss in the general area of his mama's headdress, Arden approached Davina. "How are you today, my lady?" was his cheerful greeting.

Davina thought his eyes were twinkling at her ridiculous costume and obviously contrived pose, and she respected him the more for such insight. What was her mother going to do next? Pretend to faint, and have the duchess assist her out of the room?

"I so enjoyed talking with your young brothers while they were in town, sir," Davina said, trying for a little general conversation to postpone the inevitable. "How unlucky that they had to leave so soon."

"Ah, the poor dear boys," put in the Duchess of

Arden, noticing that her son had confined his reply to an unkind snicker. He had vanquished her darlings on the second day of their visit, and in the company of his horrid secretary, Finley, thus ensuring their misery on the trip back to university. "I'm afraid their brother is overstern with them."

"My father wanted the boys to be educated at Cambridge, and there they shall stay till they can at least pretend to be gentlemen," said Arden, winking at Lady Davina.

"Well! You know Paul and Peter have the most delightful manners in the world," his mother said. "Everyone says so. They are perfect pattern-cards of fashion besides, and if their thoughts don't turn to bookish things, why they should be subjected to years of discomfort merely to satisfy an odd provision of their father's, which you as their guardian might easily overturn . . ."

Davina and her mother observed with interest as the duchess grew positively red in the face under her rouge. The real flush was most becoming to her hawk-like profile, Davina thought, giving her grace an air almost of real humanity.

The Duke of Arden made the only response possible in such a situation. "Mama, our family quarrels are best left settled in our own drawing room. I'm certain Lady Dauntry doesn't appreciate—"

"Oh, Duke, do consider yourselves *en famille* with us," the countess interrupted with a meaningful leer.

Davina bit back a rude laugh.

"Why, madam, you do me too much honor," the duke replied with a bow.

His mother, perhaps out of a wish to go home as soon as possible, thought it best to get matters under way at this point before they all sank into a sea of inanities. "Dear Belinda," she said loudly, with a pointed stare at the countess, "do take me to the conservatory now. I'm perishing to see that new species of ivy you were telling me about earlier. The children can entertain themselves for a few moments. Can't you, Michael?'' The imperious and insistent tones of her last words, directed to her son with her most speaking look, nearly finished the duke's composure.

''Perhaps we'll skip around the room and sing songs. Don't worry about your children, ladies,'' he said with an impish grin. Lady Davina muffled another giggle behind her embroidery.

The two elder ladies swept out of the room, purple and puce skirts trailing regally behind them.

The duke, somewhat to Davina's shock, immediately approached her sofa and stood staring. Not at her, luckily, but at the painting which hung above her.

''Your eyes are exactly like theirs,'' said Arden, scrutinizing Davina in his turn.

''Oh, Duke, don't be ridiculous,'' Davina murmured. She had begun to shake with horror. Such an empty compliment was surely a prelude to the dreaded declaration! She had thought he wanted the marriage no more than she did.

And it seemed rather cruel for him to be choosing this exact moment to tease her. Davina's mother wasn't the only one to have stood before the ancestral Gainsborough to wish, in vain, that Davina bore some resemblance to those beautiful sisters of long ago. Davina had even sent some childish prayers into the air that she would miraculously wake up someday with the features of her departed grandmother—at a young age, to be sure.

''No, I mean it,'' said the duke. ''The shape, the color—it's all there.''

Davina shrugged, resolving privately to take a close look at the painting, and into a mirror, at the earliest opportunity.

''And now down to the business of our interview,''

continued Arden. Davina couldn't bring herself to look up at him. She was so embarrassed to have been set before him like a bitter pill coated with sugar; and for him to be apparently set on swallowing it was too much!

"My lady, won't you look up? I'm not here to bite you, nor to secure your lovely hand in marriage."

Davina did raise her eyes, such a look of dawning hope lighting her face that the duke was, for the merest second, less flattered. "You're not?" she asked eagerly.

"Why, how could you think so? Our conversation at my mother's ball should have convinced you my intentions are strictly . . ." The duke paused, frowning. "Well, neither honorable nor the reverse. I do think we should take this rare opportunity alone to consider our position, though."

"What is there to discuss?" Davina said. "My mother and yours are determined that we marry. All we can do is continue to refuse. I am praying that this time, Duke, my mother won't come running into the room shrieking and crying, 'Unhand my daughter.' I hate to say this of my own mama, but I wouldn't put it past her to try to force a wedding."

Arden took a seat beside Davina and companionably patted her hand. Davina was particularly glad her mother wasn't by to witness this supposed intimacy, and prayed anew that the countess would not choose this moment to come back.

"My dear girl," the duke said, "I've been worried about you. With both our mothers pushing you my way, you haven't had a chance to make the most of your Seasons. This is your second, isn't it? I'd hate for the ladies' ambitions to come between you and a man you love."

"I haven't yet met that man," Davina responded. She felt her face redden, and cursed inwardly. She might not want to impress the duke, but she was still loath for him—or anyone—to see her in the blotchy and unappealing state her blushes induced.

"Well, at least your life hasn't been ruined yet," Arden said, speaking in a more cheerful tone.

Davina stared in surprise. He spoke as if the question of her happiness really meant something to him. Was the Duke of Arden actually a kind and generous man? It was so hard to see behind the mask of his constant levity.

"Sir," Davina said diffidently, "I can't tell you how much I appreciate the honor you do me. That you should be forthright with me about your absolute lack of any wish to marry me means a great deal. Even though we did have that short talk at your mother's party, I've been wondering if you hadn't changed your mind. The word is going around society that you're hanging out for a wife—"

"Word carefully planted by my mother," the duke pointed out.

"I'm glad to hear it, Duke. It would make me so happy *not* to be your wife."

"Er, thank you," said Arden with a cough. "Now, what must we do to achieve that goal for you, Lady Davina?"

"You might marry someone else," Davina suggested. Her large blue eyes took on a look of absolute longing.

"Besides that. Now, I propose, Davina . . . may I call you by your Christian name? Thanks, it seems so infernally formal to have to 'my lady' someone I agree with so completely—I propose that we play a sort of prank on their motherships."

"A . . . practical joke, in other words?" Davina asked. A sudden thought struck her. "No, Duke, that would never do. If we pretended to be betrothed, my mother would never let us escape. She'd have us down the aisle so fast, if for no other reason than that she would be afraid you'd change your mind.''

"Oh, I know my mother would feel the same. I don't say we do anything so drastic as an actual betrothal,'' the duke assured his nervous co-conspirator. ''But what say we hover on the edge for a while? See how that goes.''

Davina furrowed her brow. ''Hover on the edge?'' she repeated.

''Why, yes. You say you've no one on the string. Why don't we simply give it to be understood by our mothers that we may very well become engaged at any moment? They know nothing of our real feelings, and they think we're both approaching this marriage of convenience they've set out in their minds. Why not continue to let them think so?''

''You forget, Duke, that when they come back into this room they will expect you to have asked me,'' Davina said. ''How will I explain that you haven't come up to scratch?''

''Why, Davina, you credit me with very little ingenuity. There is the simple expediency of the choking fit.''

''The . . . the choking fit?''

''Precisely.'' Arden smiled in his most encouraging style. ''Though it will pain me to ruin a finely done Oriental, no sacrifice is too great for your happiness. And, I might add, my own.'' And with an air of great aplomb, the duke began to untie his white lawn cravat.

Davina gasped; never before had she seen such a thing. She wouldn't have been more shocked had he started to undo his pantaloons. ''Duke! What are you doing?''

''The necessary, my dear. I hear them coming— choking fit, you understand . . .'' And Arden began a masterly imitation of a man in the depths of violent coughing at the very moment the door opened and

Lady Dauntry and the Duchess of Arden sailed through, happy and expectant smiles on both their faces.

"Davina!" Lady Dauntry cried. "My God! What have you done to him?"

Mama had so little faith in her own daughter. Davina had grown philosophical about this sad situation in late years. She did not answer the countess. Instead she patted the duke on the back, at first hesitantly, then with some force. He still sat beside her on the sofa, and his half-unwound cravat lent him a wild and disheveled appearance. He continued to wheeze and snort as the two mothers stared, fascinated.

At length the choking wound down to a gentle cough, and Arden was able to open a pair of eyes that were wet with the aftermath of his ordeal—to all appearances. "Sorry, Mama, one of my deuced coughing fits. Cravat must have been too tight."

"Michael, you are a sight," the duchess said in a disapproving tone which Davina found to be remarkably lacking in sympathy. Perhaps the duchess saw through her son's ploy? Well, that was all right, so long as the lady didn't pass on any suspicions to Mama.

"But, children," the countess wailed, "do you have no news for us? We were certain . . ."

"Mama, the poor man has been choking off and on ever since you left," Davina said in a rare moment of inspiration. She immediately returned her attention to her embroidery, which she had picked up again when she had left off "helping" the duke.

"Is that so?" The Duchess of Arden fixed her son with a very suspicious stare. "Oh, do fix your cravat."

"With pleasure, Mama," Arden said, clearing his throat as he rose from Davina's side and sauntered over to the nearest mirror. "Pity I haven't a new neckcloth, not to mention my man. The Gordian knot, I think." He began to busy himself with the length of white, twisting it this way and that. Suddenly he turned from the glass and stared penetratingly at Davina, who had had to raise her eyes to observe this unprecedented sight of a man of fashion finishing his toilette. "You know the Gordian knot, Lady Davina? If it can't be untied, it must be cut."

"Yes, your grace," Davina said demurely.

The countess and the duchess looked from one to the other of the innocent pair.

"Mark my words, there's mischief afoot," muttered the duchess to her hostess. Luckily they were far enough across the drawing room that this utterance went unheard by either Michael or Davina. "Arden," the duchess added in a much louder tone of voice, "you may finish that quickly and take me home."

The duke gave a last pat to his neckcloth and spread out his hands in a gesture which seemed to demand a compliment. "Ever at your service, Mama."

"That will be the day," snapped his mother, and she collected her reticule and parasol and preceded her smiling son to the door.

A calm and innocent Davina was left to explain to her mother the lack of a declaration. By the end of her masterly description of the poor duke's ill turn, the countess was quite convinced. They must make another opportunity for his grace to speak.

He was evidently teetering on the precipice of matrimony.

7

"AUNT Poppy, I am feeling stifled," Matilda said, "and I mean to do something about it. Do you realize that we haven't seen a green field since we arrived in town?"

"I realize it every day, dear," her elderly companion said with a sigh, bending her head once more over one of Matilda's costumes, which had a tear in the minuscule bodice. Dear Matilda was such a well-endowed young lady, and so energetic in her movements, that Aunt Poppy had to spend many of her leisure hours in this manner. Not that she minded; she really did like to sew, and even if she had not, how could she cavil at these few inconveniences when her darling Matilda was making the supreme sacrifice of acting upon the stage, all to put bread on their table?

The two ladies were enjoying an almost unprecedented day of leisure, for Matilda would not be wanted in the evening's performance at the Royal George. This was a holiday she had begged for, and, for a wonder, obtained. Matilda had thought she would like to stay at home for a day, but somehow she did not feel herself on holiday, sitting in the cheerless living space she and her aunt had enlivened with all of the duke's flowers they had managed to fit into a hackney on several successive nights. These blooms were taking their inevitable course and now gave the place the air of a neglected church some days after a wedding—or a funeral.

While her aunt worked, Matilda gazed out of the window. In her mind she was going over their financial

80

state. She had earned nearly a hundred pounds since coming to town, over and above the debt to the moneylender, which was finally repaid. All of her earnings she had been investing in safe and stodgy four-percent consols. She was certain that she and Aunt could live quite well on one hundred a year, either in cheap Oxford lodgings or in a country cottage. Perhaps even fifty pounds a year would do. How much more time would it take before she could consider them settled?

She was earning money a bit faster than she had expected; why should not she and Aunt Poppy have a day's treat? They would go out to a nearby village and walk about, perhaps take lunch at an inn—no, it would be better both for their finances and for their privacy to take some bread and cheese along. But go they would.

Matilda stood up. "Get on your things, Auntie, I'm taking you out on a picnic. It's such a lovely day. Hampstead, perhaps? That shouldn't be too far." Matilda had an indefinite idea of distances in this still-strange London world, but she remembered passing Hampstead in the stage which had brought them to town, and as she recalled they had arrived at Hyde Park Corner not a great deal later.

The two ladies put on their walking things and left the house, looking rather like two crows. Off the stage, Matilda was still in mourning for her father. Though her gown was brown, Aunt Poppy had banded it in black, and her pelisse was of a black broadcloth. These drab trappings helped immensely to tone down her lush beauty. Her simple straw poke bonnet shaded her face and tied under her chin with black ribbons. Aunt Poppy boasted a small but complete wardrobe in much-worn black, having been in constant mourning for one person or another for some years, and was dressed entirely in that dusky hue.

They easily secured a shabby job-carriage and found

themselves bowling down the streets as quickly as the driver could contrive, on the way to the village of Hampstead. Matilda looked out the dirty window as they traversed London. What a great city she sensed her metropolis to be, and how dearly she would love to explore it from top to bottom! How sad that constant employment in the theater, not to mention her gender, made this impossible. She felt a pang as she realized how little she knew of London, for all she had spent nearly six months in town.

When the ladies had stepped from the carriage and Matilda had given more of the cash she had in hand than she would have dreamed possible to the rumpled, rheumy-eyed driver, both women sighed in relief. The great teeming warrens of London might be hard by, visible in fact from the hill they stood upon. But London looked pearly and majestic from this vantage point, the dome of St. Paul's rising proudly above the seemingly endless sweep of buildings. And, most important, this was a village in the country, on a beautiful May morning. How could they not be content?

"Oh, what shall we do first, my dear?" asked Aunt Poppy excitedly. "Feed the ducks or go for a walk across the Heath? It's such a very pretty place."

Matilda and Aunt Poppy decided the ducks could do very well with some crumbs of the bread in their reticules. They paced across an expanse of green to the Heath pond. There was a rustic seat for Aunt Poppy, and Matilda crouched at the edge of the pool, urging the birds to feed out of her hand while her more generous aunt simply flung large crumbs into the water.

"Careful, Auntie, you'll give away all our lunch," Matilda said, looking over her shoulder with a smile of pure affection. The sun lit her face, which was the more lovely for being totally oblivious of any attractions.

From the shelter of a tall tree, a pair of gleaming brown eyes was observing the scene.

"Miss Graham, you try my patience sorely," murmured the Duke of Arden. She was so very beautiful! It was all he could do to resist going out to her at once and provoking another sparking scene of some kind. Would it be courtship or an outright brawl if he intruded on her morning? Either way, he wouldn't risk it. He did send up a silent cheer to the man of his who had been watching Miss Graham night and day, and had given the duke the interesting information that she and a female companion had told the driver of a hackney to head for Hampstead. Arden had happened to be stepping into his curricle when his employee brought the news, and he had immediately decided that the boxing match he had set out to see would be a dead bore, and that the Spaniards Inn in Hampstead deserved more of his custom.

Who the devil was that with Matilda? An old bawd, perhaps, or a maidservant of sorts? According to Arden's spy, the two females went everywhere together. Perhaps this was one of the other actresses of the company. Arden had seen nothing but Matilda in his recent visits to the Royal George, but he remembered from earlier forays that some of the actresses were well stricken in years. And if Matilda were attached to this person, perhaps she wanted her as a companion? Luckily, all would be ready. Thinking to tease his ladylove, Arden had provided for the reception of an elderly lady at the house in Half Moon Street, anticipating a good laugh when Matilda confessed to him that the "aunt" had been a fabrication.

It never occurred to him for a moment that the other woman might be the genuine aunt of Matilda's stories. Actresses did not have aunts. This was a fact as firmly established in Arden's mind as the simple truth that any actress, once confronted by enough material goods, must succumb to the protection of a very dashing duke.

Matilda and the companion finished feeding the ducks and were walking away, leaving the duke to look after them and meditate on their extraordinary costumes. Must be a disguise of sorts. Actresses, he thought sagely, would not want to be noticed as such while taking their bucolic exercise.

Coincidentally, Matilda was giving a thought to her clothes at the same moment that the duke shrugged and tried his best to put her and her costume from his mind as he aimed his steps in the opposite direction, choosing a circuitous route back to the inn rather than risk disturbing the two women.

Matilda was noticing, for the first time in months, how very worn Aunt Poppy's clothes and her own were becoming. She ordinarily went out only in the shadowy city streets, and that for the most part at night. Today she saw the bright spring sunshine outline the shiny spots on the sagging back of Auntie's shapeless black outer garment; and there was a place on Matilda's brown dress which would have to be patched! She expected that if she took off her bonnet to examine it, she would be mortified by its tattered state. She already knew that its black ribbons were frayed.

"Aunt Poppy," she said as they wandered slowly down a path which would, a woman had told them, lead to some pretty farms in the Kilburn meadows, "we are in rags."

"Yes, dear," returned the elder lady vaguely. Her real attention had been captured by a butterfly flirting in and out of the hedgerow.

"Tell me," Matilda went on, "would you be willing to spend some of our money, to go home to Oxford a wee bit later, if it meant getting a new gown now? We can't go about in these things much longer, you know; they will simply shred around us and leave us naked."

Aunt Poppy nodded. "If we could buy a few yards of summer-weight black stuff, my dear, I'd be pleased to make us up some things."

"Oh, I can't have you tied to your sewing all the time. You do enough for me as it is," Matilda said. "If we do it, we do it right. We will have our things made up." She paused at Aunt Poppy's shocked gasp, then went on resolutely. "And . . . well, it's been over six months since Papa died. I mean to come out of mourning!"

Another gasp. Then, as Aunt Poppy presumably did some serious thinking, she was heard to murmur, "Well, half-mourning is quite proper in the circumstances, dear. You are so very young, and you haven't many pleasures . . ."

Matilda suspected that her aunt's wildest idea of the pleasure Matilda wished to enjoy was something like a gray or lavender muslin trimmed in the ever-present black. That was nowhere near the truth.

Some secrets Matilda couldn't hope to discuss with her aunt, such as the desires which her association with the Duke of Arden had brought dancing to the forefront of her mind.

Pushing to one side that shameful desire for the duke's caresses, Matilda concentrated on the other longing his attentions had generated within her.

Luxury, pretty clothes, the best modistes: he had seemed to hold all these up before her when he had promised to be generous. Matilda would be less than human if she had failed to be just a little jealous of the other actresses, those who were not saving every groat for a fixed goal. Their pretty clothes and bright ribbons had stirred up some envy in the resolutely chaste bosom of their odd friend Miss Graham.

Matilda had to admit that although she loved the good-hearted girl dearly, Dulcie Moore had horrid taste. But there were others of the company who dressed with elegance. Matilda had memorized where they had their clothes made. Perhaps she had always expected, sooner or later, to succumb to this temptation.

It seemed such a very small indulgence, too, when she thought of the much greater temptation she had resisted in the person of the handsome Duke of Arden.

"Aunt," she said, squeezing the old lady's hand, which rested within her own arm, "we will each have a new dress. You will have your summer black, and I'll have one in lavender"—thus she put aside her dream of a spring-green costume, out of deference to Auntie's sensibilities—"and they shall be made up by Madame Hélène."

Aunt Poppy blinked and nodded. She had no idea of who led the London world of fashion. And it was better that way, Matilda thought shrewdly. Aunt Poppy would never sit still for having their new garments made up by the most exclusive modiste of the Polite World!

When Matilda made up her mind, she had to act quickly or lose her courage. Thus the coachman who picked up the two shabby-genteel ladies in front of the Spaniards Inn later that morning was given the improbable destination of "Madame Hélène, Bruton Street."

Aunt Poppy spent the journey back to town in dithering over whether they should be so extravagant as to have someone else sew their clothes, while Matilda was ever more grateful that Aunt Poppy didn't know how very extravagant they were about to be.

Only one dress, she silently promised her stern and disapproving conscience. *I'll be good. I promise.*

Her conscience merely snorted and opined that Matilda was taking her first luxurious step on the road to ruin, but Matilda paid those better feelings no mind.

She had earned the money, hadn't she? And she had been so very frugal for the last months.

Earned the money? Well, there was a problem. Matilda had only enough cash with her to pay for the coach ride home, after she had settled with this jobber who was conveying them to Bruton Street. Her salary was due soon, but for now she must buy on credit. She would have to appear before Madame Hélène in her character of Miss Graham, the rage of the London stage and the newest conquest of the Duke of Arden.

Rather a distasteful duty, but Matilda made up her mind to it. She *was* an actress, and one of note, and she might as well turn the situation to her own advantage for once.

After paying the hackney driver, Matilda turned on the pavement of Bruton Street and faced the elegant portal of Madame Hélène's establishment. An uneasy glance around told her that the promenaders in this street of Mayfair, where she had never been before, were of a style and fashion totally outside her own experience.

She knew rich people, and even well-born people, and had from her cradle, but she had never seen so many of them. They were all massed together in this street, seemingly for the sole purpose of making her uncomfortable and certain, if she had not been before, that she was out of her element. Here strolled two bucks in impeccable clothing, probably of Weston's cut. Their bored eyes raked Matilda with a glance which was less than respectful. There promenaded a stern-looking dowager in fur-trimmed bombazine and an amazing Paris bonnet, who seemed to stare right through Aunt Poppy and Matilda and to give them a wide berth as she continued on her way, followed by a footman bearing packages.

"We have to go in," Matilda muttered. "We're here."

"Certainly we are, dear," her aunt said in surprise. "Where else would we be?"

Matilda gripped Aunt Poppy's arm firmly, put on the demeanor she had used to such great effect as Lady Macbeth, and sailed in through the door.

The interior of the salon was about what Matilda had expected, trimmed in gold and white and redolent of exquisite French taste and honest English money. The front room was empty, and Matilda felt herself relax. She had not even thought of the embarrassment she might have felt before elegant customers, dressed as she was and in such pressing need of new clothes.

An interior door opened and a haughty-looking young person in a severe dark dress approached the two ladies, looking them up and down. Matilda guessed this woman to be an underling. The great Madame Hélène would never, Matilda was sure, greet any but the grandest of customers in person.

"You wish, mesdames?" said the young woman in a tone which implied that she would be happy to direct them to the correct address in Cheapside.

"I am Matilda Graham. *The* Matilda Graham," said Matilda, tossing her head and managing to dislodge slightly the wretched straw bonnet. This was no time for the modest and retiring ways which became any young lady. "Tell Madame Hélène that I have arrived."

To Matilda's surprise, the shop assistant's eyes widened. "Mademoiselle! Forgive me for not recognizing you. If you would sit—but a moment—I will fetch my mistress."

She bustled away, and Matilda and Aunt Poppy settled into two gilt chairs covered in white brocade. Matilda began to fret. Astonishing that she should be so well-known! She had not expected her little show of bravado to work at all, let alone so beautifully.

Aunt Poppy had taken the encounter in her stride.

She picked up a newspaper from a table at her side and read through the society columns.

"Oh, heavens!" she said with a little giggle. "Listen to this, Matilda dear. 'A raffle for charity was held at Lady C's brilliant gathering. A certain well-known gentleman, who shall be nameless, arranged for a jest that each guest who took a ticket should receive a prize. All the lucky partygoers were soon seen strolling through the rooms laden with sundry objects such as teapots, coal scuttles, flatirons, and birds in cages which they tried unobtrusively to deposit in some convenient corner . . . ' Did you ever hear anything so funny?"

"The work of our duke, I'll wager," Matilda said, trying, with limited success, to stifle her instinctive laugh.

"Oh, the dear, amusing man," said her aunt. Matilda glanced at the old lady sharply.

"Auntie, you are not to *like* that horrid man. He wants to ruin me, remember."

"Yes, dear." And Aunt Poppy turned back to the unaccustomed perusal of a recent newspaper.

Then a female swept into the room. She was outwardly little different from the assistant who had entered a few minutes earlier, for she wore a simple dress of dark material and her chestnut hair was done up in a simple knot. By the woman's regal carriage, though, Matilda knew this to be Madame Hélène in the flesh.

"Mademoiselle, I am delighted that you honor my little establishment," the woman said in a moderate French accent. Her intelligent dark eyes were surveying Matilda and Aunt Poppy with lively interest, and the tip of her sharp little nose seemed to quiver with anticipation.

Matilda felt it only fair to disabuse the modiste of any notion she might have that an extensive wardrobe was in the question. "I have been wishing to come to

you this age, Madame,'' she said with a regal smile.
''As you can see, my aunt and I are in pressing need
of new walking costumes. Each of us want . . . one
dress.''

''A lovely light summer black,'' chimed in Aunt
Poppy with a winning smile.

''One dress.'' The modiste nodded. Either she was
a fine actress herself, or tattered women came into her
shop every day to order single garments. ''Whatever
Mademoiselle requires, I will be glad to supply.''

''I'm going into half-mourning, you see,'' said Matilda with a glance at Aunt Poppy, who gave an encouraging nod. ''Something in lavender—something
practical . . .''

''Ah, lavender! That is a color we had not thought
of, with Mademoiselle's hair . . . but we shall contrive.'' Madame Hélène's eyes glittered, presumably
with the pleasure of making a difficult color work on
a redhead.

Matilda wondered about the modiste's phraseology.
Perhaps the woman's English was bad. Why else would
it sound as though Madame had already been thinking
about Matilda's clothes?

''And now, ladies, if you will but step into the back,
where I have some lovely bolts of cloth in every shade
of *laveande*, I'm certain we will manage to flatter
you—''

The door at the back opened again, and out stepped
two fashionable women, one young, one of a certain
age. Both ladies let a shocked stare at the shabby black-
clad women escape them before they remembered to
put on bland masks.

Madame Hélène turned from Matilda and Aunt
Poppy with an apology and proceeded to take leave of
these clients, who, Matilda gathered as she shamelessly eavesdropped, were a countess and her daughter.

She had never met a countess in the flesh. I wish I'd gotten a better look at them, she was thinking as Madame Hélène finally ushered her and her aunt into a pretty back room furnished in the same style as the outer salon, but littered with every sort of bolt of cloth Matilda had ever imagined. Fashion plates were scattered about like rushes in a medieval hall, and the aura of expensive elegance about the establishment seemed to have permeated even this disordered place.

On the pavement of Bruton Street, the Countess of Dauntry stepped into her carriage with an audible sniff. "Did you ever, Davina?" she said over her shoulder to her daughter, who followed her. "I heard Madame address the red-haired creature as Miss Graham. I happen to know that that particular young person is an actress, and that furthermore—" Lady Dauntry cut herself off, for though she had indeed heard the shocking rumor that the Duke of Arden had been mesmerized by that shameless actress, there was no need to present Davina with the little interests of her future husband until the marriage took place. "Never mind," said the countess, settling herself on the plum velvet squabs.

Davina didn't demand that her mama finish her sentence. There was no need, for Davina, being out in society, had naturally heard the rumors about Arden and the actress.

"I wish I had gotten a better look at her," Davina murmured in disappointment. "And I wish—"

"What was that, Davina?"

The sharp voice of her mother brought her out of her reverie.

"Never mind, Mama," said Davina, casting down her eyes. No purpose would be served by letting the countess know what fantastic thoughts were presently having the audacity to cross her daughter's mind.

If only that young woman were a lady of the proper social sphere! Davina knew that Miss Graham must be extraordinary, and that the duke must love her. Arden's love affairs had never before captured the *ton*'s imagination to the extent of popular gossip. He had been as other men were, someone who set up mistresses and gave them their *congés* in that mysterious society of male lusts and female pragmatism, the demi-monde. If he had lost that proper reticence, he must be besotted whether he knew it or not.

Davina knew that there was no chance in the world that the Duke of Arden would forget his duty to birth and breeding and marry an actress. He might delight in playing pranks, but that would be too audacious even for him. Oh, what a perfect solution it would have been to Davina's problem had Miss Graham not been a mere actress!

Still, I must meet her, Davina thought with a guilty glance at her oblivious mother. Davina enjoyed having such a rebellious thought. Meet an actress! And why? All the meetings in the world couldn't turn such a person into a suitable bride for Arden. Davina had to see Miss Graham nevertheless, and soon.

If Miss Graham loved the duke, and he loved her, perhaps something could be contrived.

Davina had no notion what, but she began to spin a fantasy in which she and her mother might come upon the duke and his light-o'-love in a compromising position. Davina, a pure and innocent girl confronted by the worst sort of tawdry behavior from her intended, could quite justifiably be shocked by such an encounter, shocked into refusing any offer the duke might make.

A little smile playing about her lips, Davina wondered what Arden would think of her creativity. She suspected he would call her clever and go along with such a delicious joke. The gentleman did bring out Davina's devilish side.

8

MATILDA swam and drifted in a sea of fine lavender muslins, cambrics, and silks as Madame Hélène walked round her, threw one length of fabric over Matilda's shoulder, whipped it away, and followed it immediately with another. Meanwhile an assistant trotted in and out of the room with various rolls of fine black cloth, which were placed before Aunt Poppy.

"How strange it is that we did not think of lavender," said Madame Hélène, swathing Matilda's upper body in violet cambric of a peculiar, pale shade. "This is most striking with the deep russet tones of Mademoiselle's lovely hair. We concentrated, as Monseigneur suggested, on those common shades of golds and greens and such. Ah, but we should have needed you here to judge the proper shade of more difficult colors, mademoiselle, and naturally, as your schedule did not permit a visit . . . But I comprehend, when you found there were no things for the half-mourning, you made the time."

"What?" Matilda's questioning face peered out from the oddly becoming folds of violet cloth. "Madame Hélène, perhaps you're confusing me with someone else. I've ordered nothing from you." Matilda's heart sank as she reflected that it was more likely a case of mistaken identity than her far-reaching fame which had gotten her this royal treatment from Madame Hélène and her staff. Would she and Aunt Poppy be assisted out to the street once their true identity was known?

A frown flitted across the features of the modiste.

"You are not the Miss Graham who acts at the Royal George? But even I have seen you, for I went to the *As You Like It* some weeks ago, and I was certain . . ."

"I am that Miss Graham," said Matilda. "This is a tangle. Can some red-haired impostor have been ordering gowns in my name? Heavens!" She paused, catching her breath. Would she be legally responsible for such a bill?

"But no," answered Madame Hélène, "we have taken our orders only from *Monseigneur le duc.*"

"Duke," Matilda repeated in awed tones.

"And the things were only yesterday delivered to mademoiselle's house in Half Moon Street, as you know, for you have perceived the lack of a lavender costume—" The modiste was going on when she was interrupted by Matilda's choked sound of rage.

"That man!" Matilda said, rising suddenly from her chair in a swirl of varied fabrics. "Oh!"

Madame Hélène's shrewd eyes narrowed. "Something is not to your liking, mademoiselle?"

Matilda, remembering her manners and her difficult position, smiled at Madame Hélène and said sweetly, "You must excuse me, madame. The duke's generosity seems to me excessive sometimes. He really shouldn't do so much. We'll forget about the lavender dress for today, for I have a sudden desire to go to my house in Half Moon Street and reexamine my wardrobe. Oh, dear!" She put a hand to her face in pretended chagrin. "I've forgotten the number of the house. Could you help me, Madame Hélène? I haven't yet moved in there, you see, and the direction isn't familiar yet."

Madame Hélène looked very wary, but she saw no reason not to impart to the lady the number of her very own house, a house to which the modiste had just had delivered a sumptuous wardrobe worth more than the rest of her present orders combined.

"And the black dress for mademoiselle's companion?" she said in parting. "Shall we wait for that too?"

Matilda had forgotten about Aunt Poppy. She now glanced at her great-aunt, who had been sitting across the room seemingly enraptured by a wide variety of black bombazines, muslins, and sarcenets while an assistant showed her fashion plates.

At that moment the old lady looked up. "Oh, Matilda, this is the one I want."

"Let's measure for it today, madame," said Matilda with a shrug, "and if you would open a separate account for my aunt's things? I'd dislike for the duke to pay for them."

Madame Hélène looked perplexed at this economy and said, "But his grace was most insistent in his generosity to you, mademoiselle, and I am sure he would not quibble over the price of another gown or two—or even more . . ."

Matilda held up her hand in its well-worn black kid glove. "I can't allow him to be put to the trouble. If my aunt could be measured now, we are rather late for an appointment."

"To be sure, mademoiselle." The modiste proceeded with the business at hand, and Matilda felt the inclination to squirm under Madame Hélène's acute observation. The dressmaker must surely have guessed that there was something amiss between the Duke of Arden and his latest mistress.

His latest mistress! As Matilda marched her aunt out of the dressmaking establishment, hailed another hackney, and directed it to a certain number in Half Moon Street, she was considering her new position. It had become clear to her weeks ago that all her associates—perhaps all of London!—thought she had succumbed to Arden's lure.

It had simply never occurred to her to think that the

Duke of Arden was one of those who had taken her
acceptance of his *carte blanche* for granted. Indeed,
she had thought she'd made it clear to him that she
would never become his mistress. She had written a
note to state her position in plain English, and when
the duke had plagued her no further as a result of that
note, she had been certain her virtue was safe from
the infuriating peer. (Matilda supposed she couldn't
count Arden's constant presence at the playhouse as
"plaguing," for though she hated to admit it, she
looked for him every night that she performed.)

"Oh, my dear, it's been years since I had a fitting
at a fashionable modiste's," Aunt Poppy said, star-
tling Matilda out of her reverie. "It was very like old
times. My sisters and I . . . But are you quite sure we
can afford the dress?"

"We certainly can, Aunt," Matilda said tightly.
"What do you think, dear, of Arden's latest trick?"

"Trick?" The sweet lined face was a complete
blank, and Matilda recognized that Aunt Poppy had
not been listening at all during the earlier conversation
with Madame Hélène, and likely didn't realize even
now where they were going.

"Aunt Poppy," Matilda began gently, "it seems the
duke hasn't limited his attentions to me to those flowers you enjoyed so much. You remember, don't you,
how you said he must be quite a rake?"

Aunt Poppy nodded, frowning in perplexity.

"Well, it seems the duke has taken a house for me
and bought me a wealth of clothes from Madame Hélène's, all on the assumption that I will become his
mistress! He likely thinks I'll be dazzled by such
riches."

"How very devious of the dear duke," Aunt Poppy
said with a little giggle.

"Aunt! I've told you before, you're not to like that

man! Don't you realize he's made my name a byword, among the modistes of the town if no one else?''

''But, dear, I had understood that your name was already linked with his—through no fault of your own, of course. And it is only Miss Graham's name, not your dear father's. You are a pattern of every virtue, dearest, and no aunt could wish for a better grand-niece. But your work upon the stage, and all those flowers . . .''

Matilda frowned. She supposed she ought to be glad that Auntie was exhibiting this streak of shrewdness, but she wasn't. How unfortunate that such a sweet old lady was being corrupted by the evil cynicism of the theatrical profession. Matilda realized she couldn't keep her elderly relation in cotton wool, but even so she mourned the loss of innocence.

The hackney rolled to a halt, and Matilda peeked out the window. A neat brick house, much like the others in its row, with a white-painted door and window moldings. How harmless the place looked, nothing at all like the residence of a woman of ill repute! Matilda couldn't think, however, how the house of such a woman should appear.

Dismissing the hackney, Matilda took her aunt's arm and mounted the steps. She lifted the gleaming brass knocker.

A butler answered the door: a superior-looking individual in late middle age, impeccably uniformed, his balding pate seeming to gleam as brightly as the exterior of the house.

Matilda hesitated, unsure how to explain her mission.

The man, however, took that decision out of her hands. ''Madam!'' he said, bowing low and stepping aside so that the ladies might enter. ''I am Drumm, madam's butler. His grace of Arden has indicated that should Madam be displeased with the staff in any way,

Madam is free to make changes.'' His eyes glinted
with humor for the merest second. ''Naturally such a
provision has made all of us even more anxious to
please than we would have been ordinarily.''

Matilda stared at the man. She and her aunt were
now standing, with the butler, in the pretty papered
hallway of the house. Several little gilt tables and
chairs ornamented the small room, and the staircase
which led to the upper reaches was gracefully curved,
with an inlaid rosewood banister.

''You know me, Drumm?'' Matilda managed to get
out in a fairly normal voice. She could think of nothing else to say.

The butler nodded. ''I had the pleasure of seeing
Madam's performance in *Macbeth* not long ago . . .''
His bland servant's expression changed again, momen-
tarily, to one of amusement.

''I suppose it was the night of the dagger,'' Matilda
replied with a sigh. Instinct told her it would be best
to brazen out this visit. She had to see what the duke
had done in her name, and, more important, devise
some way to get back at him. If she were really to be
served by Drumm, she would first make him stop
''madaming'' her at every turn, but she decided not
to bother, since his continuing presence in her employ
was not in the question.

''Indeed it was, madam, the night of the dagger,
and if I may say so, even from the gallery the joke
was clear. The Duke of Arden is a famous joker, as I
am sure Madam knows. I must be allowed to say,
madam, that I and the rest of the staff feel ourselves
doubly fortunate to be serving not only yourself but
also, by extension, his grace. What a striking man he
is, the talk of the Polite World! But do let me summon
the rest of the staff for Madam's inspection. Beemer!''

A liveried young footman stepped from the shadows

by the stairs. At the butler's orders he bowed, then disappeared to the lower reaches of the house.

"If you intend introductions, Drumm, I am sure you remember that I am Miss Graham," said Matilda, trying for a bored expression, though she was longing to lapse into hysterics. "And this is my great-aunt: Miss Graham."

Drumm gave an extra-respectful bow to Aunt Poppy, though he did examine the shabby old lady with a special interest. It was not every day that a fashionable Cyprian dragged along an elderly companion, and though the duke had warned Drumm that this might happen, the butler was still surprised, both at the lady's presence and at her eccentric air of poverty. (Matilda's odd costume Drumm had instantly put down to a modest desire not to be recognized in the street.)

Soon the small but adequate staff of the house had filed in for the promised inspection: a cook, a housekeeper, three maids (two chamber, one kitchen), the footman Beemer, and a potboy. Matilda gave them all gracious nods, not bothering to recall their names. The respect each servant exhibited toward her, a supposed kept mistress, astonished Matilda, and she attributed it to that town sophistication that seemed to permeate to all classes in London. A little part of her did realize that persons in service would naturally treat an employer as graciously as possible, the object of the game of life in the servant class, as in many others, being to keep body and soul together.

"Thank you all," Matilda said when the introductions were over. "Now, Drumm, would you show me and my aunt over the house? You others may go back to your duties."

Matilda, whose entire staff in her father's house had consisted of a man-of-all-work and one maid, couldn't interpret the triumphant glance Drumm shot the housekeeper, who should more properly have been asked to conduct the ladies on their tour. With a fixed expression of distaste bedecking her pretty face, Matilda suffered Drumm to lay open to her eyes and her aunt's the beauties of the small house.

Downstairs there were a salon and a dining room, as well as a small back parlor, all decorated richly, but in colors Matilda would not have thought of ordering. The salon was done in soft greens, with furnishings of gold and white and a pretty Chinese paper. Touches of russet in sofa cushions and footstool tapestries delighted the eye, and there were many precious bibelots in the form of ormolu clocks, decorative screens, and the like. There was even a piano in one corner of the room, by one of the front windows.

"Oh, how charming," Aunt Poppy said at once, rushing to the instrument. "The duke couldn't know that you don't play, dearest, but how I should enjoy . . . Oh. I forget." And Aunt Poppy, looking very uncomfortable, backed away from the tempting pianoforte. "A Broadwood!" She sighed in regret.

Matilda gave her a piercing look and hissed, "Do hold yourself back, Aunt. Remember we haven't decided yet"—she shot a glance at the interested butler and moderated her tones—"whether we shall keep this decor, I mean to say."

Drumm spoke up for the absent duke at this point. "Ah, madam, his grace has labored long over these decorations. He was especially insistent that the furnishings and hangings of every room should be such as to pay tribute to Madam's lovely coloring, if Madam will forgive me the liberty of passing on such intimate information."

"You say the duke labored over decorating this place?" Matilda cut in, in a sharp tone. "In person?"

"Wasn't it odd, though, for a man in his position? But his grace explained that he was indulging himself, for he had never had occasion to design living quarters, and since you are so very special to him, madam—''

''I see,'' Matilda said. ''Shall we go on?''

The tables and chairs of the dining parlor were of a gleaming golden wood that Matilda couldn't even identify; the walls were covered in a yellow silk; and the carpet was an Axminster of the very finest quality. On the sideboard were displayed plate and china, the latter in a pretty pattern which harmonized with the colors of the room.

And so it was throughout the house: Never had Matilda seen so many rooms meant to compliment a lady with red hair. She didn't know whether to laugh or cry; she grew more disturbed by each complacent remark of the butler's and every new arrangement the duke had made for her supposed pleasure or comfort.

Upstairs, after viewing a modern water closet and a suspiciously masculine dressing room, Matilda turned to Drumm. ''That will be all. My aunt and I will go through the rest of the rooms. Thank you for all your help, Drumm.''

The butler could only respond by bowing and asking ''Madam'' to ring when she wished refreshments, though his disappointment was evident.

''Oh, Aunt,'' said Matilda when they were alone in the upstairs hall. ''Isn't this dreadful?''

''Awful,'' said Aunt Poppy, running her gloved hand over an Oriental vase displayed on a small table between two doors.

''Well, we might as well see the rest of the rooms before we leave,'' Matilda said. ''What's in here?''

The next sound was Aunt Poppy's gasp of pleasure, for Matilda had opened a door onto what was, to an elderly gentlewoman, a paradise.

A cozy little sitting room fitted out with every comfort imaginable lay before them. In one corner was a spinet; a canterbury by the instrument's side held a quantity of music. Another corner of the room was devoted to sewing implements, and Aunt Poppy ran over to open the large workbasket that stood waiting on a table beside a comfortable chair. While she happily examined embroidery threads, yarns, fringes, and all sorts of pattern books, Matilda looked over the rest of the place. A little case held books which, when examined, proved to be a collection of Minerva novels as well as some improving works by Hannah More and Fordyce. There was a long chair by the fireside, with a satin comforter for the warming of old limbs. The room had been decorated in soft blues and roses, a welcome respite to the determined greens and golds of the rest of the house. Best of all, a little canary was singing in a cage by one window. The bird was evidently well-fed and only waited for someone to bear him company.

No place could have been better designed to keep busy the elderly companion of a man's mistress while the mistress and the man were otherwise engaged.

"Why don't you look through these things, Auntie, while I go on?" Matilda suggested, and at her aunt's happy nod, she softly closed the door to the room and went on her way down the hall.

There was one chamber Matilda had not yet seen, and she had a feeling she had better not see it in the company of her aunt.

The second door she tried opened onto the room she was seeking. Matilda stepped inside and turned this way and that, taking it all in.

Mirrors! was her first impression. Her shabby brown gown and black pelisse seemed to reflect at her from every angle. Gold-framed pier glasses were set in every conceivable place. Dominating the room was a vast gold-curtained bed with a cream-colored silk counterpane.

The ceiling, a glance up told Matilda, was painted

to represent a particularly indelicate scene out of Greek mythology. And what was that glittering to one side of the *Venus and Adonis*?

Taking a deep breath, Matilda marched over to the bed and looked up through the framed curtains. "That evil man!" she exclaimed, blushing hotly.

One section of the ceiling had been left unpainted. Ornate plasterwork acted as the frame for yet another mirror, placed directly over the bed.

Pressing her hands to her hot cheeks, Matilda continued her exploration. She opened a door onto a dressing room. Hanging in armoires and folded in cupboards was what must be the wardrobe ordered from Madame Hélène: clothes for every sort of occasion, all obviously in the first style of fashion, all in colors which would set off Matilda's creamy skin and fiery hair to perfection. Dashing bonnets, gloves of softest kid, and slippers of gold and colored satin peeked out at her from every corner.

"How dared he!" Matilda cried, picking up a transparent nightdress of cream-colored tissue which lay across a chair. Beside it was a man's dressing gown. Matilda instinctively moved the gown to a footstool across the room.

She preferred not to dwell on those beautiful clothes, all made with her in mind, and left the dressing room quickly. The large bed confronted her once more.

Matilda stared at the bed. She could almost see Arden lying upon it, cradling her, Matilda Graham the actress, in his strong arms. He would be gentle with her, that she knew; he would be passionate. If she would but say the word, she could feel his kiss again, and much, much more! In return for the fulfillment of all the fancies which had been haunting her dreams, all of these beautiful things would be hers . . .

"Arden," Matilda said in a low, dangerous voice, "you'll pay for this."

He was laughing at her. He was laughing at her with this house, with these delightful trappings of a courtesan's life. Matilda was beside herself with shame. Tears rolled down her cheeks as she contemplated the real life of a woman of easy virtue. A moment's sober reflection reminded her that going down that path would mean yielding not only to the duke but also to those who would come to her when he was finished. For affairs of this sort, she knew instinctively, must come to an end.

And she would never be able to marry in good conscience if she yielded to the rakish duke now. Matilda had always cherished the hope that somehow she might find the man of her dreams. These days she tended to think of a more sober union, made in calm friendship and affection when the duke was long forgotten. But the dream was still there.

"Decadent, libertine, disgusting duke," Matilda muttered, brushing away her angry tears. "How dare he tempt me? I hate him."

She glanced this way and that, wishing she could think of something to do that would hurt the duke. Her eyes lit upon the big, evil-looking bed.

She smiled through her tears. It would be a joke on him, for certain! Maybe he wouldn't even care; but it would at least confound him.

Writing materials were set out on a small gold escritoire in one corner of the room. Matilda sat down at the desk and wrote out a note. It occurred to her that this was her second letter to the duke; and, with any luck, this one would finally get him out of her life for good.

The letter sealed and addressed to his grace of Arden, Matilda went about the next step in her plan. She took off her shoes and bonnet. Then she walked with a determined stride to the bed and pulled back the covers.

Appearances were everything, as Matilda knew from her work on the stage. If a bed were to look as though it had been slept in, someone must get into it.

Matilda climbed into the bed and writhed about from side to side, putting half the pillows down onto the floor, setting the counterpane askew, and wrinkling the fine linen sheets as much as she could. Then she matter-of-factly got out and set the note she had just written on one of the remaining lace-trimmed pillows, a colored one. She was certain the note would be noticed. It seemed to gleam at her, a white speck on salmon-pink satin.

Matilda had put her shoes back on, and was just setting her bonnet on her disheveled curls with the aid of one of the mirrors, when Aunt Poppy peeked in at the door.

"Oh, there you are, my dear. What a pretty room this is!"

"The tour of the house is over, Aunt," Matilda said. "We're leaving now. And you may be sure we're never coming back."

9

HUMMING a little tune, the Duke of Arden strolled down Half Moon Street. The watch was crying one, and Arden had just come from a particularly satisfying entertainment.

Peterborough was an awfully good sport. He had roared with laughter when Arden and some other friends had run through the halls of his mistress's establishment, crying "Fire!" in their loudest tones. His mistress, to do the little opera dancer credit, had laughed as loud as or louder than her swain after shrieking out only a few obscenities at the gentlemen pranksters.

Arden chuckled, seeing again the large rawboned Peterborough, hair every which way and dressed in only a shirt, who had burst wild-eyed through a bedroom door accompanied by his voluptuous light-o'-love, the latter clad only in one petticoat and *no* chemise. Ah, there were unexpected benefits to this habit of practical joking! Now Arden must watch carefully for what Peterborough would no doubt perpetrate in retaliation.

The sight of Peterborough's mistress had reminded the duke of his own soon-to-be lover. Not that Miss Graham was ever very far from his thoughts. Since she had moved to the forefront of his mind this evening, he had decided to inspect ''her'' house once more, to see that everything was in readiness. He intended to bring her to see it the very next evening, outwaiting the others in the greenroom if necessary to steal to her dressing room as he had that other, memorable evening of the dagger joke.

He hadn't so much as come near her since that night. Intolerable. Yet he was certain that when she looked up at his box, as she did every evening she appeared on the stage, there was affection in her eyes. She would be his, and soon.

Ah, tomorrow! The duke was thinking pleasant thoughts of the seduction to come as he rang the bell of Matilda's intended domain. The hour was very late, and when the footman finally opened to him, Arden had a good-humored word of apology for the rumpled young man.

The footman mumbled something indistinct which ended on "your grace," and busied himself lighting candles in the hall as Arden stood patiently by.

"You may go back to bed, lad, I merely want to look around," the duke said presently. "I'll ring if there's anything I require."

"Y'r grace," the young man muttered, and he stumbled in the direction of the servants' quarters. Arden noticed in amusement that one of the footman's stockings was missing. He resolved on the spot to let himself out rather than summon the young somnolent again.

Taking up a branch of candles, the duke started on his inspection of his handiwork. He had been intimately concerned with everything in this house, from the draperies to the ceiling in the main bedchamber, and pride in his artistry washed over him as he made the tour. Upstairs, he walked into his lady's future bedroom with pleasant musings of next viewing it in the company of Matilda Graham.

The dark eyes wandered over the furnishings casually; then Arden started and returned his gaze to the bed. How odd that the servants should get so out of hand as to leave a bed unmade! And why the devil had they been using it in the first place? Arden sighed over the necessity of speaking sharply to this new staff. He never enjoyed "putting on the duke," as he called it, and, being of a personality which inspired instant and steadfast loyalty in retainers, he usually never had to do so. But neither could he allow housemaids and their swains to disport themselves in Matilda's bed.

Taking a closer look at the disheveled bedclothes, he spied a piece of white laid in the center of a pillow. He reached out and snatched it and, to his astonishment, read his own name.

A moment later Arden had placed the branch of candles on a nearby table and was tearing open the letter:

> Your grace,
>   My cavalier and I thank you most sincerely for making this lovely room available for our tryst. You need not trouble me again, as I will never submit to *you*.
>
>   M.G.

"Good Lord!" the duke roared, his eyes bulging with disbelief. "How could she dare?"

His words had been of a truly stentorian volume, and before many minutes had passed the pattering of feet announced the arrival of Drumm, followed by sundry other staff members, all half in, half out of their nightrobes and slippers.

"Was Miss Graham here today?" Arden snapped. His expression was so different from that of the good-humored master they had all come to know and love that the servants quailed in a body.

Drumm, as head of the household, found courage and cleared his throat. "She was indeed here, your grace. She and an elderly companion, the elder Miss Graham."

"And who else?" the duke said in a cold voice.

"Why, no one else, your grace."

"You may all go back to bed except for Drumm," were the duke's next words. The servants scattered like autumn leaves in a gust of wind.

"Drumm, tell me all about Miss Graham's visit," Arden said.

The butler complied, his alarm mounting at the duke's high color and enraged expression. He told of Miss Graham's tour of the house and related that he had left her and her, er, "aunt" upstairs at the younger lady's request. He had not seen them leave.

The duke nodded tightly and dismissed Drumm, who went on his way back to bed in discernible relief. Arden, left alone in the bedroom, clapped a hand to his throbbing forehead.

Anything could have happened between the time Drumm left the ladies and the unspecified hour of their departure!

Arden bounded down the stairs and out of the house. In Piccadilly he hired a hackney.

"Bloomsbury Square, and hurry." He snapped out his orders in his most imperious manner. As a result, the hired chaise rattled through the London streets at a bouncing speed that would surely have sickened a lesser man.

Matilda turned on her thin pillow, trying to dislodge from her mind a disturbing dream involving a duke, a houseful of pretty clothes, and herself. Despite the clothes, in the dream Matilda seemed to be naked. She twisted once again as the duke called out to her.

"Out of that bed, damn you!" The voice was so real, and the sentiments so wrong for the dream, that Matilda opened her eyes. A dark, angry face glared at her, lurid in the flickering light of one candle. Matilda let out a little gasp.

Arden grasped his quarry by the shoulders and summarily hauled her out of her narrow bed. "Alone, are you? What a surprise, my dear. What have you to say for yourself?''

Finding herself on her feet, Matilda snapped to instant life. ''You dreadful man, what on earth are you doing here? I . . . I'll call the watch! How dare you?'' She slapped at him, and he caught her wrist in a vise-like grip, though he was forced to let go his hold on her flannel-clad shoulders.

''How dare *I?* I'm not the one who used our love nest for another tryst!''

Matilda stared at the duke in awe. He was looming over her, dark eyes brimming with fury, lips drawn back in a sneer. ''You're jealous,'' she whispered.

''Jealous? Of a slut like you? I should be so foolish,'' Arden yelled.

''That disgusting, overly ornate house is not *our* love nest, by the way,'' Matilda said, tossing her head.

''Overly ornate?'' Arden's eyes nearly popped out of his head. ''Why, you—''

''You are a snake!'' Matilda cried, getting into the spirit of his anger. ''How dared you fix up a house, buy me clothes, without so much as a by-your-leave? I've already told you I won't become your mistress!''

''But you didn't say it was because you had someone else on the string, you scheming piece! Did the two of you laugh at my taste in furnishings as you wallowed in *my* bed?''

''Matilda,'' a soft voice quavered, ''are we being robbed?''

Arden whirled around. In the opposite corner of the room was another narrow bed he hadn't noticed when he had stormed in, aided by the landlady's key, which an obliging porter had brought him in exchange for a bribe. He had seen only Matilda's red hair spilling over her white pillow. Now he made out a nightcap and a pair of startled eyes visible above a sheet clutched in trembling old hands.

"Good God," the duke said, "the aunt."

"Don't fret, Aunt, we aren't being robbed, unless his grace the duke hopes to relieve me of my virginity in front of you," Matilda said.

"Virginity," Arden jeered. "You must have left it behind you long ago, my dear."

"Oh, don't you understand, you stupid man?" Matilda exclaimed. "That note was a joke. I mussed the bed myself. All by myself. In retaliation for your horrid assumption that I'd fall into your arms when confronted by riches. Ridiculous, horrid man." Matilda turned her head to one side, unable to bear the suddenly piercing stare of the Duke of Arden.

"A joke," he said.

"Will you stop repeating everything I say and get out of here?" Matilda said, turning her eyes to his once more. "My aunt can tell you that I'm innocent of what I wrote in that note, and heaven knows I'd only hoped to get you out of my life forever by making you angry. I certainly didn't expect to be defending myself to you. And why? Why need a mistress be virtuous? I hadn't even accepted your . . . your terms, and even if I had taken a lover, it would have been within my rights. Why must you keep plaguing me?"

The words had come out in a rush, and Arden merely blinked as he stared into the flashing green eyes so near his own. "You're right," he said quietly. "You said the truth a moment ago. I was jealous. I am jealous. No other man must have you."

Matilda swallowed and stared at him. She had a sharp retort ready, but somehow she was unable to utter it.

Suddenly, to Matilda's astonishment, Arden's firm lips were curving upward, and the dark eyes twinkled in the old way. "You had me, didn't you, my love?" said the duke with a laugh. "Your cavalier, indeed!

And your joke had the charming effect of showing you how much I want you.''

"Hah," Matilda managed in a choked voice. She was longing to laugh with him, and she knew that would be fatal.

"My darling." Arden stepped forward.

Heaven help me, was Matilda's only coherent thought as she was enveloped in the duke's embrace. His lips moved insistently, demanding a response, and Matilda found herself clinging to him like a madwoman, kissing him as deeply as he kissed her and wishing in confusion that her thick flannel nightdress and his sleek evening clothes were a thousand miles away.

"Matilda! Good heavens!" came a shrill voice.

Matilda gasped and tore herself out of the duke's arms.

"The aunt," Arden muttered. "Forgot."

Throwing a guilty glance in the direction of Aunt Poppy's bed, Matilda spoke nervously. "Please, Duke. You must leave now. Can you understand if I tell you that I'm not an ordinary actress? That is, I am indeed an actress, and by my choice, but I am only working on the stage because my aunt and I have no money and I have no other talents which could earn our way. My father is dead, and he was a poor tutor who was unable to provide for us. My only wish is to return to Oxford someday and live a normal life again." She hated having to lie to him in this particular, since her real desire was to return to the stage one day, but she must keep up appearances in front of Aunt Poppy. "I *can't* begin having protectors now. I've made it nearly six months without, and I call it cruel of you to insist."

"Oxford," the duke muttered in fascination, staring at Matilda. Never had she looked so beautiful, so desirable, as she did at this moment in that flannel sack, her bright hair tumbling down her back, her cheeks glowing so hotly the color could be made out even in the candlelight. How yielding, how sweet she had felt in his arms. Her words were not making much sense to him, entranced as he still was by their embrace, but some things managed to sink through and lodge in his brain-box.

"Will you please leave?" said Matilda. She did her best to stare him down, not realizing that her eyes were doing strange things to the duke's heart. Had he told her that she looked more lovely than he'd ever seen her, Matilda would have quite sensibly informed him that it was because she was not wearing her lurid stage paint.

He didn't voice his thoughts of her beauty, though, merely reached out for her again.

"Matilda, you must not!" Aunt Poppy cried out.

"She is so right. I *must* not. Duke!" Matilda struggled out of this latest embrace.

"Must not? But we're made for each other, dear girl. Heavens, if you come from Oxford, I see no reason you may not go back there now if that's what you want. A house near the town, that's the ticket. I've an estate in Oxfordshire, a minor property, but no reason I shouldn't find many reasons to go there." The duke, speaking quickly, ended his latest assault on Matilda's virtue by kissing the girl's hand.

Matilda's eyes widened as she contemplated the extent of the duke's depravity. It was too hard that he should offer her what she most needed in exchange for what she most wished, to her shame, to give him. "Do not keep holding these plums just out of my reach," she ordered, speaking just above a whisper. "You are horrid, evil, and mean. I hate your generosity. Now, go!" Her words, despite her best efforts, had risen in volume until the last "go!" was uttered in a shout.

Arden looked at her. "Quite the respectable young

lady, aren't you? Outraged virtue and all that. I must remember you're an actress before you place me totally under your spell. A place, by the way, where I would delight to be in honest circumstances. My dear Miss Graham—Matilda—if this is only more of your coquettishness, I must beg you to give over. We're both about to go mad from desire.''

His small arrogant smile and glinting eyes drove Matilda right over the edge. ''Go, go, go!'' she shrieked. ''Do you understand plain English, Duke? Must I hit you over the head and drag you out? Leave us alone!''

Arden kept shaking his head. ''This is most curious,'' he said in that detached manner which was making Matilda angrier than she'd ever been in her life. He didn't move to go, but he turned about, examining all the details of the modest room, everything from the shabby sofa to the deal table to the cowering aunt behind that heap of bedclothes in one corner. Did two women really live in this room, as it appeared? His eyes lit on a picture which ornamented the wall next to the door.

''I've seen something like this before,'' he said, walking up close to look at the crude watercolor of five girls in a garden.

''Get out,'' Matilda intoned.

The aunt lowered her bedclothes to expose her entire face. ''Oh, Duke, do you like it? I did it myself years ago. I have little talent for painting, but I wanted the piece more as a memento than anything else. My sisters—''

''Aunt Poppy, you are not to talk to him. Out, sir!'' Matilda cried. She had crossed to the fire and picked up the poker, which she proceeded to brandish in her best Lady Macbeth manner.

''My dearest Miss Graham,'' the Duke of Arden said, turning from the watercolor, ''my apologies for

disturbing your rest. We will be in communication.''
He opened the door and went out with only one more
raking glance at Matilda and a slight bow to Aunt
Poppy.

Matilda peeked out the door after him to hiss, ''We
will never communicate again, you vile creature.'' She
said the words to his retreating back, and he responded by turning round to give her a flourishing bow
and a wink.

''Nothing out of the ordinary, good people,'' he
said, and went on his way.

Matilda noticed belatedly that more than a few
nightcapped heads were peeking from doors up and
down the long hall.

She was ready to sink. But there was nothing to do
but give the assembled company her most apologetic
smile and close herself up in her room.

Tomorrow would be time enough to deal with all
problems save that of her ruined night's rest and her
besieged heart.

The duke was right about one thing. Matilda was
about to go mad with frustrated desire.

10

❧

"YOU can't mean it, Mrs. Burnaby," said Matilda.

The landlady sniffed. "I most certainly do mean it, miss. I run a respectable house here, I do, and even if the gentlemen and the ladies have their little adventures from time to time, I can't be closin' my eyes to the kind of larks you and your, er, aunt are kicking up. One man for two of you, indeed! Never have I been so shocked, and I've been havin' theater people in my house since I left the boards myself some thirty . . . er, twenty years ago. Out you must go, and today. My Lord, miss, I've my reputation to think of!"

Mrs. Burnaby's substantial bosom seemed to swell and the iron-gray fringe of hair under her cap to waggle in disapproval.

"I can't believe this," Matilda murmured, thanking the stars that she had left Aunt Poppy in their room when the two of them had been summoned to the landlady's quarters for this interview.

"I've a dozen witnesses who can swear they saw a man leaving your room last night. That duke they say you've had on your string. Well, I don't hold with a girl throwing over a duke, to be sure, but to do it in my house! And to use your old auntie! Many's the ear that heard her screaming out last night. Though I'd wager that old bird has more experience in this game than the two of us together."

Matilda choked on a hysterical giggle. "I cannot let you insult my aunt, who is the most virtuous of women," she said with dignity, rising from the hard chair Mrs. Burnaby had advised her to take upon her

116

entrance into the room. "We will of course vacate the premises today, ma'am. And you may be sure that I will never recommend your house to anyone!"

"Much I care. A trollop's recommendation . . ." the landlady was muttering as Matilda stalked away.

"Old harridan!" Matilda cried, pausing in the doorway.

"Slut!" was Mrs. Burnaby's bellowed rejoinder.

Matilda went upstairs to her room, cheeks burning. She had to be at the theater in an hour, and how were she and Aunt Poppy to pack, transport their effects to a new place, and arrive in time for rehearsals?

They simply couldn't do it. Aunt Poppy caught her breath and shed a few tears when told that they had been asked to leave the lodging house, but she was soon industriously packing their things. The plan was to take everything to the theater, where Matilda would ask others of the company for recommendations of a place to go. The manager had been the one to tell them of this house when the Grahams first arrived in London. If they couldn't find another room, they would have no choice but to return to the only other place of lodging Matilda knew, the coaching inn where they had spent their first night in town. The expense would be ruinous, but what choice did they have?

Matilda and Aunt Poppy didn't have very many belongings; this made their task easier. There were only their two large valises and a small trunk which contained precious personal effects such as Aunt Poppy's watercolor and dear Papa's old edition of Shakespeare's plays. What made their baggage ungainly were the plants the two ladies had brought home to their room, the plants the duke had included among his floral offerings that night at the theater.

"Auntie, I think we should leave these depressing greens in the street," was Matilda's comment as she vainly tried to hail a hackney from their little forest

on the pavement. The orange tree and a half-dozen
other pots filled with flowers or ivy were lined up on
top of the trunk.

Finally a job-driver stopped beside them; from the
glint in his eyes, Matilda suspected he was more
amused than chivalrous, but he good-humoredly
hoisted the trunk onto the hack, leaving the ladies to
deal with their valises and the sundry plants.

"That duke," Matilda said, sighing, when she and
the orange tree were finally sharing one corner of the
vehicle. "It seems he's laughing at me at every turn."

"Your pardon, dear?" Aunt Poppy was cradling two
precious pots on her lap, and, if Matilda wasn't mistaken, actually crooning to them.

"Oh, nothing," was the niece's rejoinder. She tried
to look more kindly on the bedraggled orange tree
since it and its compatriots were serving the very important purpose of keeping Auntie's mind off their
troubles. Aunt Poppy had accepted without question
Matilda's reason why they must leave their lodgings,
and Matilda was not at all anxious to tell her the truth.

After many more trials and tribulations, Matilda
found herself where she had to be: in her dressing
room at the theater, with the baggage stacked neatly
against one wall. Auntie bustled about, seeing to the
plants.

"Now it's off to rehearse *The School for Scandal,*"
Matilda said briskly. "Have you enough to do, Aunt?"

"I'm perfectly fine," was the cheerful rejoinder, and
Matilda grabbed a copy of the play and ran to the
stage.

She arrived on the boards, breathless, to be confronted by the amused stares of her fellow players.

"Had a rough night, dearie?" asked the old beldam
who was doing Lady Sneerwell.

"Oh, Fanny, let the poor thing be." Dulcie Moore

giggled. "Poor Mattie can't help it if her spark likes things a bit odd."

Matilda's lips set in a tight line as she struggled to keep back a very unladylike stream of abuse. She reminded herself that, for good or ill, these people thought she was the duke's mistress and had thought so for some time. She couldn't change their minds.

She forced herself to laugh and shrug. "Would you believe it, Mrs. Burnaby booted us out of our lodging this morning. Do any of you know of a place we might try? I can't keep Aunt in my dressing room forever."

"Never say the duke won't set you up and pension off the old 'un," put in Mr. Blore in the whining drawl which so differed from his robust stage tones.

"I prefer my own establishment," Matilda said with dignity, cursing inwardly as she felt her cheeks redden under the gazes of all these gossipmongers. *The School for Scandal* seemed a particularly appropriate piece for today. Imagine news of her and her aunt's escapade having reached the company already!

Eyebrows raised at this odd streak of independence in one who enjoyed the favors of the Duke of Arden. Several of the actors, however, had recommendations to make of this or that lodging house, and Matilda calmly noted them. She might have time between the end of rehearsals and the beginning of the play to inquire at one or two of the closer places.

"Well, Lady Teazle," Mr. Devlin inquired, "have you got your business taken care of? I'd hate to interrupt . . ."

Flushing even redder, Matilda nodded and bent her eyes to her script.

The day, which had started out so badly, quickly went to worse. When Matilda went round to the lodging houses her fellows had recommended, she found that her new reputation as a perverse practitioner of the sexual arts had flown before her.

"It's this red hair," she said to herself, hurrying along Maiden Lane on her way back to the theater. The day was rainy, and Matilda's tresses were beginning to kink up in the dampness, adding to her ordinary dislike of the russet mop. "They recognize me every time. And I can hardly rent lodgings in a wig, under another false name." That sort of scheme, which had earlier occurred to her desperate and overtaxed mind, would only land her in a worse scandal broth when the prospective landlord discovered her deception. As he or she would, Matilda being so well-known in local acting circles.

Safe in her dressing room, she set before Aunt Poppy the packet of buns she had bought for their supper. "No luck, dear?" the old lady asked with a timid look into her grandniece's stormy face.

"None at all," Matilda said. She glanced about the dressing room. Aunt Poppy had spent the day making the little chamber as homelike as possible, getting out their shawls and an embroidered pillow to ornament the sofa, and even hanging up her homemade watercolor picture of the girls in the garden. "Why, Aunt. You didn't expect me to find anything."

"Well, my dear," twittered Aunt Poppy, "we know how fast news travels. And since we left Mrs. Burnaby's rather under a cloud—"

"How do you know that?" Matilda interrupted.

"Heavens, what else could it be? The very morning after the duke's visit, we find that Mrs. Burnaby has forgotten to tell us that she has promised our room to a relation? No, my dear, that excuse didn't hold water, as your papa used to say."

Matilda stared. Her aunt had been entirely corrupted by the evil city, and it was all Matilda's fault for bringing her into this ramshackle life.

"Oh, Aunt," she said, sinking weakly down on the

hard chair before the dressing table. "I don't know what to do."

"Heavens, you must not worry, child. We are quite well-fixed here for the night. I've asked one of the young men to bring us in a pallet and some blankets if he can find them, and though we must watch carefully for fleas, I see no reason why we can't move on tomorrow as easily as today. You must search for a house in which the proprietors are not privy to this dreadful scandal we seem to be embroiled in. Unless"—Aunt Poppy paused delicately,—"you would wish to ask the dear duke for help? He seems very fond of you, and now that you've made your position clear, his lust will turn to reverence. I read that in the sweetest novel."

Matilda burst out laughing. "What a practical aunt I have! But, no, I couldn't ask the duke for a thing. He still has designs on me, Aunt Poppy. Lewd, not reverent, designs. I'll find us something tomorrow. How clever of you to provide for our comfort tonight."

"And now, hadn't you better get ready to go on the stage?"

"Oh! It must be very late." And Matilda, recalled to her duty, tore out of her clothes and into the dress she would wear as the abigail in *The Clandestine Marriage*.

Matilda, with her cheerful face and bright beauty, was a natural in the comic abigail parts. Many compared her to Miss DeCamp, now Mrs. Kemble, who had also made her mark in such roles. Matilda felt much more comfortable this evening, with nothing to do but prance about and act coy, than she had in the woeful miscasting of Lady Macbeth. (Though she had already heard, to her horror, that Mr. Devlin was thinking to revive that performance, with everyone in the same roles, it having been an unexpected success.)

Were there more hoots and raucous comments than usual? Matilda furrowed her brow slightly when she and Dulcie Moore—the miscast one tonight in the role of innocent young bride—took the stage for the opening scene. Well, perhaps it was only normal, not at all an indication that the rumors of last night's *ménage à trois* had spread. Matilda and Dulcie were a striking combination, and not only was Matilda the rumored mistress of the Duke of Arden, Dulcie had just accepted the protection of the great Lord Drummond. Both of the young actresses were all the rage.

Matilda prayed for the strength not to look up at the duke's box, but her eyes seemed to stray there of their own accord. *He* was leering down at her, as usual. This evening he sat between two dowagers of daunting aspect: one positively queenly, with white wings of hair springing back from her temples, ending in a turban ornamented with diamonds and emeralds. Matilda immediately recognized the Duchess of Arden, the duke's mother. She didn't know the less striking older woman on Arden's other side, but assumed her to be of equal rank and power with the duchess. A patroness of Almack's, at the very least.

In fact, it was the Countess of Dauntry whom Arden escorted that evening, along with his mama. Lady Davina, in whose interest he had formed the party, had had to stay home with a sick headache, much to the elder ladies' disgust. It was obvious to both mothers that Arden had already set one foot in parson's mousetrap. Why, he had never asked Davina to the theater before!

Matilda, all unaware of these plots and counterplots, resolutely forgot the duke and continued with the play. On returning from the wings to her dressing room for the interval, she was surprised when Aunt Poppy flung open the door, all in a flutter.

"Oh, Matilda, we have a visitor," she cried.

A lady rose from the moth-eaten sofa: a lady richly dressed, in expensive clothes which proclaimed her to be young, as did her upright carriage. These were the only available indications of her age, for her head was shadowed by a dark veil. Over the lady's eyes was a loo-mask.

The stranger approached Matilda. "You're more beautiful than I'd imagined," she said matter-of-factly. "How fortunate. I do address Miss Graham?"

"I am Miss Graham," Matilda said, "And you?" The wild thought went through Matilda's mind that perhaps this was some member of the duke's family, come to beg Matilda, perhaps pay her off, if she would set Arden free of her silken bonds.

The veil came off to reveal rather lackluster light brown hair done in a fashionable knot. Next the mask was removed, and Matilda was facing a young lady of perhaps eighteen or nineteen, a lady with an honest pair of blue eyes and a nose of unfortunate length. A pleasing face, decided Matilda, forgetting about the nose immediately, as did the few people who were fortunate enough to view Lady Davina Lowden when she was not casting her eyes down to the floor.

"I am Davina Lowden," said the young lady. "I've come to speak to you about the Duke of Arden."

Matilda gasped and groped for a chair. "You have? I assure you, ma'am, I have no designs on his grace. You mustn't worry."

"Oh, but I do." Lady Davina sat back down on the sofa and looked earnestly at Matilda. Aunt Poppy, fascinated by the richly clad young woman, perched on the opposite corner of the couch and listened in silence.

"I'd hate for you to be in a pother about nothing at all," Matilda said. "I am not under the duke's protection, nor do I mean to be. Are you his . . . his cousin perhaps, or his betrothed?" Matilda doubted the latter

was true, for she had been shamelessly scanning the
social columns of the *Morning Post* lately, fearing to
come upon news of the duke's engagement.

Lady Davina sighed. "I'm not the duke's betrothed,
but things would seem to be heading that way. Marriage with the duke would be a dreadful fate, Miss
Graham, and one I won't submit to."

Matilda stared. "You won't?" That any young lady
should spurn the legitimate attentions of the Duke of
Arden struck Matilda as nothing but a mistake. "We
are talking about the same duke?"

"The very duke who's sitting out front now with my
mother and his," Lady Davina said. "I was to go
along, but I stayed home so I might come to you in
secret. The duke and I are being pushed together by
our families, Miss Graham. I have no desire to wed
him."

"No desire to wed the duke," repeated Matilda,
absolutely fascinated by this glimpse into the private
life of the man she had thought must be irresistible to
all women.

"No desire." Lady Davina let the phrase echo
around the room for the third time. She got up and
walked about, coming to a stop in front of the dressing-
table mirror. "Look at me, Miss Graham. I'm not
exactly a beauty. A loveless marriage is bad enough,
but a loveless marriage with a handsome devil like the
duke? Intolerable! A lifetime, Miss Graham, of listening to people explain to one another that of course he'd
married me for my bloodlines, and on his mother's
orders. A lifetime of standing up at balls with a man
I don't love, appearing at court with him, and being
invisible." Davina's lovely blue eyes filled with tears
as she stared into Matilda's still-incredulous face.
"You can't know what it's like, Miss Graham, to be
invisible."

"My dear Miss Lowden," Matilda said, rising from her chair to clasp the young lady's hand in sympathy.

"Lady Davina," said the other, sniffling into a handkerchief. "Please call me Davina. I've come to you for help, Miss Graham."

"Help?" Matilda frowned, totally at a loss. She guided the other girl back to the sofa and sat her down, taking the hard chair across from her as before. "You must call me Matilda . . . Davina. But how can I possibly help you? If you don't want to marry the duke, simply tell your mother and his. Unless . . . Does the duke wish to marry you? Is that the problem?"

"He doesn't. We've agreed to bide our time. He asked me very kindly if there was a man in my life, for he didn't want me to waste my second Season as his almost-betrothed. I'm afraid, though, that I haven't yet met the man I could love. The duke and I decided, since my situation wasn't desperate in a romantic sort of way, to act as though an engagement might take place at any time, meanwhile avoiding being left alone. I don't trust my mother, you see. If we were left alone, she would cry 'compromise.' But it seems to me that this avoiding of the problem doesn't solve anything."

"It does seem a weak plan, given that you have desperate mothers nipping at your heels," Matilda said with a little smile. "Perhaps the duke does want to marry you, and doesn't know it." She felt her heart sink at this prospect.

"I'm certain that's not it," Davina proclaimed, furrowing her brow, a habit which was much deplored by the Countess of Dauntry, who said Davina had enough problems with her looks without adding wrinkles to the tally. "I do feel some sympathy with Arden, and I suspect that he wants to make a love match if he can. As I do. With a plain man." Davina sighed a little, thinking of her most romantic fantasy. "A man who matches me in looks."

"I see," said Matilda, who did not really see at all. Trying to think of the duke as a stranger, not as the dashing and eminently desirable man she knew, she conceded that perhaps a young woman could wish to avoid marrying him. Young girls did dream of love, even, to Matilda's surprise, young girls of rank whom she had thought impervious to such a weakness of the common classes. How, though, could any young woman set out to fall in love with a plain man? That course seemed as riddled with perils as that of a girl who wished to love a man with money. Surely love was ruled by no such externals. Neither funds, nor looks, nor . . . nor rank could stop love in its inevitable course. Matilda knew that as well as she knew anything. Why, she wouldn't be in love with the duke, would she, if rank were to be considered? . . .

"My heavens," said Matilda. She was in love with the Duke of Arden! She hadn't consciously realized it until this moment.

Lady Davina and Aunt Poppy were looking at her curiously, both pairs of expressive blue eyes filled with true concern.

"My dear? Is something wrong?" Aunt Poppy asked gently.

The sympathetic looks of the two women undid Matilda. Overwrought and nervous as she was with all the day's problems, and now on top if it, an interview with the duke's reluctant intended, Matilda burst into tears. "I'm in love," she sobbed, her face in her hands. "How can I keep resisting him? And he won't love an actress. He'll merely bed me and leave me with a . . . a s-settlement."

"Oh, my goodness," Aunt Poppy cried, patting her niece on the back.

"My dearest creature!" Lady Davina reached forward to clasp Matilda's hand.

Matilda quieted down, for she had to go back to the

stage in a few minutes. How was she to act the care-
free maid while the Duke of Arden watched her with
his cynical, admiring gaze? His mocking eyes would
be the death of her, now that she knew the state of her
own heart.

Lady Davina was smiling now. *Heartless creature!*
thought Matilda in resentment. At least sweet Aunt
Poppy continued to emit coos of distress at her niece's
confession.

"Miss . . . Matilda, this is better than I'd hoped
for," Lady Davina said. "I came to you hoping I'd
find a jealous mistress, one who would be glad to en-
act a plot to stop the duke's marriage. If you are really
in love with him, you must be willing to go to any
lengths to stop his being wedded."

"Why?" Matilda asked. "To me, he can never be
more than a . . . a temporary protector." Large tears
rolled out of her eyes, and she brushed them away.

Davina frowned at the sad truth of this. "What a
pity it is indeed, my dear. But he would be more truly
yours if he wasn't sharing his favors with a wife, even
so."

Matilda sighed. "Davina, do tell me what your plan
is. I can hardly speculate about something I haven't
been told. And please don't believe everything you
hear. I am not now the duke's mistress, and I will
never be that to him. Never."

Davina looked doubtful at the last remark, but she
obediently outlined the plot which had come to her
after her first sight of Matilda at the modiste's. Davina, Mama, and the Duchess of Arden would come
upon Matilda in the abandoned embrace of the duke.
Davina would be shocked, as any innocent young
creature must be by such a display, and both haughty
and unbendable mothers would understand Davina's
refusal of the libertine duke's offer.

Matilda shrugged. "I can't say that I would willingly be in the duke's company ever again, Davina. Perhaps some other actress would be a better choice, and I can recommend—''

''Oh, but I had such high hopes of you, the very one who's his mistress already, according to gossip. Then Mama and the duchess would be bound to understand that I'd heard the rumors and was now confronted by the dreadful truth.'' Davina's beautiful eyes sent an appeal to Matilda. ''Whereas it would seem that his simply embracing some strange woman would be something they'd want me to overlook.''

''I have a friend, the heroine in tonight's play,'' Matilda said in determination. ''I'm certain she would go along with this. I simply can't.'' Another tear ran down her cheek as she tried to smile. ''I want to stay away from that man. Forever.''

''My word.'' Davina gazed earnestly into Matilda's face. ''Is that what it's like to be in love?'' She had somehow assumed that people who loved would wish above all else to be in each other's company.

Matilda noticed that both Aunt Poppy and Lady Davina were waiting for her answer.

''It's many things,'' she said with a sigh. ''I'm too far beneath him to have any of it happen. I want to grow old with him, and walk in gardens, and have babies, and all sorts of distressing things I've never thought of doing until this moment. And I want to make l—'' Catching herself on the edge of the last dread confession, she reflected that making love was something she had thought of before she had found her emotions as well as her body to be under the spell of the rakish duke. There was no need to shock the ladies.

''Have babies,'' Davina said in awe. ''It makes you *want* to?'' Davina had been bred up almost from infancy to know that her eventual fate would be that of brood mare to some uncaring peer who would be induced to marry her for the sake of the Conqueror's blood, and she had never looked on the prospect of children with any emotion stronger than indifference.

"Well, it isn't the very first thing I thought of," Matilda amended her rash confession, even while in her mind she clasped a miniature Duke of Arden to her breast.

"Oh." Davina was still fixing Matilda with that searching look. "How lucky you are, Matilda."

"Lucky indeed," chimed in Aunt Poppy. "I have always wanted to be in love, my dear."

"Lucky?" Matilda surveyed the two ladies in astonishment. "I can't see that. Well, Davina, I must bid you good-bye now; the interval will be nearly over. Good luck, and I . . . I hope you don't have to marry him."

"Oh, how I wish *you* could," Davina said fervently, touching Matilda's shoulder with an elegantly gloved hand.

Wild horses could not have dragged from Matilda the fact that she wished the very same impossible thing, but as she left the dressing room and made her way back to the wings, she was certain that both Lady Davina and Aunt Poppy could see right into her heart. In love, indeed!

How much simpler life had been only an hour before.

11

LADY DAVINA had to struggle to contain her disappointment at the outcome of her meeting with the notorious Miss Matilda Graham. Nothing had come of this brilliant idea. Davina had been looking forward, before meeting Miss Graham, to the successful conclusion to all her own difficulties with the duke.

Davina had had such high hopes from the encounter. She had not doubted she would find a crude and jealous beauty who would be happy to take part in a scheme to part Arden and the mousy Davina.

"Whatever you say, m'lydy," Davina had expected the voluptuous redhead to utter with no trace of her cultivated stage accents. "What's in it for me?" (Or words expressing such a sentiment, delivered with an outstretched palm. Or perhaps a thumb rubbed against two fingers in the time-honored manner.)

Davina had, of course, been prepared to pay Matilda Graham for the favor of the deception. Instead she had found herself warming to the young woman, asking an actress to call her, the daughter of an earl, by her Christian name. What was it about Matilda Graham?

Davina had never dreamed that she would find in that forbidden den of all iniquities, the backstage of a London theater, a truly cultivated young woman chaperoned by an obviously well-bred aunt. Matilda Graham could have been shamming the accents of a girl of gentle birth in order to fool Davina; she was an actress. But could she have pretended, as well, her sad emotional state?

Davina's heart went out to the poor girl who labored in the grip of a hopeless love for Arden. It was no wonder the young actress wouldn't let herself be caught acting out a compromising position with the duke. As Davina understood it, Matilda was fighting with all her willpower to keep out of such a position in reality. Sadly Davina contemplated Matilda's dilemma, and Davina's own problems receded for the moment to the back of her mind, where she heartily hoped they would stay.

"Child," the sharp voice of her mother broke into Davina's thoughts, "sit up straight."

Davina repositioned her spine and tried to concentrate on where she was and what she was doing—not as tempting a prospect as even a gloomy daydreaming, since where Davina was at present was her mother's barouche-landau, which was engaged in a tedious circuit of Hyde Park at the fashionable hour.

At least the weather was clement, a welcome respite from the past few days of spring rain. Still, no pleasure brightened Davina's eyes as she looked around at the brightly hued crowds, riders and drivers and pedestrians, and wished above all else that she were at home with a good book.

"The duke!" Lady Dauntry hissed into her daughter's ear. "Quick, girl. Straighten your bonnet. Fluff your pelerine. Twirl your parasol. Smile!"

Davina complied, obedience to the last order coming readily to her lips as she reflected that, all over the park in similar carriages, other mamas were giving similar instructions to their daughters.

Then Arden was beside their carriage. Attired in striking riding clothes, his dark crop of hair slightly tossed by the wind, he sat a magnificent black stallion with all the ease of a superb horseman.

"Lady Dauntry. Lady Davina." He executed a smooth bow from the back of his steed. "You remember my young brothers?'' With a casual glance over his shoulder.

Davina followed the direction of his eyes and saw Lords Peter and Paul Beresford, mounted on identical grays, approaching at a little distance behind their brother. ''I thought they were in Cambridge,'' she said.

''The dear, sweet boys, the duchess must be so very glad to have them home with her,'' put in Lady Dauntry with a fond look at the handsome lads.

''Ahem! Let us say that Mama's happiness far exceeds my own,'' the duke responded. His black brows drew together. ''Their second escape this term! It's shackles for them this time, ladies. Ah, Paul. Peter. Here you are. Make your greetings to the ladies. We were just this moment discussing your futures in the iron industry.''

The boys exchanged exasperated looks before turning their vaunted charm on the countess and her daughter.

''I was calling on your mother, Duke, when she received the letter from Lord Julius. How happy I was to hear of his escape at . . . what was that place called?''

''Badajoz, Mama,'' said Davina softly.

''Yes, Bad-something. A German place. Eudocia must worry so, having a son in the army. And him the next heir!'' The countess shot a conscious look at her daughter, who glared.

''Plenty more where he came from,'' said the duke with a shrug, waving his hand in the general direction of the twins. He made a practice of hiding from the world his own anxieties about his military brother, finding his solicitude as well as his affection old-womanish. It would be best to ignore the dratted woman's hints about him and Lady Davina setting up a nursery.

The twins, to do them credit, had been chatting with Lady Davina about their latest vaulting of the Cambridge ramparts. "If we keep coming out, old Michael will tire of returning us," Lord Paul was saying as Arden and the countess turned to join the conversation.

"You may be sure I would never tire of such an amusing prospect," the duke contradicted his brother. "You must know, ladies, this time I'm going back with the lads myself, so as to have a word with their proctor. Then, not to be outdone in my touring of the halls of academe, I'm off to Oxford on a matter of private business."

"Oxford? Extraordinary. But aren't you also a Cambridge man, Duke?" Lady Dauntry inquired. "You won't be making a long stay, I hope? We do look for you at the Carlton House rout, and we quite depend upon you to partner Davina at her cousin's ball next month."

"A few days at most," the duke assured the predatory mother with his most entrancing smile. "How could I remain for long away from your side, my lady?"

Lady Dauntry was teased into the flutters under the eyes of the handsome young man. Her daughter, looking on in disgust, reflected sourly that it did not take much to put the countess into such a state. How had Mama managed to retain a spotless reputation all these years? Perhaps—a little smile lifted the corners of Davina's wide mouth—no one had wanted Lady Dauntry.

That idea did much to cheer Davina as she said a bland farewell to the duke and his fair-haired brothers. Seeing Arden looking so abominably cheerful this morning, and remembering Matilda Graham's tears and vexations on his account, Davina was more than half-inclined to snap at him.

"You could have been more forthcoming, you impossible girl," Lady Dauntry grumbled out of one side of her mouth when their carriage was on the move once more. Graciously she nodded and waved to an acquaintance over the way.

"Oh, the duke and I understand each other," Davina replied with an insouciant shrug. No matter how her suddenly avid mother plagued her, she could be induced to say nothing more.

Before conducting the twins back to Cambridge on short leashes, Arden unbent so far as to take them to one of his clubs in St. James's. The boys were content to stride about, puffed up in their own consequence as dandies and brothers of a duke, while their older sibling sought out Lord Peterborough.

"You're an Oxford man, Perry. Give me the name of someone to see there. I'm looking for a tutor. A dead tutor," Arden said, sinking down into an armchair opposite his friend.

Lord Peterborough blinked and passed a large hand over his head. "Must be the wine last night," he muttered. "I could swear you just said you were looking for a dead tutor."

"So I did."

A rough laugh escaped Peterborough. "My old tutor's in that condition. Heard from my young cousin that Glendenning went off some months ago. Sorry to hear it, for I liked the old party. Would he do?"

"That's not the name," Arden muttered. "What I wish from you is the name of some don or other to go to with my questions about this departed chap I'm looking for."

"You know, I shouldn't bother if I were you. Dead men are remarkably difficult to engage in conversation," Peterborough said cheerfully. "Is this one of your jests, Duke?"

"No, damn you. It's . . . private," the duke said. "I wish to dig up the dead man's family."

"Sounds unappetizing at best."

The duke was too good-natured to give that line the quick burial it deserved. He let out a laugh. "The name of a man at Oxford?" he reiterated his request, still in good humor, but with a certain edge to his voice which made Peterborough sit up and take notice.

Perry came up with the name of an old clergyman, a distant relation of his own family, and "a dashed bore when it comes to prosing on about the history of the colleges. He's the man you want."

"I don't doubt it. Thanks." And Arden had already risen, and was about to leave in search of his brothers, when Peterborough stopped him.

"I say, old fellow, it ain't sporting to leave me out of this one. 'Specially when I've not gotten back at you yet for the 'fire' business."

Arden could certainly see the justice in this. Yet his business was private and he meant to keep it that way. It occurred to him, however, that one aspect of his association with Miss Graham was common knowledge. The world believed her to be his mistress, and he had been fielding envious gibes from the bucks and gallants for some time now. There would be no harm in a simple reference to her. It might be thought odd, in fact, that he hardly ever did mention her.

"What do you think of Miss Graham, old boy?" he asked, sitting back down. "What's your impression of the lady?"

"I take it you're not referring to her looks," Peterborough answered. "No one can doubt her beauty. And you know I was one of the ones tried to capture her before she gave in to you." He sighed. "The flowers and baubles I sent that girl's way! Enough to tempt a saint. Tossed the baubles right back at me, of course."

Arden nodded. This information simply confirmed his original ambiguous impression of the girl; her fastidiousness in turning off Peterborough could denote either the virtue she claimed or a pragmatic holding out for the highest bidder. "You've never spoken with her, or heard anything about her?"

"No. What makes you ask?"

"There's something about her," Arden answered with a shrug. "The way she talks and certainly the way she behaves. Not your typical actress."

"Indeed?" Peterborough looked at his friend carefully. A fleeting expression of something very like affection had crossed the duke's face. "You're not being indiscreet with this one, are you?"

"Indiscreet? No. That's part of the problem," Arden said with a sigh, rising again. He clapped his friend companionably on the back and went on his way in search of two preening curly heads.

Meanwhile Matilda Graham was beginning to believe that she had been beached during the tide in the affairs of men, as her father used to say of his more useless pupils. All her arrangements seemed doomed to failure. She, a virtuous young woman, was sinking in a mire of scandal.

It had been three days since she and Aunt Poppy had been thrown out of Mrs. Burnaby's, and in that time Matilda hadn't succeeded in finding them a new place to live.

Tales of their scandalous proclivities had flown before her; even the meanest of theatrical lodging houses refused to give house room to a "pair of bawds," "wicked, perverse strumpets," or "odd, unnatural whores," as they were variously described.

Strange it was that in the loose theatrical circles which had at first shocked Matilda with a lax disregard for the strictest principles, she herself should now be doing the shocking.

Curiously enough, it wasn't the mere fact of a threesome in love that had raised universal hackles. Aunt Poppy's age, and the lack of discretion the three had employed, were the criticisms Matilda heard. She wasn't a stodgy girl, and considering that the rumors were lies, she would have thought the situation funny if it hadn't resulted in her homelessness.

The only comfort left to Matilda was that her aunt never went along on these forays to hunt for lodgings and didn't have to hear the names she and Matilda were called. Unfortunately, Matilda could not avoid Aunt Poppy's knowing that they had not yet found living quarters. Every night spent in the cramped theater dressing room made that clear.

The situation came to a head one day when the manager informed Matilda in no uncertain terms that she couldn't continue to billet in the theater. He ended this ultimatum by pressing into the actress's hand a slip of paper which proved to contain the number of a house in Monmouth Court, which, he said with a cough, would no doubt accept the ladies as lodgers.

"No doubt?" asked Matilda, shocked. "Is it that bad?"

"Er . . . a bit unconventional, ma'am." And though Matilda pressed him, Mr. Devlin would say no more.

Matilda returned to the dressing room and presented the problem to her aunt. "I hate to try this place, but it seems we have no choice if we're to be out of here by tonight. At least the street is close by."

Aunt Poppy's eyes were thoughtful. "But, dear, there is another choice. We might apply for help to some of our great connections."

Matilda laughed. "Great connections? Us?"

"I mean the duke, of course, dear. Or perhaps that sweet young lady who came to see you the other night.

She gave me her card before she left, you know, and said that if we needed anything—''

''No. We will survive on our own, Aunt Poppy. And that is final.'' Matilda found herself swallowing hard, for her aunt's suggestion was tempting. Impossible, but tempting. Pride and thwarted love tied Matilda's hands in the matter of the duke; though she trusted that he would indeed help them, she couldn't stand the thought of begging him for that aid.

And as for Lady Davina! Not for worlds would Matilda expose their new shame to that innocent and cultivated young lady of quality.

''If only it weren't for the shameful associations,'' Aunt Poppy said with a sigh, ''we might walk right into that pretty house in Half Moon Street.''

''Aunt Poppy!''

''Sorry, dear. It's merely that I've heard the duke is gone out of town. I read it in the *Morning Post* society column, which Mr. Blore lent me this very morning. So if we were so lacking in decorum as to go to Half Moon Street, we would be in no danger of meeting with him—''

''Out of town?'' Matilda asked sharply. She immediately colored up, ashamed at having betrayed any interest in That Man's movements.

''Why, yes, dear, for I would never have suggested removing to Half Moon Street if I thought it would place you in an uncomfortable interview with a seducer.''

''That's a mercy,'' Matilda said, resolutely putting from her mind the hollow, lonely feeling which had come over her on hearing the duke was not in London. ''Aunt, I must have Lady Davina's card. It's not that I don't trust you—''

''All the same, you don't trust me not to contact her. How right you are, dear Matilda, to save me from temptation,'' said Aunt Poppy. She fished in her tattered reticule and came up with the card, which she pressed into Matilda's hand.

Matilda kissed Aunt Poppy's forehead, patted her shoulder, and immediately crumpled the card into a small white ball. "Why don't you busy yourself with packing our things, dear? I'll go out and make arrangements for us at this newest lodging house."

Matilda got into her drab pelisse and went out into the day, trying not to think about the sumptuous appointments of the house in Half Moon Street. How difficult it was to be independent! She had a sudden vision of herself, clad in a lacy nightdress, peacefully asleep—alone—in the big gold-curtained bed in that jewellike bedchamber.

It had been most unkind of Aunt Poppy to bring up that particular temptation.

12

THE Duchess of Arden was awake upon every suit. Nothing could slip by her that had to do with her sons or the consequence of her family, which latter she guarded as jealously as she might have had she been born into the house of Hanover.

She had known for some time of her eldest son's intrigue with a certain actress at one of the minor theaters. She had not even raised her eyebrows; the many years out in society, and, more important, marriage to a philandering husband, had taught the duchess not to refine too much upon the little adventures of her menfolk. A liaison with an actress had never hurt anyone, the duchess had been thinking in some complacency. In fact, she had noticed how Arden's practical joking appeared to have slowed down as the actress presumably took up more of his time.

The duchess was ensconced in the morning room of Arden House one day, writing a rather subdued letter to another son in which she mentioned the liaison, when Lady Dauntry was announced.

The countess twitched into the room importantly, her round face purposeful and serious, and came right to the point. "What do you think of *this*, Eudocia?" she said, slapping a large paper down in front of her old schoolmate, smudging the paper the duchess was crossing and coming very near to upsetting the inkpot in the process.

The duchess drew back slightly; she and Belinda pretended a great friendship for one another, given

140

their plans for their respective children, but was quite
this much familiarity warranted? Lady Dauntry was
obviously too upset for the amenities.

The duchess turned her eyes to the paper and found
herself looking at a new cartoon.

"Rowlandson, is it?" The Duchess of Arden was of
an artistic turn of mind, and she quite naturally regarded the style of the drawing before passing on to
its content.

"Cruikshank," the countess said. "I have never
seen anything so scandalous in my entire life. Look at
it, Eudocia!"

The duchess did, and at first glance shrugged. "Another start of Arden's? Why make a fuss about it, my
dear?"

"Look at it!" the countess nearly shrieked.

Her hostess scrutinized the piece more carefully;
despite all effort to keep her old friend from seeing
any sort of emotion flitting across her aristocratic lin-
eaments, her eyes widened and she drew in her breath
audibly.

"How could he?" she said through set teeth.

The Duke of Arden, with his narrow, classic features and fine, well-proportioned figure, was a natural
subject for the pen of either of the Cruikshank brothers. The scion of the house of Arden was represented
at his ease in a large tufted bed; on one side of him
leaned a lush, beautiful girl, nearly naked. Both these
figures were leering awfully at a cowering old lady in
a nightcap, who was under the covers at Arden's other
side. A very large sword hung over the duke's head,
bearing a Latin legend the duchess would wager was
obscene; and among the tangled bedclothes a verse
could be made out, describing the scene:

Come young, come old, come shy, come bold,
So says our D. of A.;

Ah, love can be no slight ennui
With only two to play!

Do hear my plea, dear Miss M.G.,
Though our amours are strong,
Respect my plight, enhance our night,
Bring your old bawd along!

"I had to pay a pretty penny to get *this* removed
from the print-shop window in Bond Street," Lady
Dauntry said. "There must be dozens more flying
about the town, but I simply couldn't leave it there for
every shopper to leer at. Should Davina see it! The
poor girl would be so disillusioned. We have had a
little talk, naturally, Davina and I, and she understands perfectly well that men will have their little interests. But this! I wouldn't blame the child for being
scared off from a marriage to such a hardened, shocking libertine, even if he is a duke."

The countess's words washed over the duchess as the
latter lady tried to think. How odd that Michael should
turn to the perverse in his eternal quest for amusement! A pity he hadn't simply continued to play jokes
on his friends. "Have you heard any details about this,
Belinda? I presume the young woman here is that actress he's been keeping. But an old lady? A pity Michael isn't in town so I can question him. Drat the boy!
This is probably some dreadful mistake. You know
how quickly these *on-dits* get out of hand."

"No doubt," Lady Dauntry said in tones which betrayed her complete disagreement with such sentiments. "I've made it my business to learn the shameful
details, Eudocia, and a sordid tale it is. It seems Arden
was seen late one night leaving the lodgings of the
actress person, a room she occupied with an old
woman she passes off as her aunt. But before the duke
left, all the other lodgers were treated to a . . . a very

noisy scene of passion though the walls! And so the disgusting tale got out.''

''My word,'' the duchess said. ''And what do you suggest we do about it, Belinda? It would seem the proverbial cat has been let loose from its concealing sack already. Do you think Davina will not hear of this? We might shut her up in her room for the rest of the Season, but I don't see what else we could do. She must simply be told that this scurrilous cartoon is a lie. And that only if she appears to have heard the story.'' The duchess's eyes narrowed. ''It would be convenient, though, for the Arden name, as well as for dear Davina, if Michael should break off with this horrid actress creature.''

Lady Dauntry sighed. ''I don't see how that could be managed, but I will tell you the truth, Eudocia, that would be the best gift a young girl could receive from her future husband. How romantic! To change his ways for the sake of his future duchess!''

''I would hardly expect Michael to change his ways to any great extent,'' the duchess remarked dryly, ''but to rid him of this particularly loathsome actress would be doing a service to all of us. Well! What time is it?'' She rose to her full majestic height, straightened her gown, and pulled forth the watch which hung from her belt on an intricate arrangement of several chains. ''Two o'clock. Excellent. Wait for me here, my dear, and I'll return shortly in my walking things.''

''Where are you walking to, Eudocia?'' the countess asked, totally bewildered.

''I'm not walking anywhere, you ninny, I'm taking the carriage. And you are coming with me. To the Royal George Theater.''

The countess gasped, and then her eyes began to gleam as the duchess's meaning sank in.

''Precisely,'' the Duchess of Arden said. ''No little stage strumpet will be able to withstand our combined

wills. *Ménage à trois* indeed! Have you any money
with you? Oh, no matter,'' as the countess fumbled
for her reticule, ''I'm persuaded the little tart will be
bought off as easily with a note of hand.''

Matilda hummed in harmony with her aunt's singing
as that dame warbled ''A Red, Red Rose'' over her
knitting. Aunt Poppy was engaged in making bed socks
for both herself and her niece; the attic chamber in
their new lodging house was drafty even in the summer, and should they have the bad fortune to be there
still when winter rolled around, Aunt Poppy was certain they would both freeze to death without proper
gear. She had unraveled the most moth-eaten of her
shawls for this important project.

The ladies were sitting where they still sat most often: in Matilda's dressing room. Though they had been
living at Mrs. Peck's in Monmouth Court for several
days, they spent as little time there as possible. They
were fulfilling Mr. Devlin's requirement that they not
sleep at the theater; that was the important point.

Matilda hadn't realized that any place on earth could
be as tawdry as their new address. She suspected every
one of the female residents was a woman of easy virtue; she was certain that Mrs. Peck was, she with her
cheap satin dressing robes barely held together, and
her winking acceptance of Matilda and Aunt Poppy as
lodgers.

Sad to say, Matilda couldn't have had much respect
for any woman who would rent to herself and Aunt
Poppy, considering their vile reputation, which seemed
to have permeated all corners of the town.

The situation was truly desperate. Aunt Poppy cried
herself to sleep every night, and Matilda spent all her
leisure moments in trying to find somewhere else to
live. Each evening they pulled most of the furnishings
of their new room over to barricade the door; and more

than once the handle had rattled and some raucous voice had called out for "the pair o' ye, and name yer price."

Only at the theater could they relax; hence their sunny mood this day. Matilda was putting on her stage paint for her first night in the role of Lady Teazle, an experience she was eagerly anticipating. *The School for Scandal* had done its part in taking Matilda's mind off her troubles. Never in her life had she been so grateful to have employment as an actress. For several hours a night she could forget she was Matilda Graham, principal in one of the seamiest scandals in London, and become someone else.

Matilda was applying blacking to her eyelashes—the last touch—when the door was summarily flung open.

"Y'r la'ships," muttered the voice of the porter.

"Barker, how dare you?" Matilda cried, turning about on her stool.

She nearly fell off the rickety seat. The elderly porter had already disappeared, and standing before Matilda were two middle-aged ladies clad in the first style of elegance. The taller, more regal-looking female stirred some vague feeling of discomfort in Matilda's breast; the other lady, rounder and less prepossessing, though no less sumptuously gowned, caused her no alarm. She rose.

"Ladies? Can it be you have the wrong room?" A curtsy might have been in order, but Matilda was not about to essay such a maneuver in her old wrapping gown, which might well gap open and disgrace her.

"Miss Graham?" the taller lady intoned, fixing Matilda with a haughty stare.

"Yes, madam." Matilda eyed her in return with as steely an expression, though it was much less effective coming from a young lady only half-clothed.

At this point the shorter, rounder stranger had an

attack of the flutters. "It *is* the creature!" she cried.
"I recognize her from the cartoon."

"Cartoon?" Matilda looked from one lady to the
other in query; then her glance hit on Aunt Poppy,
frozen behind her knitting in a corner of the room,
only her wide blue eyes and her cap visible above the
needles. "Ladies . . ." she began lamely, wondering
how to get them to leave so that any shocking statements wouldn't be uttered in front of Aunt Poppy. They
were obviously indignant about some new horror concerning Matilda and the Duke of Arden. Were they
Evangelists? Relations of the duke's? Matilda was wild
to get them away from her aunt, but she could hardly
accompany the women to another room in the theater,
dressed as she was in her revealing robe.

The short, round lady had followed Matilda's gaze
and spied Aunt Poppy. "Good Lord! The old bawd!"
she shrieked.

Aunt Poppy twittered something indistinct and burst
into quiet tears.

"Madam!" Matilda said. She still maintained her
regal stance before the two ladies; Aunt's tears would
have to take care of themselves until Matilda could
manage to clear the room. "Watch your language before my aunt, if you please. I have not had the pleasure
of making the acquaintance of either one of you, and
that you should stand in my dressing room and abuse
my dear aunt—"

"Aunt! Do you dare to perpetrate that charade?"
The taller lady sneered. "We know who she is, and
what you are, you vile, disgusting woman of the
streets! And we're here to insist that you remove your
claws from my son."

Matilda blinked and stared harder at the lady. Peer-
ing under the fashionable bonnet the woman wore,
Matilda could barely discern two white wings in the
raven hair. "Your son?" she whispered in fascination.

"I am the Duchess of Arden," the lady said, favoring Matilda with a certain look she usually reserved for vermin and housemaids caught in indiscretion.

"And I," the duchess's companion, not to be outdone, said, bustling up a bit closer to Matilda, "am the Countess of Dauntry. The mother of the poor creature you're wronging."

Matilda was silent. For a moment the only sound to be heard in the room was Aunt Poppy's faint sobbing. Matilda's mind was whirling busily. If she was not mistaken, there stood before her not only Arden's mama but also the reputedly dreadful mother of the sweet and kind Lady Davina Lowden.

Matilda straightened her shoulders proudly and gave a gracious nod to the duchess. "Your grace would wish that I remove my . . . my claws from the Duke of Arden? What have I done, pray tell, to provoke such a request?"

"Don't play the innocent," the countess interjected before the duchess could open her mouth. "You've done *this.*"

Matilda found a paper slapped into her palm. Eyes widening with horror, she stared at the awful sight of herself, the duke, and an anonymous withered old lady caricatured in bed together. At least they hadn't come by Aunt Poppy's likeness. Her face now stained with a blush other than the stage red, Matilda looked over the verses and nearly choked.

A guilty eye slid to Aunt Poppy, who had quietened and was now looking at both the noble ladies as though they were wild beasts.

"Ladies, I have not done this," said Matilda quietly. "Now, if you would please leave—"

"Not without your promise to discontinue your black liaison with my son," the Duchess of Arden said firmly. In one hand she held a parasol, and she tapped it on the floor for emphasis.

"We're prepared to pay you, you wicked creature," Lady Dauntry said, putting up her chin in an effort to approximate Eudocia's queenly air.

Matilda was astonished into a continued silence.

The duchess cast an annoyed glance at her friend. "We are indeed prepared to pay you off, you painted terror. Anything to get my sweet son out of your clutches."

"Your . . . sweet son?" Matilda succumbed to a hysterical hoot of laughter while the two ladies looked on in exasperation.

"Dear Matilda, did the ladies say they would pay you? For promising to leave the Duke of Arden alone, I presume?" spoke up a reedy little voice from the corner of the room.

"Aunt, stay out of this."

"The person is urging you to be practical," the duchess said to Matilda. "And it would be wise. My son never keeps any ladybird for more than a month. Your time is running out in any case. But in order to soothe the feelings of the countess's dear daughter, my son's intended, we will pay you to get out of London. Having broken off all relations with the Duke of Arden."

"How much?" piped up Aunt Poppy.

"Mercenary old harridan," murmured the Duchess of Arden. Speaking to Matilda, she answered the question. "Two thousand pounds."

Matilda actually stopped to think. To be offered more money than she could hope to put away in years of stage work, and for leaving off doing something she hadn't even done!

She looked straight into the duchess's hard eyes. "You and your son are much alike, madam. You offer propositions that are very tempting to a woman in my position."

The duchess started.

"How dare you speak in such tones to her grace?" put in Lady Dauntry.

Matilda turned to this lady. "Do you not think I dare anything, ma'am? I am not a woman of easy virtue, though I admit that appearances are deceiving. I can hardly help what the gossips are saying. And as for this"—she held up the cartoon and crumpled it before the ladies' eyes, then threw it at their feet—"I deny this scurrilous libel absolutely. And now, your grace, my lady, you will oblige me by leaving my room."

The countess and the duchess simply gaped. A painted redheaded little actress stood in front of them, a cheap creature whose ripe bosom was nearly falling out of a ragged dressing gown. And she was standing up to two of the most powerful ladies of the *ton*.

Lady Dauntry was the first to crack under the hate-filled stare of Matilda's green eyes. "Perhaps we should be going, Eudocia?" she asked meekly.

The duchess had been returning Matilda's gaze with her own challenging glare. "We do not go without this creature's promise."

"You need no promise from me. There has been nothing of an immoral nature between me and the duke," Matilda said. "If you wish to stand here forever, I suppose it is no business of mine. Would you excuse me, though, while I change for the play?"

She marched behind the wobbly screen in one corner of the room. Within seconds her wrapper had been tossed up over the screen.

"The creature is undressing! In front of us!" the countess gasped.

"A drab of that class would stick at nothing," the duchess reminded her friend.

From behind the screen came a sound of exasperation.

"I have never been one to meddle in my son's little

diversions,'' the duchess said, speaking in a slightly raised tone of voice to be heard over the screen, ''but in the case of you and your, er, elderly companion, Miss Graham, I have forgotten the dignity due my rank and consequence and come here to plead with you. It isn't that the Duke of Arden's name is not a byword. He has always cared more for his horrid jokes than his reputation. So it will be, whatever you and he do. But think of the broken heart of an innocent young lady. Picture her shock on hearing—and she will hear, the world is cruel—that the man she loves and is to marry is nothing more than a perverse scoundrel!''

A muffled giggle came from behind the screen, provoking an indignant exchange of looks between the visitors.

Matilda was thinking, as she struggled into her costume, of Lady Davina's honest eyes and trembling voice as she had declared that marriage to the duke would be a ''dreadful fate.'' Matilda suspected that Lady Davina would greet with glad cries the news that the duke was figuring in a scandal too horrid for a respectable young lady to countenance. Matilda resolved on the spot to help a young woman she considered her friend, separated though they were by walls of rank and consequence. She herself would see to it that this latest scandal came to Davina's ears.

''You would be so cruel as to laugh at the plight of my poor wronged daughter?'' Lady Dauntry cried.

Matilda appeared from behind the screen; she was fully attired in her Lady Teazle costume, but it was not fastened in the back. That her aunt must do for her. She made a strange, wanton picture in the loose gown. She was the very image, in both the duchess's and the countess's minds, of a fallen woman.

''I wish nothing but good to your daughter, ma'am,'' Matilda said with a nod of her head to the countess. ''And as for you, your grace . . .'' She paused, and, holding her gown together awkwardly, moved closer to the duchess. She took in the cold eyes and the stern, unyielding expression of the haughty face.

"I wish you liked your son better," Matilda said with a helpless little shrug.

"You dreadful, disgusting *courtesan,*" burst out the Duchess of Arden. "Do you persist in your stubborn refusal?"

"I won't take your money, if that's what you mean," Matilda said.

"Oh, Matilda," Aunt Poppy sniffled. "We might move into better lodgings had we money enough to bribe a landlord—"

"Nothing is worth giving in to these harpies, Aunt."

"Why, how dare you—" began the countess.

"Get out," Matilda said. "I seem to be saying that to members of your family frequently, your grace. And I mean it. Get out now. I must leave soon, and I won't have you remain to harass my aunt."

"Your procuress, you mean," the duchess spat before she turned on her heel, signaled to the countess to follow her, and opened the door. "You haven't heard the last of this," was her parting shot as she sailed out of the room.

Matilda sank down onto the dressing-room sofa, trembling in mingled pride and indignation. The audacity of those women! And she had routed them, in a way. She, an actress, had ordered about a duchess and a countess.

"Aunt Poppy, I am sorry that you have to keep observing these sordid scenes," she said a bit later, smiling over her shoulder at the old lady, who was presently engaged in doing up Matilda's buttons and hooks.

"Belinda Lowden has certainly grown coarse; I wouldn't have known her," was Aunt Poppy's only comment. Matilda shrugged it off, assuming her aunt had glimpsed the countess years ago and remembered her name.

As, indeed, Aunt Poppy had.

13

THE spires and ancient walls of Oxford were particularly appealing when caressed by the yellow sunshine of a perfect summer's day. The Duke of Arden, as he wandered down the High Street, was glad he had decided to walk out upon his errand. He could feel the quiet, scholarly tradition of the town permeating to his very bones. He had to remind himself that he should, by rights, feel no such enchantment. He was a Cambridge man.

The house the duke was seeking was the abode of that old clergyman, distantly connected to Lord Peterborough's family, whom Perry had extolled as the last authority on Oxford matters. As he walked, Arden tried to imagine Miss Matilda Graham traversing these same streets. Her radiant and very noticeable beauty would stand out against these old buildings; therefore the duke was confident that if she had actually lived in Oxford, and was the child of a tutor, he would be able to find it out.

A creaking manservant ushered the duke into a low-beamed sitting room in a crooked little house which looked to date from the fifteenth century. "Mr. Beresford," the man announced, for Arden had decided to visit Oxford incognito.

From a chair near the unseasonable fire rose a short, round old man—an ancient dressed in knee breeches and frock coat, with what remained of his hair powdered and worn in a tail. Spectacles perched on his long nose, and in one gnarled hand he held a fusty-looking book, the place marked by one of his fingers.

"Mr. Beresford? How d'ye do." Behind the spectacles, a pair of piercing light eyes was glinting with intelligence and query.

The duke bowed. "Mr. Pettigrew, it is kind of you to receive me. I bring greetings from your kinsman, Lord Peterborough."

"Young scamp," the old man snorted. "Well, sit down, sir, and tell me why you're really here. Crump!" The manservant looked in. "Wine and biscuits."

With a nod, the servant shuffled away on his errand. The duke accepted a hard seat across from the leather armchair where his host had been ensconced and now proceeded to resettle.

Mr. Pettigrew was eyeing the young man over his spectacles with what appeared to be suspicion. The duke cleared his throat and, with no preamble, began.

"Peterborough has lauded your ability to recall the doings of Oxford in every particular, sir. As I'm, er, a Cambridge man, I had to ask his help in finding a resident of this town. I am trying to locate someone, you see, the daughter of a deceased tutor. I don't even know the college he was with, merely his surname, and I am hoping you will be able to—"

"Help you seduce a friendless young woman?" croaked out Mr. Pettigrew, glaring mightily from under a pair of bristling gray brows. "Cambridge man, indeed!"

The duke was slightly taken aback. Mr. Pettigrew had hit on his visitor's foul purpose. Or had he? Arden was the first to admit that his fantasies of Miss Graham didn't end outside the bedroom door. Since meeting her, however, his plans had undergone several changes. When he had seen her for the first time, from his theater box, he had lit up with the possibility of making the lovely creature his mistress. A woman who was still holding out for the right rich protector had seemed a certain conquest. A duke, after all! Arden was lacking in that personal modesty trained into those of lower station and lesser looks, and his confidence was usually justified.

When his sterling qualities of rank, riches, and seductive prowess had not resulted in the immediate catapulting of Miss Graham into his eager arms, the duke's first thought was that he hadn't made a generous-enough offer. Hence the house in Half Moon Street and its accompanying luxuries.

That measure having failed, he had no choice but to look at the problem from another angle. Virtuous behavior in an actress wasn't unheard-of. Miss Graham's looks were against her, to be sure. She had the appearance of a young woman made for amorous delights. If Arden had made a mistake in thinking her his for the taking, he had been abetted in that error by Miss Graham's delightful beauty. So he would not hesitate to tell her, if he ever had the chance, though the idea that she looked made for love would doubtless infuriate her.

Arden was hoping that this visit to Oxford would either dig up the news that the Grahams of whatever college were respectable people or that they didn't exist at all. Certainty was what he wanted. If he exposed Miss Graham in her lies, perhaps she would finally break down her reserve, laugh with him, and fall into his embrace.

He was longing to get her into his arms again, and next time, he swore, he would not be interrupted by a squawking aunt or a false uprightness on his lady's part.

If she were respectable, though . . . The duke spent much of his leisure dwelling on such a possibility.

The Duke of Boulton had, long ago, married an actress, the immortal Lavinia Fenton. There were like cases. Such things as had been tolerated in the last century, however, were seldom done in the present day.

Yet visions of his mother's angry face tempted Arden sorely. Then there was Matilda's angry face. Suppose she was respectable. Would she turn from the duke in disgust, saying he hadn't trusted her word in the first place?

She would be well within her rights to do so. Arden hadn't trusted her word in the least.

Remembering the very angry, distractingly lovely Miss Graham of that last interview, in her Bloomsbury lodgings, Arden reminded himself that there was nothing like a challenge.

The duke cleared his throat again. Mr. Pettigrew was still frowning at him in moral outrage. Arden opened his mouth, but no sound came out. He coughed and tried again.

"I assure you, sir, that my intentions toward the daughter of a reputable tutor are all that is honorable."

Thus did the Duke of Arden declare, for the first time in his life, his willingness to shackle himself in the bonds of matrimony.

He let out his breath in relief once the words were out, for he knew he had spoken the truth. His intentions were indeed honorable. He wished nothing more than to make Matilda his duchess, and he hoped with all his heart that his inquiries in Oxford would prove her to have been telling the truth about her origins. He wouldn't foist a practiced adventuress on his ancient family—much though his mother's prospective ire urged him on in that scandalous course—but he wouldn't hesitate to bring any other sort of girl he might find Matilda to be into the ducal fold.

He didn't want his wife to be a liar. That was his only requirement now.

"Honorable intentions?" Mr. Pettigrew snapped.

"We'll see, young fellow. Well, let me have the name of this tutor."

"Graham," the duke said. "I know that and nothing more. He would have recently died, within the last year, I believe. He would have had one daughter and perhaps an elderly female relation living with him. The young lady doesn't speak of a mother."

"Graham." Pettigrew mulled this over as he sipped at a glass of Madeira. The duke lifted his own glass, scrutinizing the old man. A serious, sharp face. Arden didn't doubt that his friend Peterborough had sent him to the right party.

His heart sank when Pettigrew said with a shrug of black-clad shoulders, "No Graham. There's a live one or two: one a bachelor, tutors at Trinity, one a man with a large family, a master of Greek out of Balliol. There ain't a recently dead Graham in the town."

"Oh." Arden was dismayed at his own reaction to this news. She didn't really come from Oxford, at least not in the guise she had claimed. She was presumably of more dubious origins. He might resume his pursuit of the lovely Matilda with every hope of wearing her defenses down to the point of becoming his ladybird.

Why, then, did he feel so unhappy?

"Now, if the name weren't Graham, I could help you," Pettigrew said reflectively. "There's a well-loved gentleman recently dead. Well, not too recently either, it's above six months now. A classics tutor with a daughter. In fact, Glendenning was that loose screw Peterborough's tutor. I shouldn't like to see his lovely daughter fall into the wrong hands." Another forbidding glare from under the shelf of bushy brows.

"Tell me about the Glendennings," the duke said.

"Not much to tell. The old chap died. Hadn't married young, and so left no parents or other relations of his own that Miss Glendenning could turn to. If there had been people of his, they would have been off in

Scotland, at any rate. Glendenning came to us out of Edinburgh. Well, he left her nothing but a parcel of debts and a flock of great relations on her mother's side that she couldn't have approached had she wanted to, they having cast her mother off when the lady married Glendenning. The girl had no choice but to find a post.''

The duke nodded. This was a common-enough story. The faint suspicion which had been growing in his breast died a quick death. Naturally the daughter of a tutor would find a post: a post as a governess or some such. No woman of scholarly, respectable background would tread the boards.

''Did she find a post? Miss Glendenning?'' he asked, more out of politeness than anything.

''Yes, and had to leave town to take it up,'' Pettigrew said. ''She couldn't find anything here, you know. Glendenning would have done better to see the girl was taught some of that useless female drivel rather than make her into a classics scholar. No one would employ her to teach their daughters, and why should they? She knew none of the things that people want their daughters taught. Didn't play a note or embroider a stitch, as Glendenning often bragged. But a young lady classics tutor is out of the question—at any rate, one with Miss Glendenning's looks. Out of town was her only choice. She must have answered an advertisement, exaggerating her qualifications, I shouldn't wonder. I wish her well, but I must say I miss her. Used to come in to see me sometimes, for we shared an interest in the writings of Aristophanes that she couldn't discuss with her papa. Glendenning was a good man, but the humorless wretch persisted in seeing no use in Aristophanes. Ah, he was a Scot, though. Must make allowances, mustn't we?''

The duke was beginning to lose interest as the old clergyman's reminiscences grew lengthier and more rhapsodic. Arden jolted to attention, though, midway through Pettigrew's description of a typical visit from Miss Glendenning.

"What did you say?" he asked sharply.

"Why, you must forgive an old man running on, but beauty and wisdom are rarely conjoined, as Petronius says, and that made Miss Glendenning a special joy."

"What did you say about her? Her red hair all in a cloud? Her *red* hair?"

Mr. Pettigrew lost his faraway look and frowned. "Hair of that color is a trait of the Scots and the Irish, true, but in Miss Glendenning's case it was far and away her most striking beauty."

The duke sat straighter in his uncomfortable chair. "Had this Miss Glendenning red hair and green eyes? A shape to drive men mad? A face to rival any goddess you care to name?"

"Shape indeed! Matilda Glendenning is a lovely creature," said the clergyman with a reproving snort. "I wish her every—"

"Matilda?" the duke shouted. He sprang up from his chair, overturning it in the process.

"Young man," Pettigrew said severely, "your manners are unseemly. A Cambridge education did this, you say? I cannot approve such—"

"Mr. Pettigrew," Arden interrupted, smiling from ear to ear. "You must forgive me. You have just helped me to discover the girl I . . . love."

The last word had come out wrapped in a strangled half-choke. The old clergyman thought back to the days of his courtship of the late Mrs. Pettigrew and remembered that very word issuing from his own lips, and sounding about the same.

He was all genial heartiness as he answered further questions from "Mr. Beresford." The duke was feeling quite exposed, but not altogether unhappy about it by the time he left Blue Boar Lane on the next stop in his tour of Oxford.

Arden had been directed by Mr. Pettigrew to a certain young gentlemen's lodging house across town, where the Glendennings' former maid had taken up the position of assistant housekeeper to the elderly dame who owned the house.

Within the precincts of a house not unlike the lodgings where he had but the other day left the twins in Cambridge, "Mr. Beresford" accepted a cup of tea from a lively middle-aged lady with snapping dark eyes and an intelligent face which softened as she reminisced about her late employer and his daughter.

"Happy I was to be in the service of such a family, sir," said Mrs. Brown, speaking in the consciously genteel tones common to those in her position. (She had confided to her handsome visitor that she had taken the courtesy title of "Mrs." upon her elevation to the rank of housekeeper. The Glendennings had known her as Nan.) "Dear Lady Violet, Miss Matilda's mother, was such a sweet lady. I was only working in the scullery when she died, poor creature, much before her time. There was good blood in her, some say too good for the master, for all he were of a good family in Scotland. That's the thing, sir, Scottish he was, and those of us what don't have a personal acquaintance with Scottish people can tend to be prejudiced—"

"Lady Violet?" the duke interrupted. "Oh, I beg your pardon, madam, and I do agree that there are those unfortunates who harbor unreasoning prejudice against the Scottish race. I am surprised to hear that Miss Glendenning's mother was . . . the daughter of an earl?"

"Oh, a marquess, sir, but cast off by her family." It needed no more encouragement for Mrs. Brown to be off and running on the sad tale of Lady Violet, who

had romantically fallen in love with her brother's aging
Scottish tutor, Glendenning, and married him over her
parents' objections. Lady Violet had been of age, and
her family had had no control over her movements,
though they naturally never spoke her name or received her again. They had given the same treatment
to Lady Violet's sweet maiden aunt too, a dear creature who had taken the young lady's part against her
parents, the result being that the aunt came to live with
the Glendennings and was probably with Miss Matilda
still.

What a sweet-looking lady Miss Matilda's mother
had been, not in the style of her daughter, who must
take after the Scots line, but blue-eyed and golden-
haired like her mother before her. And Lady Violet's
mother, for whom she was named, was one of those
famous sisters. Not the Gunnings, there were only two
or so Gunnings, if Mrs. Brown remembered aright.
There were five of these others, and two had married
dukes. Lady Violet's mama had caught the marquess,
and one had wedded an earl. Then there was the
maiden sister, who, though very elderly now, was a
sweet lady too. Never had there been such a nice, unaffected old gentlewoman to work for as Lady Poppy
Parmenter.

The duke blinked. In the far reaches of his mind,
several things clicked into place.

He was standing in Matilda's room the night he had
rushed over there mad with jealousy at what he had
considered her infidelity. He was about to leave, having once again failed at putting Matilda under his protection, when a simple watercolor painting caught his
eye. The old aunt chirped out something about having
done it herself, and Matilda admonished the old lady
not to exchange pleasantries with the duke. *Aunt
Poppy, you are not to talk to him*, Matilda shouted in
the duke's memory. It crossed his mind that he would

have to get back to town posthaste—he so longed to hear her shout at him again.

The duke stared at Mrs. Brown in seeming fascination, mulling over all these vague impressions. Why did Lady Davina Lowden next sneak into his thoughts? He seemed to see her pretending to embroider, of all things. The duke knew Lady Davina well enough to be aware that she hated needlework. Except when her mother insisted . . .

Mrs. Brown grew a touch uncomfortable under the intense gaze of the handsome young man.

"I have it!" the duke cried. "Gainsborough. Ma'am, your Miss Matilda has played the greatest joke ever on me. And on London."

"Miss Matilda was one for playing pranks as a small girl," Mrs. Brown said doubtfully. "Gainsborough, sir? Where is that?"

"Never mind, my dear lady. May I kiss your hand?" The duke rose, bowed over Mrs. Brown's chair, and suited his action to the word. "No, that's too cold," he said, dropping the trembling fingers. "A kiss on the cheek it must be." And he matter-of-factly plucked the amazed Mrs. Brown from her place and proceeded along these lines.

Mrs. Brown held one hand to the honored cheek and gazed up at the young man. "I hope Miss Matilda's well, sir, wherever she is. London, or the other place you mentioned?"

"Miss Matilda is well. I will ask her to write to you," the Duke of Arden said, grinning widely.

When he left Mrs. Brown's house he was nearly running in his haste to get to the Mitre Inn and thence to his horse. London! the Oxford church bells seemed to chime.

"Matilda," the duke murmured back, chuckling.

14

LADY DAVINA Lowden had gotten into the habit of breakfasting in her room. She was not by nature a person who slept late; nor was she antisocial before her morning tea, as were many of her friends. The reason for her seclusion was nevertheless simple enough.

The longer she stayed in her own apartments, the later she would have to face her mother and, though this was rarer, her father. Neither parent ever failed to make some comment regarding the progress of Davina's relations with the Duke of Arden—or, to be more accurate, the lack of such progress. Once she emerged into the day, that sort of inanity couldn't be avoided.

Sometimes Lady Davina would be saddened by the fact that she was consciously staying away from her parents. More often, she simply enjoyed the peace of being alone.

She was in the latter mood, basking in luxurious solitude in her silk-hung bed, when a maid arrived with her tray. The morning post lay beside the pot of chocolate and two slices of buttered bread which commonly got Lady Davina through until luncheon.

Davina had drunk her first cup before she languidly picked up her letters. There were only a few, and they were bound to be unexciting. Since Davina's bills went in with her mother's, and her invitations came under the aegis of cards to the whole family, the only personal mail she ever received was from cousins, aunts, or the occasional female friend. Davina was not the sort to receive *billets-doux* from eager suitors, a fact she often deplored.

As she read through an insipid, gushing invitation from Miss Smytton to a morning waltzing party, Davina's eye strayed to the letter next in the pile. There was something odd about it; for one thing, it was bulkier than the others, and it had come by the two-penny post, whereas Davina's young lady friends in London were more likely to have correspondence transported in the hands of a family footman. Putting aside Miss Smytton's note, Davina opened this second, vaguely mysterious letter, hardly daring to hope it would be something to interest her.

A folded paper tumbled out when Davina broke the wafer. Well! That accounted for the unusual bulk. The text of the outer leaf was brief and to the point:

My lady,
If you are sincere in your wish *not* to marry the D. of A., the enclosed will help you settle the affair with your parents. Who could expect you to marry such a libertine? And if you were not quite candid with me, and it should really be your wish to become his wife, do rest assured that the enclosed is a disgusting and completely false libel. You have met my aunt!

M. Graham

Quite naturally, Davina's next act was to open the enclosure. She noticed as she did so that it appeared to have been crumpled up at some point, then re-smoothed. When she saw the drawing, she was not surprised.

''Oh, poor Matilda,'' she cried out, glad that the maid had already left the room and was not by to hear the anguish in her voice. ''How terrible.''

Davina had heard rumors of Arden having figured in a particularly scandalous episode with the actress,

but luck and her mother's care had kept her from seeing the famous cartoon until now. Her heart went out
to the poor young woman who was sketched in beside
Arden in an evil-looking bed. To add insult to injury,
Mr. Cruikshank had made Matilda very plump.

Davina couldn't have been more certain that whatever the source of this revolting cartoon, there must
be some reasonable explanation. Now the question remained: Was she to do as Matilda suggested?

Davina toyed with the idea for a moment. She would
run to her mama's room in tears, before she got
dressed, so as to assure a wild and disheveled appearance. The infamous cartoon would be clutched in her
fingers. Mama had probably seen the thing already,
for she had taken great care that a scandal which must
be the talk of the town had not come to Davina's ears.
Therefore Mama could be counted upon to understand, if not approve, Davina's hysterical decision
never to marry the duke.

Even Mama couldn't say that a peccadillo of this
magnitude—supposing it were true, which Davina
knew it was not—should be excused as one of those
little situations in which men (weak creatures!) will
embroil themselves.

Like all young ladies of rank, Davina had naturally
been warned to expect a marriage of convenience.
Destined to be bedded only for the sake of the line,
she would avert her eyes from her husband's adventures. Lady Dauntry had added to this typical speech
her own view that Davina, as a plain young woman,
would need this show of dignity more than her prettier
fellows, since her husband would have every excuse
for any indecent behavior.

Davina had been very hurt by her mother's asper-
sions on her undoubtedly plain appearance. But she
had also gleaned from this uncomfortable conversation
the fact that husbands, loathsome as they were in their

rampant physicality, must return discretion for their wives' polite ignorance. In the eyes of the world, Arden had broken that bargain already.

"I won't do it quite yet," Davina murmured, her lip curling in naughty pleasure as she contemplated Mama's certain horror at the spectacle of Davina hysterically declaring she would not become the Duchess of Arden.

She decided to keep the drawing safely in the secret drawer of her little French escritoire, and to use the ploy only in the event of a real emergency. The cartoon would come in very handy should the duke change his mind about the marriage of convenience!

Davina, since meeting Matilda Graham and finding out about the girl's affection for the duke, had been considering the possibility that Arden might feel the same tenderness for Matilda. Since he couldn't marry a young woman of Matilda's unfortunately low station, he might forget Davina's wishes and accede to those of his mother and her own, counting on Matilda as a mistress. And what a dreadful fate that would be! Davina thought herself a strong young lady, but there were limits to the resistance she could put up. If the duke himself joined with her own shrill and opinionated mother and the Duchess of Arden to stand against her, might not her resolve crumble before the force of those combined personalities?

Davina shuddered. For the thousandth time she wished that she would meet a gentleman who touched her heart. The duke would likely not decide to marry Davina even if he were sure that Matilda would be by to act the loving courtesan. He would more probably stay single in order to drive his mother into Bedlam. Unattached, he was a danger. Only by marriage to others could Davina and the Duke of Arden ever be truly safe from the dreaded union.

Davina opened the third letter in the pile, noticing

as she did so that it was addressed in a spidery handwriting.

Much later on that same day Matilda trudged backstage after her performance. She hadn't slept at all the night before, and the role of a spirited and perky young matron had had to be wrung from her this evening. And she couldn't even look forward to a good night's rest! Mrs. Peck's seedy lodging house, with its myriad indignities, seemed too much to face. If not for fear of incurring the manager's wrath, Matilda would definitely keep herself and Aunt Poppy at the theater for the night.

Matilda's lack of repose hadn't had much to do with her horrid living arrangements, though she tried to convince herself that she had quite naturally lain awake solely because of the noisy party going on in the room beneath hers. In truth, she had been thinking about the duke.

She had been considering, as she often did, how much nicer the luxurious bed in Half Moon Street would feel than her thin, moldy cot; only this time she had not been able to picture herself in the bed alone. That impossible duke had held her close all night in her fancies; and she had arisen as tired as though he had really been with her and allowed her no sleep. The satisfaction arising from a night of love, the sort of catlike, contented languor described to the wide-eyed Matilda by Dulcie Moore, had been all that was missing.

In place of that warm feeling was a smoldering resentment of the Duke of Arden. That, added to shame over her own thoughts, which the duke had nothing to do with, made Matilda snap at Aunt Poppy before breakfast was over and send the old lady into tears.

The rest of the day followed along those lines. The only bright spot was the performance. As usual, Ma-

tilda gloried in the opportunity to forget her troubles
and take on Lady Teazle's. It had been such a strain
to do so, though, that she was now in a very weakened
state.

To make matters worse, Arden had been leering
down at her from his box all during the play. He had
been absent ever since the appearance of that dreadful
cartoon, and Matilda had nourished the fond hope that
perhaps he was staying away out of delicacy for her
feelings. But he was on the spot again, and no doubt
determined to plague her.

Matilda closed the dressing-room door behind her
and leaned against it, sighing and putting a hand to
her throbbing head. She had to admit it; she had been
so glad to see the duke in his theater box that she had
nearly run off the stage to join him.

"What? Out of sorts, my love?" said a too-familiar
voice.

Matilda found herself looking into Arden's sparkling dark eyes. He had been sitting on her dressing-
table stool, and now he rose and came toward her.

"What have you done with my aunt?" She spoke in
a hoarse whisper. The strain of throwing her voice out
into the audience had taken much more than its usual
toll this evening.

"Your aunt." Arden was quite near her now; if he
put out his arms, he might imprison Matilda between
himself and the door. "Oh, I asked her to give us a
little time alone."

"And she agreed?" Matilda's eyes widened in disbelief. It had finally happened; Aunt Poppy had run
mad.

"She did. She understands that you and I must be
private for the interview I have in mind." The duke
gave Matilda no opportunity to respond to this. He
merely reached out and took her into his embrace.

A gentle, searching kiss followed, and Matilda

didn't even bother to feign indifference. She was too tired. He might as well know that she wanted his kiss; it would make the decision she felt herself slipping into all the easier.

"My dear girl," the duke muttered, releasing Matilda's lips to plant his own on her hair and each of her eyelids, "do I understand this to mean that your sentiments toward me have undergone a change since we last spoke? Or should I say, shouted?"

His humor broke the sensuous spell that had held Matilda. "I . . . No, I can't say that," she answered, shrugging.

"Then what is it? I would have expected to be clubbed over the head with that candlestick before you'd allow me such liberties."

His words were teasing, affectionate. Matilda gazed desperately into his eyes and saw only goodwill there. He wouldn't hurt her; he would help her aunt immeasurably, filling the good lady's last days with comforts, not indignities and privations. Matilda was living under the cloud of scandal already, and no action of hers could be worse than what the gossips said she had done.

If she gave up her honor now, she could never marry, of course. She wouldn't foist a duke's discarded mistress on any honest man.

"I've thought over your proposition, Duke," she began.

"Why, what a coincidence. I've done the same. And I have some news for you, my dear."

"News?" Confused, Matilda kept on staring at the duke's face, wondering how soon he would initiate her into what Dulcie Moore maintained were the delights of the bedchamber. Not tonight, surely. Nobody could expect a woman to do that sort of thing through a haze of fatigue. . . .

"News indeed, my dear Miss Glendenning," Arden

said. He smiled widely and bent to her for another kiss.

This time Matilda pulled back, shocked beyond measure at his use of that familiar name she hadn't heard in so many months. "What on earth?" she cried. "Do you . . . ? How could you possibly know?"

"I went to Oxford and asked questions," Arden explained. "You see, my dear, I was quite curious about your story. How many actresses come out of the scholarly world of Balliol and King's?"

"You went to Oxford and spied on me?" Matilda's voice was suddenly cold. "I told you what sort of a background I came from and you doubted my word?"

"Ah! I was afraid this sort of thing would happen. My dearest Miss Glendenning . . . Graham . . . Matilda. Try to look at things from my side." Arden was enjoying the familiar flashing eyes and flushed cheeks of his love even as he sought to soothe her. The encircling arms came into play once more.

Unfortunately, the gesture that had made Matilda feel safe and warm but a moment before now roused her ire. "How could you have a side in this, you . . . you fiend! Since when does a mistress need her credentials verified? Oh, do get away from me." Impatiently she flung her arms out to the side, trying to displace his.

The ducal arms did not loosen. They did quite the opposite, and Matilda found herself crushed embarrassingly close to a muscular body, her breasts, nearly bare in the costume of a dashing baronet's wife, pressing against a white shirtfront while, behind that crisp linen, something was thumping loudly. It was the duke's heart! And if she could feel his, he could doubtless discern hers.

"Physical contact, my dear," the duke murmured. "Works wonders."

To Matilda's surprise, he made no move to initiate another troubling kiss; he merely held her, running his hands over her back in a gentle, soothing motion. She sighed and leaned against him.

"Famous joke you've been pulling on society, by the way," Arden said, speaking into her hair. "The granddaughter of a marquess to be sporting herself on the stage! It will be the talk of the town."

Matilda choked in surprise. "Do you know everything?"

The hands kept stroking and the voice kept on in that same friendly tone. "Everything," the duke said.

"Then you can see what my dilemma is," Matilda said. "My wish is to play in London while I save my money, then go back home to care for my great-aunt. A false name was necessary. I also wished to hold on to my virtue, so that I might marry someday. But it's become too difficult. The gossips have us intriguing together already. You know everything about me, and there is no harm in it, Duke. I can't hold out any longer. I'll be your . . . your . . ."

The stroking hands suddenly clamped down onto Matilda's shoulders as she struggled to make her tongue get out the word.

"You, a lady of birth and breeding, you would consent to become my mistress?"

An odd half-smile lit the duke's face, and his eyes! Matilda, looking up into them, couldn't tell if they were glittering with anger, lust, or something else.

Matilda quite naturally thought she heard disapproval in his awed tones. "Yes, I would," she snapped, breaking out of his embrace with a strength she hadn't known she had. "That is, unless I accept your mother's very generous offer of two thousand pounds if I will let you out of my Jezebel's clutches!"

"My mother? What?" Arden fell back a step. "You've met her?"

"She came here. And she had the goodness to introduce herself to me before calling me a trollop, slut, and worse. Then she offered me the money, she and her friend Lady Dauntry."

Arden broke into hoots of laughter at the picture Matilda was painting. "My dear girl, are you in need of funds? It would serve Mama right if you took the two thousand."

"I've considered it," Matilda said tightly. "There would have been no little satisfaction in taking that amount of money for leaving off doing something I'd never even contemplated."

"Until now?" The duke's query, spoken through the laughter which was just winding down, hung in the air for a moment.

"Until a few minutes ago," Matilda said. "I've changed my mind again."

"Have you, now?" Arden's hilarity had diminished, and he looked at Matilda with a serious-enough expression. "I'm sorry for what Mama and that detestable Lady Dauntry put you through, my love. And I'm sorry that my pursuit of you has driven you to these straits. Accept me, forsooth! I don't wonder you've decided, upon reflection, not to go through with it. For a young woman of your background—"

"That's right," Matilda said. "I have been found to be a formerly respectable young lady; therefore, becoming a man's mistress would be unseemly. Whereas a few days ago, when you thought me a *common* actress, no degradation was too bad for me."

The duke, having feared that something like this would happen, was not surprised. From her quavering voice, Matilda would be on the edge of tears. Perhaps if she cried it out in his arms . . .

Matilda did begin to cry. In her nervous state she had held off the tears for a remarkable time. The salty drops ran through her Lady Teazle paint and continued down her neck. But she stayed far away from Arden, stepping behind the sofa.

"Have you seen that dreadful cartoon?" she flung at him.

The impossible man's eyes lit up. "Cartoon?"

"It's too demeaning. My aunt, you, and I *in bed*. With a disgusting poem about you liking more than one—" These words, uttered between sniffs, ended when Matilda broke into earnest, noisy sobs. "Get out!" she cried.

"That's more the Matilda Graham—pardon me, Glendenning—whom I've come to know and love," the duke said with a bow. He smiled. "A cartoon, you say? Your poor aunt."

"She hasn't seen it, thank God," Matilda said. "And I wish to spare her the sight of you in the next little while. Go now. Please. And forget what I said earlier, about being your . . . your . . ."

"My dear girl, you really ought to learn to say the word before taking on the position. I do intend to forget it. But may I say it's very amusing? Give in to me! Very tempting. For—what was Mama's figure?—two thousand pounds I'd take you up on it. The thought of you in my arms tonight is nearly overpowering. But I'm going. For now."

"Oh!"

The duke, without one parting touch or gesture save a little half-bow and a broad wink, was gone out the door. Matilda sank down on the couch, more confused than she'd ever been in her life.

He knew everything! He was acquainted with the particulars of her mother's as well as presumably her father's family. The knowledge had made him give up his pursuit of her. A man in his position was doubtless shocked that a gently bred girl was cavorting upon the stage for a living, and that such a girl could consent to become someone's mistress had surely turned whatever admiration he had for her into disillusionment. Matilda was certain that only the duke's good manners and habitually genial pose had made him laugh at her acceptance—and nearly instantaneous refusal—of his prior offer of protection. She would never see him again despite his parting phrase.

Now what was she to do? She was terribly glad that Arden hadn't taken her up on the offer she had so rashly made under the drugging influence of his kisses and her fatigue. She couldn't really become a kept mistress, live in that lush house in Half Moon Street, attended by those outwardly respectful servants who would nevertheless know all about her bedroom activities with a nobleman who visited only now and then. She couldn't feed and shelter her great-aunt by forgetting the principles taught her since childhood, some of them by that very aunt.

Matilda knew that there was only one thing she could do: continue as she had been for the past months. She would work, save her money, and somehow find herself and Aunt Poppy another, better place to live. Scandals were always nine-day wonders, weren't they? They must simply wait it out. The respectable boardinghouses would surely open to the Misses Graham again before too many weeks passed. . . .

"Oh, my dear, is the duke gone?" Aunt Poppy bustled into the dressing room. In her hand she held her now ever-present knitting. The time for fancywork was past, said Aunt Poppy's needlework lately. The warm, the practical, was needed now.

Matilda had a sudden vision of herself and her aunt encased in mountains of knitted wraps. She let out a hysterical giggle. "Yes, the duke is gone, Aunt. How could you leave me alone with him?"

"Why, my dear, even I know that privacy is warranted when a gentleman makes his offer."

"Good heavens, Aunt Poppy, the sorts of offers he

makes require a chaperone. Although I will concede you're probably tired of being put to the blush by these scrapes of mine—or I should say his. I wasn't the one to start it.''

''Oh, Niece, that would have been most improper. No lady—''

''No lady. A fitting description of Matilda Graham, actress. Aunt, I'm so tired of not being a lady. I'm sorry the duke misled you into thinking he was making an offer in form. I know you must be as eager as I to get into a better place to live, and . . . and a few minutes ago, when the duke was here, I thought of that lovely house in Half Moon Street—''

''You must forget that pretty house, Matilda, I am sure the duke has bigger and better things in mind now,'' Aunt Poppy said. ''So you did accept him, then? I've been rather worried.''

''Accept him?'' Matilda let out a long rattling sigh. She wished it were easier to make Aunt Poppy understand that the duke had not come here to offer matrimony. And even had he . . . ''No, dear. I can never accept that horrid man.''

''You've taken an aversion to him? But I thought that what you said about love the other night, when dear, sweet Lady Davina was here . . . But it's no matter,'' Aunt Poppy finished brightly. ''You're overwrought, poor child. Everything will look better in the morning.''

Somehow Matilda doubted that homely wisdom. She was too careful of her aunt's feelings, however, to give vent to her cynicism out loud.

15

ALTHOUGH Mrs. Peck's house in Monmouth Court was not far from the theater, Matilda and her aunt still took a hackney to and from the place in the interests of security. In her gloomier moments, Matilda was wont to say in bitter jest that she was spending her whole salary on hackney fares. This was not true, but she often reflected that though two women must always take a conveyance at night, it would be much more comfortable if they could walk to the theater in the daytime. They had been able to do that in their other, more respectable lodging.

Such was the lot of scandalous women! Matilda leaned back in the smelly job-carriage shortly after her trying interview with Arden, endeavoring not to let her head touch the filthy squabs while at the same time she avoided putting her worn slippers on the ancient straw which covered the floor. After all the excitements of this evening, all she wanted was her bed.

"Perhaps you didn't understand the dear duke's offer," Aunt Poppy ventured from the opposite seat. She had been unnaturally silent for some time, immersed in thought. "He meant marriage, my child."

"Did he?" Matilda said in a curiously flat voice.

"Well, it is quite understandable, from all that has gone before, that you should understand it as another offer of a . . . a slip on the shoulder."

Matilda laughed to cover her depressed spirits. "Auntie, you must stop talking to Barker. He has you speaking in cant! And of course I understood where the duke was leading tonight, once I had time to think

about it. You would have left the room only if he'd
said he was going to make a respectable offer—which
may have been his intention until I said something that
shocked him. I'm afraid he's only given me a disgust
of him. The one thing he seemed to retain from his
arrogant research into my background is that I am the
granddaughter of a marquess. Oh, Aunt. Why couldn't
he have wanted to marry *me,* as he saw me, not that
girl I used to be?'' Matilda began to cry, though, as
her eyes were already swollen from the earlier bouts,
every tear burned her.

Aunt Poppy's face drooped in sympathy. ''You
know, dear, a duke couldn't possibly marry a loose
woman.''

''What do you mean, Auntie? The only reputation
I've ever had for being a lightskirt concerns him! And
he knows I didn't do *that.* '' The more she thought
about it, the angrier Matilda was, and the more protective of Matilda Graham, actress. Why should that
respectable woman, doing work she loved for honest
wages, be considered beneath the notice of the great
Duke of Arden? A simple change of name and the pure
luck of a couple of ancestors of rank had done what
she could never have done on her own if she had spent
a lifetime trying.

''I wish I had been the one to win the duke's good
opinion instead of my mother's kin,'' Matilda explained, applying a handkerchief to the tear tracks on
her face. She doubted whether her aunt would understand such a wish; for all her good qualities, Aunt
Poppy was a product of the aristocracy.

''Oh, dear.'' Aunt Poppy fluttered, then subsided,
for they were coming to a stop.

It was never a pleasure to come back to the place
both ladies disdained to think of as home. Stepping
over the street offal, they entered the front door of the
squalid house and made their way upstairs to their rea-

sonably priced attic chamber. The cheapness of the lodgings was their only advantage; Matilda calculated that the difference between this and the nicer living quarters they had had at Mrs. Burnaby's nearly paid for the cost of the constant hackney rides in and out of the despicable neighborhood.

Mrs. Peck's house struck Matilda as a caricature of a run-down brothel; the ancient silk wall coverings of the hall, and the threadbare carpet which Matilda recognized as a good Turkey pattern, proclaimed that the place had seen better days.

Had the house ever been respectable? Matilda didn't know. She was grateful for one thing: though she suspected all the lady lodgers of taking custom, she had at least managed to ascertain that Mrs. Peck was not their abbess. Mrs. Peck probably had her clients as well as her lodgers! It would have been too much to live in an official house of ill repute.

The two women were only halfway up the stairs, nearly feeling their way by the light of the one tallow bed candle they had found in the downstairs hall, when a door opened in the upper corridor and a tall man emerged, fastening his pantaloons.

Matilda rolled her eyes; another typical evening within these genteel walls. She tried to remember the woman who lived behind that particular door, and failed. They all seemed to merge in her mind, though she could tell that more than one of the ladies were friendly and knew most would be able to relate very interesting stories about many gentlemen of the *ton*.

Unfortunately, Aunt Poppy was not as inured to depraved sights as was her niece. She emitted a shrill— "Oh, my goodness!"—as her eyes lit on the man.

"Why, ladies," the visitor said with a mock bow. Matilda remarked, to her disgust, that he spoke in the accents of the gentry. "Did you miss the show?" He was blocking their way, and he proceeded to undo the buttons of his nether garment.

Lady Macbeth, Matilda thought, drawing herself up to her full height. "If you will excuse us, sir, we will not detain you further. Good evening."

So haughty was her voice, so frigid her demeanor, that the man actually did fall back a pace and pause in his lewd motions. In that split second Matilda motioned her aunt around her back. Aunt Poppy scrambled up the remaining stairs and through the small space in the corridor that their large tormentor wasn't blocking. Then, with no further ceremony but a last frigid glare, Matilda followed her aunt.

"Hurry," she hissed, hustling the old lady along the hallway toward the very narrow staircase which led to their room.

"Well, mesdames," the would-be displayer of masculine charms called after them, "I know who you are. Can't the two of you take me, or are your hours all reserved for his grace?"

"Good Lord. Don't pay any attention, Aunt," muttered Matilda, newly annoyed by the cultured accents of the man. Why could he not at least be ill-bred? Then she might find an excuse for his behavior. Matilda breathed a sigh of relief when she was finally outside their door, manipulating with shaking hands the large key to the chamber.

Matilda opened the door and gasped. Rather than the usual darkness, a small aura of light greeted her. A candle was already glowing on the bedside table. Suddenly a shadow moved.

"Please, Miss Graham . . . Matilda," said a soft, cultured voice, "I've come to help."

Matilda found herself confronted by Lady Davina Lowden.

Davina was garbed in what she no doubt hoped was an effective disguise: the plainest pelisse she owned, with a dark cloak thrown over that, and her head shadowed, not only by a hood but also by the same dark veil she had worn when she visited the theater.

"Lady Davina!" Matilda said, thinking that the poor girl must be roasting in the sultry heat. "You shouldn't be in a horrid place like this."

"Neither should you," Davina returned. "I've come to help you get away. I find it easier to escape my house after dark. Otherwise I would have come to you in the morning. At night, I merely tell my mama I have the headache and can't accept whatever invitation is in question, but in the daytime she controls my every moment."

"You came here alone?" Matilda was still too shocked to think clearly. *"Here?"*

"Why, yes," Davina said. "I couldn't risk putting myself into the power of one of the servants. Even my abigail is totally under Mama's thumb."

"Lady Davina," Matilda said severely, "this is no place for you. Why, Aunt Poppy and I have but this moment escaped from a lewd gentleman who was lurking in the hall. You must get away. And quickly."

Davina shook her head. "My dear Matilda, do call me simply Davina. And you don't realize how it is *not* to be a female of remarkable beauty. I need have no fear of being accosted. See, I even took care to wear my plainest things so I wouldn't look wealthy."

Frowning, Matilda answered, "You know very little of the world, Davina. First of all, you're a very attractive lady. And no female is safe in a neighborhood like this. Now, do let me . . . well, I can't ring, for we have no bell, but I can go down to the kitchen and see that Mrs. Peck's scullery boy escorts you until you can get a hackney. And I will go with you as well."

"Dear Lady Davina," came Aunt Poppy's thin voice, "I had no idea you would come in person. Or so soon."

Matilda had forgotten about her aunt. She whirled about. "Aunt Poppy, what have you done?"

Aunt Poppy's lip trembled. "My dearest Matilda, I know I gave you Lady Davina's card so that I wouldn't be tempted to ask her for help. But you really cannot blame me for having committed her direction to memory. And try though I did, I couldn't forget it. So I wrote. But it never crossed my mind that dear Lady Davina would *personally* come to this horrid place."

"What did you think she would do?" Matilda asked harshly. "Send a servant with a basket of pork jelly? Really, Auntie, you've gone too far. Here you've put our friend into the gravest danger. Why, what if that horrid man downstairs should have unbuttoned himself to *her?*"

Davina gasped, and Aunt Poppy started to cry.

Matilda immediately regretted her sharpness and put her arms around her aunt, making soothing murmurs. When Aunt Poppy had quietened, Matilda said to Davina, "You needn't fear, we didn't see anything. That is, he started to undo his . . . I mean, we got away in time." She paused. "Thanks to Lady Macbeth."

Davina looked completely confused.

"I pretend I'm Lady Macbeth when I need to be imperious," Matilda explained. "And I intend to be imperious now, Davina. You must go home. Only the kindest of impulses could have brought you here, and I do thank you. So does Auntie. But we must stay here until we can find another place to live, which I hope we can do shortly. We've only become scandalous because of that . . . that paper I sent you, and such notoriety can't last forever. I expect to find us another lodging by next week." She spoke with false courage, for as the days went by it seemed as though they would molder away forever in this bare little room.

"Matilda, I beg to differ with you," Davina said,

looking straight into the actress's eyes. "I have a hackney waiting for me in the next street. It's ready to take you to my old nurse's cottage in Paddington. You may stay there as long as you wish, and every day I'll send a carriage to convey you to the theater. I must insist. You have been a good friend to me. Why, that cartoon you sent can be my salvation if ever my mother begins to insist too strongly that I marry the duke."

Matilda had never been so tempted as she was by this kind and generous offer. "Oh! Dear, sweet Davina. I can't let you do that. Aunt and I must live near the theater, and we can stand this place very well. No harm comes to us, though it is uncomfortable."

"It must be that," Davina said, looking around at the room. She had had more than a half-hour to explore it before the Grahams had arrived, and in that time she had learned more about poverty and want than she had in all the years of carrying round soup to the cottagers at her papa's country estates, or even observing, with helpless wishes of charity, the poorer denizens of London from the safe position of her mother's carriage.

Matilda and her aunt lived in this small attic chamber, really lived, whereas Davina had felt stifled after five minutes and longed to go back to her comfortable house in Hanover Square.

There was a rickety bed, on which Davina was forced to sit as she waited. What felt like a straw mattress was covered only by a thin quilt and did not seem to take kindly to Davina's nervous shiftings. Besides the bed there was a very narrow cot in one corner of the room, a hard chair which Davina had not cared to try, so unstable did it look, and a bureau under the one tiny window. The walls had been papered once, but were now peeling, as Davina could see by the light of the one candle the landlady had allowed her. There was no sign of comfort anywhere to be seen, save for a few good cushions and one painting on the wall, a painting Davina didn't look at closely. It hung in a shadowed area of the room which she was certain housed spiders. As for the mice, she could hear them scurrying about and only hoped they were inside the walls.

Another disadvantage of the accommodations was that the raddled, overpainted female who had finally answered Davina's calls in the hall downstairs had been quite ready to let anyone into the Graham ladies' room, for a price.

"You must come with me," Davina said. Her large eyes looked sadly into Matilda's. They slowly filled with tears. "I won't leave you here."

"Perhaps if it would make Lady Davina happy, dear . . ." Aunt Poppy faltered, plucking at her niece's sleeve.

"No, we simply can't," Matilda said.

At that moment the door crashed open, nearly hitting Aunt Poppy. Matilda's eyes narrowed with displeasure, and she resolutely hid her fear. There, on the threshold, was the big, beefy man who had just harassed them in the hall. Flanking him were two other males, one short and thin, one even larger and more daunting than the first one. Each was dressed with a care and attention to fashion which proclaimed gentle birth. None of the three could be more than forty. They were all at the peak of their strength and vigor, and their eyes were all glinting lewdly.

Matilda called on all the forces of drama and said in an icy voice, "Gentlemen, you must have the wrong room."

"That we don't, miss," said the biggest man. "My friend here thought we ought to teach you ladies a lesson. You're used to sharing one man between you; why not give you the chance to branch out and serve three of us? Ah, but I see you've thought ahead and

brought in a third whore to even things up. Well, gentlemen? Shall we draw straws to see who takes the old
one first?''

Aunt Poppy gave a faint shriek and crumpled to the
ground.

Matilda resisted the impulse to run to her aunt's aid.
She stood her ground, looking murderous. ''Now see
what you've done, you drunken hellions! You have the
wrong room, I tell you. Leave now or I'll . . .'' She
paused. What was there to do, scream? Matilda knew
from experience that there were often screams heard
in this house during the night, and no one paid any
attention. She was still blushing over her first night in
these lodgings, when she had pounded on the landlady's door to report the frightening sounds she heard
coming from someone's room, only to be told by a
leering Mrs. Peck that that was simply Miss Tipper's
way when her gallant was with her.

''You'll what?'' the beefy man taunted, reaching out
for her.

Matilda was agile enough to evade his grasp, but
with his two friends also rounding on her, she knew
she wouldn't be safe for long. ''Run, Davina!'' she
cried, hoping the girl would take the opportunity to
duck past the three men, all concentrating on Matilda,
and go for help. Meanwhile, Matilda shuddered as the
arms of the leader clutched at her again, and in des-
peration she scrambled for the bureau and the sewing
scissors buried in Aunt Poppy's workbasket.

''It will hardly be necessary for me to run,'' the
clear voice of Davina broke into this confusion. ''Will
it, Sir Frederick?''

''What the devil?'' The large man released his hold
on Matilda's waist, causing the girl nearly to catapult
into the bureau facefirst. ''Lady Davina! You here?''

Davina threw back her veil and the hood of her
cloak, exposing her finely coiffed head of brown hair

and her pale, narrow face. "Would you leave now, gentlemen? Or would you prefer to answer to my father for this insult? Or to the Duke of Arden?" Having run disgusted eyes over Sir Frederick, Davina turned to the other two men.

"I say, Lady D., no need to recognize us," piped the thinner of the two strangers.

"Get out," Lady Davina intoned coldly. "These are my friends, and I will tolerate no further harm to them."

"I say, we didn't harm 'em in the least, m'lady," Sir Frederick said. He tipped his hat in an awkward gesture. "Have you come to buy the women off, then? I know you're to wed the duke. No need to waste your blunt, the talk's going about that Arden's dropped these two. Think you the duke would leave 'em in a place like this if he was still having 'em?"

Matilda, now kneeling at the side of her slowly reviving aunt, shook her head. Men!

Davina snapped, "Sir Frederick, I repeat, you are free to go. You and your friends, whom I do recognize. Need I mention that I won't fail to use this incident against you if need be?"

The gentlemen—if such creatures could be dignified with that title—cleared the room in a remarkably short time.

Davina helped Matilda get Aunt Poppy to the bed. The lady hadn't been injured by her swoon and was soon assuring both the anxious girls that they mustn't fuss over her.

"Do you see now, Matilda? You can't stay here," Davina said. "Do get your things and come with me to Paddington. I will help you engage lodgings nearer town as soon as can be."

"Matilda?" quavered Aunt Poppy.

Matilda was still half in shock. If Davina hadn't routed those men, what might not be happening to her—and the other two—by now? It didn't bear thinking of, and Matilda's pride couldn't stand up to the vision of her aunt injured and frightened, Lady Davina and herself raped . . . It hadn't happened this time. Such luck might not come their way on a second occasion.

"Very well," she said. "It won't take a moment to pack our things. Auntie, you stay lying down. I'll get ready."

Lady Davina clasped her hands in pleasure and demanded to help. Matilda protested at first, but after she had dragged their one trunk from its corner, she set Davina to removing the picture from the wall and putting it with their few other personal effects into the trunk while she folded their meager supply of clothes.

"How extraordinary," Davina said, looking at Aunt Poppy's watercolor. "I know this is a famous work, but it does seem coincidental."

"Auntie did it herself," Matilda said, folding Aunt Poppy's new "summer black" from Madame Hélène's into some carefully hoarded silver paper.

"My parents have the original," Davina said, smiling as her eyes lingered on the crudely painted figure representing Lady Rose Parmenter, her grandmother.

"They would," Aunt Poppy said. She uttered nothing further, though she smiled on Davina with what anyone might have recognized as auntlike affection.

Matilda was too busy packing to take much note of her aunt's remark. The thought crossed her mind that she was glad the painting, which Aunt Poppy had always told her had been lost long ago, was safe in the keeping of Davina's family.

Sharing her father's disdain for their harsh treatment of her mother and her great-aunt, she had never had many questions about her mother's family. She had no idea what had happened to any of the sisters of *The Garden of Flowers*, save for Lady Violet, her own grandmother.

And, of course, Aunt Poppy.

16

"MAMA, I am going to be married," the Duke of Arden said.

The duchess emerged at once from the haughty torpor a visit from her son always induced. "Oh, darling boy!" she cried. "My prayers have been answered. Do pull the bell for me. I must summon my dresser at once. Wait for me while I run upstairs and change, and you may accompany me. I must go to Hanover Square this instant and clasp dear Davina to my bosom."

"Most kind of you, I'm sure, Mama, but as Lady Davina is not the woman I'm marrying, she might be hard put to understand your violence," the duke returned, smiling his slyest smile.

It was a bit premature of him to talk of his marriage to Matilda as a settled thing, but Arden had decided to give the projected wedding a hint of legitimacy by announcing it to his mother. He had made the right decision, too; he already felt more hopeful about the campaign. He would succeed with Matilda, for he must.

"But of course you're marrying Lady Davina! Who else could be worthy of an alliance to our family?" the duchess said, her temper firmly in check as she fumbled for the restorative salts on an adjacent table.

"I tell you, Mama, it's not Lady Davina. It's a Miss Glendenning," Arden replied.

"Sounds Scottish," the duchess murmured darkly, applying the salts to her aquiline nose before treating her son to a glare from snapping dark eyes. "And who," she asked in a deceptively sweet voice, "is this Miss Glendenning?"

"Oh, someone totally respectable. A pity, really, that I had to fall in love with her, for I'd hoped to journey further afield for my bride when the time came. An Italian, perhaps, or an Irish girl. We need some fresh blood. But what could I do, Mama, when captured by Miss Glendenning's bright eyes?"

"Who is she?" the duchess said through set teeth.

Arden waved a casual hand. "Oh, nobody you'd remember. She has lived rather a retired life until recently. A granddaughter of the last Marquess of Deane. Oldest blood in the world, I believe. Pity that title reverted to the crown."

His mother put her head to one side. Oddly enough, this did not sound so bad. "Old Deane must have had twenty grandchildren, what with all his daughters breeding like rabbits," she said with a sniff. "He married the first Lady Violet Parmenter, one of the sisters in the Gainsborough, so this girl must be a connection of the Dauntrys too. Good blood there, no doubt about it. Now, who is on her other side? Some clan of Scottish tinkers?"

"As I understand it, an eminently respectable family long established in Edinburgh. Clerical folk and university people. No titles, but no tinkers either."

The duchess snorted. "I must meet this young woman and pass judgment. You will not be announcing the engagement until I do so?" Her question was more like a command.

Arden shrugged. "My dear mother, I have a small task to perform before I can trot the unfortunate girl round to have you look at her teeth. I must make Miss Glendenning love me."

"What?" His mother's incredulity expressed itself by a sharp intake of breath. Arden was gratified. He remembered that though he might not be her favorite son, she still considered him the most eligible *parti* in the kingdom. "Are you saying the girl won't have you? She must be mad."

"Thanks, Mama. The truth is, I've been somewhat undiplomatic in my pursuit of her. The arrogance of rank and all that. And since I've been captured by her charms, I wish to have the same effect on her. I will not simply inform her that she has had the great good fortune to have caught my eye as duchess-ware."

"How very odd." The duchess paused, and her finely arched eyebrows drew together. "Are you sure, Michael, that this isn't one of your little jokes? Marrying a young woman I've never even heard of, throwing over poor Lady Davina, who has been expecting your declaration daily . . ." She let her words trail away under her son's amused eye. He *was* up to something! But what?

"Lady Davina will dance at my wedding with all her heart," Arden said. "And as for Miss Glendenning, Mama, you've not only heard of her, you've met her! Granted, you might not recall the encounter, but it was quite vivid in her mind."

"Well! Is that so?" The duchess was not surprised that an obscure young lady would recall a meeting with her majestic self, nor that she had not noticed the chit in question. So much the better! If the young female was colorless and not a "coming" sort of girl, she would fit in more readily with the duchess's plan. Her own absolute control of the Arden dignities would not end with the duke's marriage. But there was still Lady Davina. "What will I say to Lady Dauntry about this?" she demanded. "She as well as her daughter is counting on this marriage, whatever you seem to think. And while the girl is so retiring and well-bred that I am willing to guarantee you'll never hear a word of reproach from her, the mother is quite a different case."

Arden shrugged. "What can Lady Dauntry do in the face of true love? Mark my words, she'll simply go one brother down the line and throw her daughter at Julius' head next, if the wretched lad ever comes home." His lips twitched. "Or perhaps her ladyship would think it more expedient to drag her daughter over the Peninsula looking for Julius. There are all sorts of camp followers, although, since her ladyship appeared to confuse Germany with Spain in our last conversation, it might be a long and fruitless trip."

"Horrid boy! Must you insult my friends and make light of your brother's danger in the same breath?" the duchess burst out.

"Rotten of me, wasn't it? You know I have every regard for my brother." And the duke rose, kissed his mother's powdered cheek, and took his farewells.

"What about this Glendenning person?" she fairly shouted at his back. "When am I to see her and make up my mind?"

Arden turned and gave the duchess a devilish wink. "Why, after she passes judgment on me, Mama. Hold yourself in readiness. You are bound to enjoy the encounter." He went out chuckling at the very thought of his mother's second meeting with Matilda.

It remained to persuade his love that she held first place in his heart. Armed with a bouquet of flowers, Arden made for the lodging house where he had burst into Matilda's room on that memorable night she had fooled him into believing another man had enjoyed her charms in the Half Moon Street love nest. The duke drove his curricle; it was likely too early in the day for Matilda to be at the theater, and he would try to persuade her—and her aunt, if need be—to come for a drive.

He would be courteous, distant, and unfailingly mild, he was planning as he drove through Blooms-

bury. Matilda would find no fault with his behavior.
And by taking her driving in the park he would pave
the way for the *ton*'s reception of their marriage plans.
Yes, the aunt should certainly come along on what
would be a drive of eminent sedateness.

Unfortunately, this sterling demeanor had no chance
for display. A gray-haired landlady, nearly tripping
over her skirts to get to the duke once she was brought
his card, informed him that the Misses Graham had
left quite a while ago to take up residence elsewhere.

"Extraordinary," Arden drawled, employing his
best ducal manner in combination with a winning
smile. "And I don't suppose you know where they've
removed to?"

Mrs. Burnaby looked a touch uncomfortable. "Begging your grace's pardon, but I would have expected
you to be the one to tell *me* that. The situation being
what it is, very odd folks have been calling it . . ."
The woman paused, gulped, and sank into confusion.
"Not to be calling your grace niggardly by any means,
but most men sets up their, er, I am making a mull of
this. Your pardon, sir. I recollect now I've heard the
gossip. You're finished with the pair of 'em. Quite
kindly to stop in to see how they're getting on, and
awful sorry I can't help you."

The duke frowned at these revelations, but he wasn't
in the mood to spend time enough with the woman to
convince her she'd been misinformed about the whole
affair. Once he was satisfied Mrs. Burnaby was in ignorance of the Grahams' new address, he plunked the
bouquet of flowers into the astonished woman's hand
and took his leave. He was just disappearing through
the door when an elderly man caught at his sleeve.

"Couldn't help overhearing, your grace," the old
party said, sketching a low bow. "You want to know
where the Grahams went after the Burnaby kicked 'em
out?"

Mrs. Burnaby was still standing in the front hall, gazing after the duke in a very bold way which juxtaposed oddly with her matronly appearance. "Hold your tongue, Manders," she said in a shrill tone Arden hadn't heard before.

The aged man returned a pithy oath. Mrs. Burnaby gave one last raking glance at the duke, turned on her heel, and slammed out.

The duke thought he recognized his new informant. The old chap was an actor long established in comic roles. "You did the porter in *Macbeth*, didn't you, sir?"

"To think of your grace remembering that!" Manders said, and preened a little.

"Well, I was at every performance," the duke explained. "Now, tell me where Miss Graham and her aunt have gone, if you would."

Manders related a colorful version of Matilda's ejection from the house, provoking in the duke a strong wish he had not given Mrs. Burnaby those flowers. Mr. Manders had not believed those vile stories about the ladies for a minute, and he called the cartoon outright libel. Downright illogical to think that if a man of the stature of the Duke of Arden were to set up a mistress, he wouldn't provide her a house of her own.

Manders was certain there was some reasonable explanation for the duke's presence in the Misses Graham's room that night (this he posited with a sidelong look at Arden, who declined to take the bait and remained mute). The old actor shrugged this off, then mired himself in flustered commendations of Miss Graham's many virtues and beauties.

Some coin changed hands, and Manders got down to cases. He gave the location of Matilda's new lodging and the name of her landlady.

The duke was startled. That was not a neighborhood he liked to take the horses into. Neither was it a place

Matilda should have taken her old aunt to live. Thanking Manders, Arden hurried out to his vehicle and went on his way.

Mrs. Peck's house, in the grim light of even a sunny, warm day, looked like what it was: the abode of women of doubtful virtue. "Is the girl out of her mind?" the Duke of Arden was grumbling aloud as he left his tiger to guard the horses and mounted the steps of the tatty residence.

Here also he was destined for disappointment. A very young maid in a stained dress and oversize clogs answered the door and nearly fell over in surprise at the tall, handsome gentleman who stood before her—and in the daytime! She ran for Mrs. Peck with a dazzled glance over her shoulder, not even pausing to ask the gentleman's identity.

The duke stood near the staircase and waited, his eyes running critically over the decayed splendor of the hall.

"Your lordship, what may I do for you?"

Arden blinked at the spectacle of a large, bosomy woman with brassy curls. She was attired in what might kindly be described as negligee. She was of indeterminate age, with a complexion which showed the ravages of years of lead paint, but she was smiling at him as flirtatiously as though she were a dairymaid of fifteen summers.

"My name is Arden," the duke said. "I am looking for a lodger of yours. A Miss Graham."

The smile instantly faded. "That one! I'm looking for her myself, sir, for she up and left during the night. Never was I so put out. In the dead of night, if you please! Well, it's always the same when you rents to theater folk, and so I shall remember from now on. Couldn't pay the shot, I suppose." Mrs. Peck conveniently forgot that Matilda had left the month's rent on the old bureau in the vacated room. "I don't suppose you'd be willin' to make it good for her, sir? Ah, treading the boards is a hard life, and can't say I blame the young lady for taking the easy way out, but I'm a businesswoman, and I'll be forced to set a magistrate on her . . .'' She paused delicately.

Arden matter-of-factly got out his purse and handed over the amount the woman quoted him, double the real cost of the attic room. He reasoned that the less trouble Matilda was in, the better. He had seen only the hall of this place, but it was easy to imagine the rest. He didn't blame Matilda for leaving, though running out in the middle of the night didn't sound at all like her. And where the devil had she gone?

Lacking another place to hunt, Arden resolved to be at the theater in the evening, where Matilda must put in an appearance. He spent the rest of the day regretting the fact that his situation with Matilda had set the *ton* talking. In the eyes of all, she was not just his mistress, but his discarded mistress! Could such damage to her peace of mind ever be repaired?

If a lifetime of his affection could effect such a miracle, Arden would consider himself the happiest of men, he told himself with a pardonable touch of conceit.

In White's that afternoon he accosted Lord Peterborough by the simple measure of picking that large peer up by the back of his coat as he was sitting down to cards. ''Excuse us, gentlemen,'' the duke said cheerfully, nodding to the incipient whist table as he dragged his friend away. The card players shrugged, being more or less used to such behavior in Arden and Peterborough, and flagged a new fourth for their game.

The duke came straight to the point. ''Perry, why the devil didn't you tell me that Miss Graham is the daughter of your old tutor at Oxford?''

Peterborough's mild eyes boggled. "Which Miss Graham?"

"The lovely, flame-haired actress, you clunch."

"You've mistaken the matter, old boy," Peterborough said after a moment of thoughtful silence. "Miss Glendenning had red hair, true, but she was only a plump little schoolgirl. Couldn't have been more than ten or twelve. Besides, why would a girl in that sort of family go on the stage?"

"Schoolgirls aren't preserved in amber, Perry. Somewhere along the line Miss Glendenning grew into a beauty. And she became an actress because she was orphaned and desperately poor and also, I suspect, because she liked to act."

"Well, say it's true. What's it to do with me?"

Arden frowned. "Nothing. Merely had the urge to tell you what a blind idiot you've been."

"Much obliged to you, Duke," Perry said with a touch of irritation apparent in his voice.

"Don't take my words amiss, old fellow, you were no blinder an idiot than I. And I'm to be treated kindly in my condition." Arden took a deep breath and came out with his secret. "You see, I'm busy getting leg-shackled."

"Lady Davina? Must felicitate you," Peterborough said in his best style, inwardly grimacing at the thought of Arden riveted, at long last, to that mousy thing.

"She's not the lady."

"Well! Things are looking up for you then, Duke?"

"Take care how you speak of Lady Davina in my presence, friend. I have every regard for the lady. You might do well to take a second look at her yourself, one of these days. Dashed attractive girl if you can get her to lift her eyes from the ground," Arden said with some vehemence.

"Hmm. She must be a fifty-thousand-pounder, what?" Perry actually seemed to consider Lady Da-

vina. His own family had been after him for some time
to marry. "That nose, though—"

"That nose," Arden said, "is nothing out of the
ordinary. Poor Lady Davina has been much maligned.
Now, you are as fashionable as I by some quirk of fate,
Perry. As a favor to me, why don't you dance attendance on Davina for the next little while? Might help
to ease her out of the trap she's been in these past
Seasons, with everyone and his wife thinking she's to
wed me. I'm not really saying you should marry the
girl. She might want a few more brains in her tenant
for life. But a few dances? A drive in the park?"

Perry's open face turned shrewd. "The name of that
highly secret stud farm where you bought Black Jet?"

Arden clapped his friend on the back and came up
with the name, location, and probable stock of the
farm in question. Then he went back to the Albany to
dress for the theater, his step growing ever jauntier as
he contemplated a sight of Matilda.

17

MATILDA sparkled and glowed in her role of Titania at the theater that evening. Only someone who knew her very well indeed would have guessed that her unusual brightness was the result of a tremendous mental strain.

She was actually happier than she'd been in a long while, or so she had been telling herself all day. A tremendous burden was lifted from her shoulders now that Aunt Poppy was settled in the cottage at Paddington, with Lady Davina's nurse—a woman of about Aunt Poppy's age—for company. For the first time since she had started her career upon the stage, Matilda had been able to leave Aunt Poppy behind when she set out for the theater, taking the nurse's little maid-of-all-work as chaperone instead. Aunt would get to bed at a decent hour, which lessened Matilda's guilt over the old lady's health. And it was pure bliss to be living in a quiet little cottage instead of a noisy, disreputable lodging house.

Why, then, did Matilda's nervous spirits bounce off the wings and come to rest, thank goodness, in the energy she brought to her part? She couldn't admit that it might have something to do with the Duke of Arden, who, as usual, was leaning over the edge of his box as if to see her more closely.

The things she had said to him at their last interview were still ringing in her ears. She had actually considered becoming his mistress, and had told him so!

And then there was the fact that he, alone of all the spectators, knew her for what she was: Miss Glenden-

ning from Oxford. Matilda had never realized the
depth of her role within a role as Miss Graham. She
felt dreadfully exposed, though she would defend to
the death the right of a respectable Miss Glendenning
to tread the boards if she wished it.

Lady Davina, in Lady Peterborough's box across the
way from Arden's, was enjoying herself immensely.
She had not been to the theater since meeting Miss
Graham. Davina was astonished at the pleasure she
felt on being acquainted with the performer she was
watching. The unexpected invitation from Lady Peterborough, delivered by her son, had also pleased Davina. She was not a popular young lady except among
some members of her own sex; her shy demeanor kept
her from the notice of everyone but the Duchess of
Arden, whose invitations were offered for purely dy-
nastic reasons.

When Lord Peterborough had called earlier in the
day with his mother's compliments and the assurance
of his own pleasure in acting as escort, Davina had
had her suspicions. Peterborough was a great friend of
Arden's, his partner in many pranks, and might this
not have been engineered by Arden, in his kind design
to help Davina enjoy her Season?

She had decided it didn't matter. Peterborough was
witty, charming, and *not* divinely handsome. He didn't
cause her heartbeat to quicken, but no one in the world
had yet done that. His mother, whom Davina had met
before, was friendly and unaffected; and to give the
invitation an extra fillip, Lady Dauntry had been in
the room during Peterborough's call and had emitted
a squawk of protest at the plan before remembering
her manners and presumably reflecting that there could
be no harm in her daughter spending the evening with
a viscountess and her eligible son. The countess re-
monstrated with Davina once mother and daughter
were alone, however, cautioning her not to play fast

and loose with the Duke of Arden, all the while looking at her with a new respect. Davina had never in her life attracted an admirer.

Not only was it pleasant to vex Mama. Davina had dared to cast her eyes about the theater and notice that her appearance under the wing of anyone but the Duchess of Arden or her mother was causing talk.

There was another joy in store for Davina at the interval. Walking out upon Peterborough's arm, she came face-to-face with Sir Frederick. Rather than look at the floor, she stared straight into Sir Frederick's eyes in a sort of challenge. He positively quailed, and Davina's spirits lifted even higher as she contemplated her power over the lustful wretch.

Davina began to hold her head very high indeed, remembering what Matilda had said about pretending to be Lady Macbeth when in a difficult situation. Davina couldn't feel much like Lady Macbeth, no matter how she tried. She decided, instead, to pretend she was the Duchess of Arden.

Lord Peterborough, committed as he was to hanging by Davina's side all evening in payment of Arden's information about the stud farm, began to enjoy himself. He noticed that Lady Davina wasn't the plain dab of a girl he had always considered her. He never remembered seeing her eyes before; he surely would have remembered that they were so large and luminous. And he would certainly have recalled such a dashed fine figure, he considered, looking surreptitiously at the young lady's bosom, which was shown to best advantage by her erect posture.

In the second interval Peterborough and Davina walked out again, and the first person to accost them in the crowded corridor was the Duke of Arden.

"Perry! And Lady Davina, upon my word. What a pleasure," the duke said. Davina made her curtsy and listened as Arden and Perry exchanged some masculine banter which seemed to involve matters equestrian.

She noticed that the duke looked rather worried under his habitual good humor. His eyes flitted here and there, and every once in a while his lips would tighten. Davina suspected he was worried over Miss Graham.

As it happened, Davina had had an illuminating talk with the elder Miss Graham before she left the ladies in Paddington. Though she hardly dared hope that Miss Poppy Graham's information was correct and that the duke really wished to marry Matilda, there would be no harm in aiding the gentleman a very little. Should his purpose still be indecent, he would get nowhere in the home of Davina's starchy old nurse. Should he really wish matrimony, though, Davina must help him to the best of her ability.

At a pause in the gentlemen's conversation, Davina took courage and said, "Duke, I hope you've been getting out to the country on these fine days."

Arden looked at her in total bewilderment, and Peterborough joined him.

"Lady Davina," Peterborough said gently, enjoying in his condescending, masculine way the young lady's failure to pay heed to the conversation that had been going on, "we were speaking of a horse race. Dashed impolite of us, I suppose, not to include you."

Davina fell victim to one of her horrid, unattractive blushes, but she held her ground. "But it would be tragic if the duke didn't get out into the countryside for a reason other than horse racing. I know how his grace loves the country, Lord Peterborough. Especially the area around Paddington." A heavy pause, while Davina looked straight into the duke's dark eyes and decided, from his at-sea expression, that subtlety would be wasted. "My old nurse lives in that village, so naturally I know it well. I go often to visit her and her two guests, a young lady and her great-aunt."

Arden stared. "Are you trying to say, Lady Davina, that Miss Graham and her aunt are under your protection?"

Davina looked sideways at Lord Peterborough, motioning the duke to say nothing further.

He paid no attention. "You have hidden depths, my lady. I wouldn't have believed it of you."

"You should have seen the horrid place they were living," Davina excused herself. She was unable to tell from the duke's expression whether or not he was angry with her.

Peterborough was grinning widely. "This sounds intriguing. Would both of you explain it to me?"

"There's nothing to explain," Davina said. "Some friends of mine were in uncomfortable quarters, and I took them to live in my old nurse's cottage. She is lonely in her retirement, and she loves helping me and them. Her cottage is on the green, Duke. Ask anyone for the house of Mrs. Summers."

"And these friends include Miss Graham, the actress?" Peterborough's awed expression foretold his next words. "Didn't know you had it in you, m'lady."

"No indeed," the duke said. His face cleared and he let out a laugh of pure enjoyment. "You're a great gun, Lady Davina. How on earth did you two meet in the first place?"

"I went to see her," Davina murmured, casting down her eyes.

"And dare I ask why? To beg her to give me up, perhaps?" Arden fairly snickered at this. He would have winked at Davina had she been looking at him.

Lord Peterborough moved a hair closer to Davina. "I say, Arden, no need to go teasing the lady."

Davina looked up, smiling. "His grace knows that would not have been my errand, Lord Peterborough. And as a matter of fact, Duke, I went to her to ask her *not* to give you up. I didn't know, you see, that the rumors about you and her were false."

"Lady Davina and I have a secret agreement not to become betrothed, you see, Perry," Arden said in clarification. How amusing it was to note that Perry's cheerful face had actually darkened with something like protective chivalry.

Peterborough hooted with laughter at this, and Arden joined him. Davina looked about the crowded corridor and saw with pleasure that many people, ladies especially, had their eyes on Davina and the two gentleman. Why, onlookers might even assume that the gentlemen were laughing over Davina's cleverness! That would be something new, for Davina hardly ever said a word in company, and never anything witty.

"Well, Duke, will you go to see Miss Graham?" Davina said when the gentlemen had recovered themselves. "I had a conversation with her aunt which led me to believe, er, that you had a question to ask of Miss Graham and that the answer was not to your taste."

"Right you are. She says she won't marry me," the duke said, a pained expression crossing his handsome features.

Peterborough said, "You want to *marry* her? Oh . . ." —after a pause—"that's right, she's really Miss Glendenning, the little girl from Oxford. Well, that might help put a clean face on it, Arden, but I doubt if it would wash all the same. An actress! It simply isn't done."

"I could draw your cork in the middle of the room here, Perry, and that isn't done either," the Duke of Arden said in a low voice, all the while maintaining his pleasant expression. "Why should I not marry the girl of my choice, no matter what her identity or profession? No use being a duke, is there, if I can't please myself?"

"Oh, I think you're splendid," Davina said eagerly. "But what did you say, Lord Peterborough, about her being someone else?"

"Only that she took a stage name, ma'am," interjected the duke. "You may ask her about it yourself. And she would probably not take kindly, Perry, to having any other name than Graham bandied about."

"Is that so? Would have thought the opposite," Perry said with a shrug. "Anything you say, Duke."

"There is one unfortunate detail in this happy romance yet, Lady Davina," the duke said. "Your friend Miss Graham has found that she, like her character tonight, has fallen in love with an ass. That is, if she harbors feelings of tenderness for me at all, which I am beginning to doubt."

"Oh, Duke," Davina said with a brilliant smile, remembering Matilda's confession of her love for this man, "never doubt that."

"No?" Arden's eyes lit up. Feminine confidences? There was hope here.

"Go out to Paddington, Duke," Davina said. "Please."

"Glad to go with you," Peterborough suggested with a quizzically raised eyebrow.

"Go with me on a mission of courtship? You won't live that long, Perry," the duke said. He and the two parted then, for the audience was beginning the migration back into the boxes and the pit. Arden's step was jauntier, much jauntier than it had been before he had spoken with Lady Davina Lowden.

He had thought that he would have to storm back to Matilda's dressing room after the performance to prize out of her or her aunt their new place of residence. Now that he didn't need to do that, he decided to break with his tradition of invading her privacy after performances and invade it, instead, in a country setting.

* * *

Paddington was hard by London, a pleasant village the duke had hardly visited before and thought of merely as a place to pass by when traveling on ancient Watling Street. The very next morning, much earlier than he would have considered correct for a social call, he found himself pulling up his new, highly bred stallion, Black Jet, at the Red Lion there and inquiring of the ostler the way to Mrs. Summers'.

He was directed to a little half-timbered cottage fronted by a garden cheerfully blooming with every flower from sweet pea to columbine. Arden smiled in relief; bless Lady Davina! This was a much more proper place for the ladies to live.

A rap at the shining brass knocker brought a plump young maid to the door. Arden gave her his card and asked for either of the Misses Graham. The maid, saucer-eyed, ushered him into a little sitting room and disappeared.

Arden hadn't finished with examining the many charms of the room, from the neat braided rugs to the old dark wood furnishings so highly polished that he could see his reflection, when a sound turned his attention to the doorway. Face alight with happy expectation, he turned.

Staring at him from behind little square spectacles was a very small old woman whom he had never seen before, a woman in an outsize mobcap, a black dress, and an apron. "Mrs. Summers?" he said with a bow. "I'm—"

"You!" burst out the old lady, speaking in theatrical tones. "How dare you set foot in this house, you rake!"

"Er, I . . ." Arden, not sure how he did dare, was hard put to offer his excuses.

"So you think you can break that poor girl's heart, then come sauntering out here to claim her favors again? Oh, I've always known the quality were a vile lot, for all I've spent my days serving them. Aye, a few years in the house of Lord Dauntry was enough to convince me that you're all a pack of devils, even if I hadn't known it already. The little chambermaids he used to trap in the closets, then have them turned off when it suited his lordship's convenience not to see their faces—''

Arden, while fascinated by these glimpses into the private life of Lady Davina's father, could not in good conscience let the woman continue. ''Mrs. Summers?'' he therefore interjected into the middle of her tirade. ''Lady Davina sent me.''

The little woman clapped her mouth shut instantly, glaring at the duke. After a moment of thoughtful silence she spoke again. ''My lamb set you on the trail of poor Miss Matilda? No, that I'll never believe. My lady is the sweetest creature in the world. She would never do Miss Matilda harm.''

Arden frowned, wondering how he might best get past this small dragon and attain his goal. ''I mean to marry Miss Matilda,'' he said in a confidential tone.

''Beast!'' returned Mrs. Summers. ''And why is that, might I ask? Because you admire her? Because you think she's a fine young woman? Or, you dreadful boy, is it that you've found she's of respectable birth, and you want to channel your lusts into marriage?''

The duke blinked. It had been years since anyone save his mother had called him a dreadful boy. And it was evident from the old woman's tirade that his situation with Matilda had been much discussed in this little house. By Matilda herself? Arden thought it unlikely. More probable was an exchange of confidences over the teacups between Lady Poppy and this small virago, whose likeness in age might make them kindred spirits. However his main impediment to Matilda's hand had gotten into Mrs. Summers' mind, there it was: he stood accused, by yet another person, of snobbery.

He hadn't wanted to marry Matilda Graham, the actress of obscure origins. Suddenly he found out she numbered among her relations some of the most aristocratic names in the kingdom, and he rushed to her with an offer of marriage. Legitimating his lust—was that what they thought he was doing?

The duke continued to stare at the angry old nurse. A terrible thought occurred to him. *Was* that what he was doing?

"I must see Matilda," he said. "Her aunt or you may chaperone her, Mrs. Summers, but I must talk to her. How do I know she would refuse my offer? I've never made it in form, as it were. How do you know she hasn't changed her mind about me in the day or two she's been here?" He smiled in his most ingratiating way, the same smile he used to employ to lure a woman into his bed.

Mrs. Summers said, "Humph," but her eyes appeared to soften a very little behind the concealing glasses. "I'll tell her you're here, but I make no promises." She left the room and slammed the door hard enough to set the little pottery figurines on the mantelpiece to tinkling, a force the duke assumed was meant to put him in his place.

Arden reflected that the ingratiating smile was still in top form, whatever his success with Matilda. He resumed his wanderings about the room, his eye lighting on a sampler that was displayed on one wall, painstakingly worked in cross-stitch and signed in the same, "Davina Marianna Elizabeth Lowden, aged ten years."

"I won't doubt, m'lady," he murmured. Then he turned toward the door so as to be ready when Matilda came in, as he did *not* doubt she would, if only for the pleasure of raking him over the coals.

She entered within five minutes of Mrs. Summers' going out. Matilda was wearing a simple white muslin dress sashed in black ribbon, and her hair, which Arden had never seen without wanting to bury his face in it, hung loosely down her back except for the few curly tendrils which framed her pale face. She was glaring.

"I know that look," the duke said, stepping forward. "What a comfort it is that some things never change."

Matilda held out one hand to stave him off. "Don't touch me."

"Whatever my lady wants. She knows I am hers to command," Arden said suavely. "Will you walk with me? Bring your aunt or that delightful Mrs. Summers if you will."

Matilda's mouth dropped open. "Walk with you?"

"Yes, a turn about these pleasant country lanes. Nothing but a walk, and in addition to an old lady, you may bring your parasol to defend your virtue. It's a lovely day, and I have every reason to believe that you don't get enough fresh air." Arden spoke lightly, but he was willing her to come with him.

HIs mental pleadings seemed to work. "I'd be delighted to go for a walk," Matilda said, still with that bewildered look on her face. "It won't be necessary to disturb the ladies, but do excuse me for a moment, Duke, while I get my hat. And my parasol."

Within a very short time the two were walking stiffly down a footpath which took off from Mrs. Summers' back garden across a field. The old nurse said they would be going between hedgerows after crossing the field, and eventually, though she wouldn't advise going so far, they would come out upon a lovely view over the north end of the park. Aunt Poppy and Mrs. Summers waved them away at the back door and exchanged

pleased looks before heading for the kitchen and a restorative dish of bohea.

"Duke, I haven't much time to devote to you. I must
leave for the theater shortly," Matilda said. "What do
you want of me?"

"I think you know, Miss Glendenning. I want your
next role to be that of my duchess," Arden said. The
two were walking side by side, of necessity very close
together since the path was narrow, but he didn't take
advantage. There would be no groping about in each
other's arms for this interview, Arden resolved. He as
well as Matilda must remain free of the spell induced
by their embraces.

Matilda's heart sank. He had said exactly the wrong
thing. "Duke, we have a fundamental difference of
opinion here," she said, stopping in her tracks to face
him. They were in the exact middle of the field of
clover, and Matilda made a very lovely picture, everything from her earnest expression to her simple costume causing Arden's heart to thump oddly. "You
don't want to marry *me*. That's the trouble."

"Excuse me?" the duke said. He appeared mesmerized by the lovely girl before him.

Matilda had been leered at many times, and she saw
no difference between the duke's face now and his face
the first night of their meeting, when he had been bent
on seducing her. So she was pretty? Why should that
open all doors, or any doors at all? She had always
been rather disgusted that her looks had got her into
the Royal George, not her shining talents, but she was
usually practical enough to take the help her face gave
her and be glad of it.

She knew, however, that she must not be so weak
for this, the most important decision of her life.

"Duke, you wanted to seduce Miss Graham. I saw
the house in Half Moon Street. It was a very kindly
meant *carte blanche* from a duke to a ramshackle ac-

tress of low origin. I tried to explain to you why I couldn't do what you asked, and that set you on the trail of my real name and family.'' She paused to overcome a catch which had been creeping into her voice.

"Do go on. You fascinate me," the duke said. Was his purpose merely lust with a license? He must find out. But how? Not by kissing her, but perhaps by listening to her. He had always known she was an intelligent young lady. Her interpretation of her stage roles had told him that. Now he knew that there was another side to her brilliance. This decorative young woman before him had been wont to discuss dry subjects with that old scholar of Oxford, Mr. Pettigrew!

Matilda, somewhat vexed by the duke's intent look, continued with her complaint. "On finding out my blood wasn't as base as you thought, what did you do? Change from seduction to marriage! Oh, I know you'd like to irritate your mother, and this would certainly do it. I know further that most *ton* marriages aren't much more than polite strangers bedding each other to perpetuate their silly lands and titles. I think you only want me, if you know what I mean—"

"I certainly do. I know what you mean and I want you, sure enough. But it's more," Arden cut in.

"Yes, I'm sure it's more. In one fell swoop you can set society on its ear, which has always been your pleasure; annoy your mother beyond all reason; and have me in your bed. If I were you, Duke, I'd be tempted too. But it won't do. If I hold out, I'll get over what I feel for you. And in my levels of society, both acting and university, there are marriages of a different stamp. People are companions to each other. I might be able to achieve that if you will but leave me alone."

It was a lengthy speech, and Matilda's voice had risen as she gave it, until at her last words she was nearly shouting. She had to turn away from Arden's quizzical face. She had spoken her mind, true, but now she was as embarrassed as she'd ever been in her life. She had as good as confessed her love.

"My dear." Arden had sworn to keep his hands to himself, but somehow they landed on her white-clad shoulders. He spoke very near her ear. "Is there nothing I can do?"

"No," Matilda said. In her fright at his nearness, the syllable came out in a squeak.

"You're wrong," Arden said. He knew for a fact that there was always something to be done. He removed his hands, seeing how his touch upset her, and let out a deep sigh. And she had said something just now which made his spirits soar. *What I feel for you,* she had said. She was not indifferent! "I'm asking you to share my world," he continued. "Why not ask me to share yours?"

Matilda didn't know how to react. "What do you mean?"

Arden wasn't certain. "We might read Greek together. Your friend Mr. Pettigrew was admiring of your skill. Aristophanes, perhaps, for Mr. Pettigrew confided that your father really couldn't share your sense of the playwright's humor. I suspect, my dear, that you and I share a definite, if sometimes perverse, sense of humor. Or"—he held up one finger as a brilliant thought struck him—"I could be Petruchio to your Kate in a private production. What would you say to that?"

"Only that you've taken a very clever way to call me a shrew, sir. And there is another point. Your duchess could never act upon the stage but in some little private amateur play. Why would I give up what I have, acting in a professional company in London, the greatest stage in the world?"

"Well, because you loved me. I'd give up whatever you suggest for a similar reason," Arden said. "No need to be unfair about it." He hoped, uneasily, that she would only ask him to give up raking, not something important such as his practical jokes.

Matilda did not suggest he give up anything. She only glared at him.

"My dearest girl, I swear I'll find a way out of this. Trust me," Arden said. He was beginning to look excited. "You'll love me and marry me or I'll know the reason why." And he turned on his heel and walked away with only a parting wave of his hand, leaving Matilda alone in the sunny field, gazing after him.

"I already love you," she said to his retreating back. "But marry?" She shook her head. She could see such a marriage too clearly. The ironclad disapproval of the duchess, who would doubtless become more unbearable than ever once relegated by an actress to the position of dowager; the birth of one child a year if Matilda proved fertile, even more disapproval from all if she turned out unable to perform that duty; stultifying social events crowding upon one another—it sounded horrid when added to the prospect of never again seeing a stage but from the house.

She knew that her feelings for the duke should outweigh all these disadvantages. Her body insisted she accept the duke, and her heart cried out that it might not be such a bad idea, whatever his feelings for her—and she couldn't believe those feelings ascended as high as love. But she must trust in her mind in this case, that ordered and logical brain which her father had molded so proudly.

"Our marriage would be a dreadful fate," Matilda said to herself. "I would be a fool."

18

IT would be stating the case lightly to say that the two old ladies at the cottage were dismayed by Matilda's return home, alone, and looking very depressed. They hadn't seen the duke striding past the little house on his way to the Red Lion and out of Paddington.

"It's very simple." Matilda answered their kind questions with a little shrug. "I told him why I won't have him, and he left." She thought it politic not to tell Mrs. Summers and Aunt that the duke's parting words had been of hope, not despair.

Nor did she tell them of her own doubts. It would be useless to explain to either of the ladies—Aunt Poppy, with her aristocratic background, or Mrs. Summers, who had spent her life in the service of the nobility—that the life of a duchess sounded too tedious to be borne, unless it could be sweetened by a husband's honest love.

Oh, she believed with all her heart that the duke wanted her. She had always known that as well as she knew that her desires matched his own. However, she suspected that such passions couldn't last forever, and if there was nothing but politeness to take their place, what a bleak life would stretch before her! Why, it was no wonder the present Duchess of Arden was such a sour old thing.

Wistfully Matilda wondered if the duke would even share his sense of humor with her once they were wedded. If they wedded. It seemed a very long time since the atrocious dagger joke.

"Dear Matilda is very troubled in her mind," Aunt

Poppy said to Mrs. Summers when her niece had gone on her way, accompanied again by the maid, to the theater.

''Green sickness,'' was the old nurse's somewhat old-fashioned diagnosis.

The next days passed pleasantly enough for Matilda, for the duke was to be seen only at night, in his theater box. His admiration arrived daily, both at the Paddington cottage and at the theater, in the form of flowers, bonbons, and a basket of assorted delicacies obviously sent with the elderly ladies in mind. Each offering was accompanied by a short note, usually of one line, expressing love, devotion, and the usual things. Matilda brushed off the notes as nonsense, which behavior would have upset the duke mightily. He labored over each missive, finding it particularly difficult to pen the word ''love.''

Matilda, however, had been receiving *billets-doux* featuring that word since her first appearance on the stage; she couldn't know he really meant it any more than a score of other gentlemen had.

A Midsummer Night's Dream was enjoying an unprecedented success at the theater. The play being so fanciful, the manager had seen the opportunity to fit in numerous extra songs, dances, and acrobatic acts, which delighted the tasteless spectators if not the players.

Matilda was happy in her small but pivotal role as Titania, and this was just as well, for the receipts continued so bountiful that the management couldn't afford to change to another play. In her floating and revealing fairy robes, a small crown glinting in her bright waves of hair, Matilda won rapturous applause from the bucks of the *ton* and not a few disparaging sniffs from society's leading patronesses. There were those who continued to count her scandal with the duke the Season's most shocking tidbit, though other antics duly recorded by Messrs. Cruikshank and Rowlandson had superseded it on the lips of many.

Mr. Devlin was cagily aware that it was to his advantage to keep Miss Graham in a position of prominence; many still came to gawk at the debauched young mistress—or was it former mistress?—of the Duke of Arden.

Matilda had yet another advantage: the *Monthly Mirror* had come out with a glowing review of her unusual Lady Macbeth, with its overtones of hysterical child, such a refreshing change, so distinct from the traditional and still-unsurpassed dark tragedy of Mrs. Siddons.

So it was with a pardonable pride that Matilda made her first entrance one evening for her opening confrontation with Mr. Blore in the role of Oberon.

She was, as usual, deep in her character, but she did notice that the house was full to bursting and that her appearance was greeted with more than the usual cheers. Well, perhaps another scurrilous cartoon of her had come out, she thought in the tiny corner of her mind which wasn't obsessed with keeping the changeling boy from her philandering fairy husband. She stood waiting in the wings after her first scene, for it was only a short time until the fairies would sing her into that sleep which Oberon would take advantage of by squeezing the juice of the magic pansy on her eyes, causing her the indignity of falling in love with the clown Bottom, he in the guise of an ass.

The play progressed. The fairy song was one of the opportunities the judicious manager had taken to insert much more entertainment than was appropriate to a lullaby; Matilda, busy falling asleep, always had to hold back a laugh. How could anyone drop off into dreamland when a troupe of jugglers hired from Astley's were plying their trade two feet from the would-be sleeper's couch? Matilda's major care during this innovation was to avoid ducking in her concern over the safety of her head. The jugglers were succeeded by a troupe of tumblers, and then a raucous song was sung by a frowsy female in fairy's garb. When the boisterous acts finally wound down into real lullabies, Matilda fell gracefully into a fairy slumber, reflecting that there was much good to be found in a role that required the actress to feign sleep for much of the action.

Matilda spent the interval in trying to calm down Dulcie Moore, who was having a tantrum because of the ill-fit of her costume for Hermia. Matilda suspected the hysterics were really on account of a quarrel Dulcie had had with her protector, which had been well-documented in a cartoon of one of the Cruikshanks. Matilda's sad experience of Cruikshank's satire put her in a good position to offer sympathy, and so she did, not even noticing a good many curious and amused stares that other members of the cast were sending her way.

Act Three required Matilda to open the scene asleep, in the wood. The troupe of players would enter and go through quite a bit of action before she was required to wake.

Matilda arranged herself on the rustic couch and duly pretended to fall asleep. What hoots and cheers greeted the entrance of the clowns! Matilda couldn't sneak a look at them from her position. Was one of the actors missing an essential part of his costume? Had the understudy for Bottom made a tremendous gaffe already? Someone had told Matilda earlier that day that her partner in the satiric amours of the third act, Mr. Kennedy, had been called to the sickbed of a rich uncle and couldn't afford not to go. In this perverted version of the Bard's work, anything was possible.

She cocked her ears to hear the lines over the crowd's vocal delight, for she must not miss her cue. So far the scene had been progressing without her being able to hear it. She must suppose that all was well and that Bottom had exited and reentered on schedule, ass's head in place, for a snatch came through of one of the other clowns saying, "Bottom, thou art changed!" Matilda stirred; very soon she must awake and love an ass.

The house quieted down, presumably with the exit of the other clowns. The spectators were always fairly attentive for the spurious love scene. Matilda, holding herself in readiness for her cur, nearly fell off her leafy couch as she heard an all-too-familiar voice declaim in ringing tones, "I will sing, that they shall hear I am not afraid."

Matilda's eyes flew open of their own accord. Titania was forgotten. Downstage from Matilda was the large figure of the duke, back to her, ass's head on his shoulders, but unmistakably the duke. He began to sing a Cambridge drinking song which the orchestra joined in on quite as if they had rehearsed it. Matilda realized, of a sudden, that they had. And she made instant sense of those sly looks which had been directed to her all the day and evening. No wonder Mr. Devlin had told her that today, of all days, she might miss rehearsal and come in late!

"What angel wakes me from my flowery bed?" shouted Matilda. The spectators roared with delight.

Arden looked over his shoulder; at least Matilda supposed he did. The ass's head seemed to leer at her before he turned back to finish the song. It was rather lengthy, and Matilda had no idea when it would be over. And the other song which was usually brought in to replace Shakespeare's brief ditty—was Arden going to sing that too?

He was. The Duke of Arden possessed a fine, strong

baritone, and he hadn't displayed it since his school days. He quite evidently reveled in this opportunity, even giving an encore performance of the drinking song when the happy spectators roared out their insistence.

Ages later, he bowed his monster's head. Matilda realized that she would have to get up and go on with her role, though every instinct demanded she storm off the stage and out into the London streets.

She was too mindful of her duty, though, and tripped up to the beast—and that was an apt description for more than one cause!—and began, " 'I pray thee, gentle mortal, sing again,' " only to have her maddening "Bottom" shout to the housetops, "Delighted, sweet lady," and move to the front of the stage again, where he warbled yet another drinking song.

Matilda lost all pretense of staying in her character. She folded her arms and tapped one foot, to the ecstasy of the crowd, until the duke had finished. Then she pulled him by the sleeve and snapped out the fairy queen's words of love.

The audience nearly split its collective side laughing at these maneuvers, and Matilda obligingly dropped them a curtsy. She was too much of a professional not to try to turn this disaster to account.

" 'Methinks, mistress, you should have little reason for that,' " the voice of the duke boomed out of the sizable hole in the ass's mask, ostensibly referring to Titania's love for Bottom. Somehow, Matilda could tell he was speaking right to her.

"You can be sure of that," she therefore snarled in an undertone before proceeding with the rest of the scene.

Seething, she bade her fairy retainers make her love comfortable in every way, critically watching the duke's delivery. His motions and speeches were crudely done, but there was a certain flair, much as

Matilda hated to admit it. And his enjoyment of the role came through every clumsy motion to endear him to the spectators. Or were they only cheering on his every word because he was the Duke of Arden?

Matilda had never meant anything so sincerely as the line she gave near the end of the scene, an order for the fairies to quieten Bottom and thus avoid being caught out by Oberon.

" 'Tie up my lover's tongue,' " she said sweetly, with an edge of meaning that did not pass by the audience, whose clapping and stamping resounded in her ears as she led the way offstage.

Matilda paid no attention to the duke, who, she could hear, was seized on by congratulatory actors. She walked straight through the wings to a corner and leaned her head against the wall, laughing uncontrollably. Luckily she had till the fourth act to compose herself.

Some of the players had caught at her as she passed by them, commending her on her aplomb. Matilda wondered, through her hysterics, if she would ever be able to finish out the play.

A hand descended on her shoulder. Matilda gulped back another hoot of laughter and turned to look into the glass eyes of the ass's head.

"My dearest girl," came the echoing voice from behind the huge face. "Did you like it?"

"Did I like it?" Matilda's words came out in a shriek, and she started to laugh again. She felt, rather than saw, the duke's arms circling round her, for she couldn't see through her giddy tears. "Why?" she gasped out.

The duke patted her back and soothed her out of her laughing fit before he answered. Removing the concealing mask from his head, he stood revealed, a rumpled but very handsome man with a tender look in his eyes. "Why, how could you doubt the reason? I wish to prove that we can share a life. I've done a lot of thinking in the past few days. I didn't know if what you'd accused me of was true—legitimated lust indeed! It sounded absurd, and I've come to the conclusion it is absurd. Why, my dear girl, I'd marry you if I could never take you to bed. I love your courage, the way you fight a thing through, your quick mind. And so I decided to come into your world in an attempt to get you into mine. And don't I make a charming Bottom?''

''No proper player would dare take such advantage of a role,'' Matilda responded with what she hoped was a severe look. His confession astounded her. Perhaps he really was in love as she was! But she couldn't descend into sentimentality yet, and thus she took refuge in satire.

''Well, I never said I was professional. Devilish lot of fun, being up there. Glad that this farcical piece was on, by the way, for I'd never have done in the part of Richard III or Romeo. Nor would your complaisant manager have been so ready to turn the evening over to chaos, however much I'd offered him.''

Matilda nodded. ''But since this muddled version of the play is chaos already . . . yes, I understand the choice. But please stop plaguing me now with your fanciful talk of marriage and . . . things. You must go back out on the stage. And you must promise to help me stay in character.''

''Will you marry me in return?''

''No!''

Arden shrugged, ''Not much of an incentive, m'dear. Don't you see? The Duke of Arden can marry Miss Graham now. She may have trodden the boards, but so has he!''

Matilda was dumbfounded by this reasoning. ''You think that five minutes cavorting across the boards by *your grace* is equal to my career upon the stage?''

"On, no, my love," he was quick to respond.

"Well, tell me this, then." Matilda took a deep breath and looked into his eyes. There was something she must know, a final test she must give him. "May the Duchess of Arden act upon the public stage?" she asked in a voice which nearly shook. Her answer to his proposal depended upon his response to this outrageous question.

He pretended not to understand. "Mama? Absurd to think of it, dearest Matilda. You can't expect to take the whole family into your profession, though I'd dare swear my young brothers . . ."

Matilda sighed. "You know what I mean."

"I do," he said, "and I have an answer ready."

There was a pause.

"Well, what is it?" Matilda asked in irritation.

"Only one Duchess of Arden may act upon any stage in the world she wants, and that is yourself." Arden shrugged and gave a somewhat crooked smile. "I like to set the *ton* talking as well as the next man and better than most. My wife is free to do the same. Though I think it would be prudent if you gave your salary to charity."

"What? Be completely under your power for every penny I want to spend?" Matilda's relief caused her to catch hold of one detail and beat it into the ground. "I shall do no such thing. My salary will be my own to do with as I will, though I will let you give an equivalent sum to charity if you so desire. And furthermore—"

"And furthermore, you're to marry me," Arden said. Carefully placing the ass's head upon the ground, he took Matilda into his arms again.

As she rested against his chest, Matilda smiled. A duchess upon the boards! What a thought. She wouldn't do it, of course, but she had his word that she might. It was enough. She had nothing more to ask of him, no more objections to raise. He did wish to marry Miss Graham as well as Miss Glendenning. "I'll marry you," she said, "but only because I love you."

"And I love you, stubborn creature," Arden responded. His dark eyes searched her face. "You wouldn't really act, would you?"

"If I'm really to be your duchess, I believe my genuine emotions will be keeping me busy enough from now on," Matilda said, not really answering his question, yet letting him know by her bright and tender smile that the Arden dignity—what was left of it—was safe with her.

"Precisely what I was going to point out, my dear." Arden's eyes gleamed. "No need for acting anymore. We're really going to be married." His arms tightened around her.

Married! This heady thought gave new spirit to their kisses. Matilda knew at last that the time would come when they would be able to go forward in their lovemaking, secure in their promises to each other. The duke, who had never exactly doubted that outcome, was more fervent than ever in his relief that all was resolved.

The sound of applause brought them to their senses.

"Titania! Sir Bottom, your grace! Remember we've a show to do," the voice of Mr. Devlin intruded into their dream world.

All the players who weren't onstage were standing in a circle round them, smiling gleefully at the scene in progress.

"Good people," the Duke of Arden said, "you are all the first to know . . . well, the second, for I've informed my mother. Miss Matilda *Graham* has consented to be my wife."

"But not before the curtain," Matilda added, blush-

ing furiously under her paint. "You must carry this joke through, Duke, now you've begun it."

"No need to be so formal, dearest. Do call me Michael." And he put back on the ass's head, covering up his brilliant smile.